IMMUNOLOGY
A Short Course

IMMUNOLOGY
A Short Course

Eli Benjamini

Department of Medical Microbiology and Immunology
University of California School of Medicine
Davis, California

Sidney Leskowitz

Department of Pathology
Tufts University School of Medicine
Boston, Massachusetts

Alan R. Liss, Inc., New York

Address all Inquiries to the Publisher
Alan R. Liss, Inc., 41 East 11th Street, New York, NY 10003

Printed in the United States of America

Second Printing, March 1988

Third Printing, December 1989

While the authors, editors, and publisher believe that drug selection and dosage and the specifications and usage of equipment and devices, as set forth in this book, are in accord with current recommendations and practice at the time of publication, they accept no legal responsibility for any errors or omissions, and make no warranty, express or implied, with respect to material contained herein. In view of ongoing research, equipment modifications, changes in governmental regulations and the constant flow of information relating to drug therapy, drug reactions and the use of equipment and devices, the reader is urged to review and evaluate the information provided in the package insert or instructions for each drug, piece of equipment or device for, among other things, any changes in the instructions or indications of dosage or usage and for added warnings and precautions.

Library of Congress Cataloging-in-Publication Data

Banjamini, Eli.
Immunology.
Includes bibliographies.
1. Immunology. 2. Immune response. I. Leskowitz, Sidney. II. Title. [DNLM: 1. Allergy and Immunology. 2. Immunity. QW 504 B468i]
QR181.B395 1987 574.2'9 87-2739
ISBN 0-471-61002-X

CONTENTS

CHAPTER 4: ANTIBODY STRUCTURE

CHAPTER 5: BIOLOGICAL PROPERTIES OF IMMUNOGLOBULINS

CHAPTER 8: COMPLEMENT

CHAPTER 9: THE CELLULAR BASIS OF THE IMMUNE RESPONSE

CHAPTER 10: TRIGGERING THE IMMUNE RESPONSE

CHAPTER 11: GENETIC CONTROL OF THE IMMUNE RESPONSE

CHAPTER 14: DELAYED TYPE HYPERSENSITIVITY: T-CELL–MEDIATED IMMUNITY

PREFACE

Why was this book written? At a time when so many excellent, extensive, and beautifully illustrated texts flood the book stores, why offer another one? The reasons are fairly simple and rather unsophisticated. In our collective 30 some-odd years of teaching all kinds of students, we have become convinced that most texts fail their purpose because they overshoot the mark.

Anyone coming into contact with these students year after year cannot fail to appreciate the burden under which they operate. If they are to graduate, they must learn an enormous amount of material on an exceptionally diverse series of subjects, each increasing in scope yearly. As any student can tell you, every faculty lecturer considers his/her particular topic absolutely essential for future graduates, and so the pile of required "essentials" grows and grows. This is a manifestly untenable approach to curriculum.

A second cruel observation arises from long years of questioning students: many of them are not really that interested in immunology! As exciting, dynamic and all-encompassing in its passion as we practitioners of immunology find it to be, the students have many other interests and concerns, one of which is to pass the five or six other subjects usually taken simultaneously with immunology.

This book was therefore conceived along the lines of the noted architect Mies van der Rohe's dictum, "less is more." We have devised this text to present the bare essentials of immunology in a palatable form that will enable most students to grasp the essential principles of immunology sufficiently to pass their course. For those developing a deeper interest in the field, numerous advanced and more complete texts exist to further their interests.

The book follows the outlines of most immunology courses and is divided into chapters that approximate the length of an average lecture reading assignment. A short introduction setting the stage precedes each chapter, the end of each chapter contains a summary, and a series of study questions appears at the very end. The questions are designed to enable students to evaluate their own progress and comprehension; the appended answers are meant as a further learning experience. As new terms or concepts are introduced, they are italicized and defined for easy recognition and recall.

It is our hope that students using this text will avoid that choking sensation so common in a course in immunology and even conceive a curiosity about the subject that will lead to further study.

ACKNOWLEDGMENTS

The authors are deeply indebted to a number of colleagues and students for valuable contributions to this text.

Dr. Demosthenes Pappagianis, University of California School of Medicine at Davis, contributed Chapter 20, which provides useful practical insights into the application of immunology to the prevention and therapy of infectious diseases.

Drs. Linda Werner and Jacqueline Maisonnave of the University of California School of Medicine at Davis and Drs. Geoffrey Sunshine, Peter Brodeur, and Lanny Rosenwasser of Tufts University School of Medicine were most helpful in reading and contributing valuable suggestions to portions of the text. A number of other colleagues reviewed portions of the text, and we are grateful for their criticisms and comments.

Finally, we applaud the forbearance of our wives, Joy and Thelma, who tolerated our constant whining during the writing of this book.

CHAPTER 1

INTRODUCTION AND OVERVIEW

INTRODUCTION

The field of immunology has been in the limelight since the late 1960s, when successful transplantation of the human kidney was achieved. More recently, the spectacular but not always successful transplantation of the human heart has been the focus of much publicity. In the 1970s, public interest in immunology was intensified by the potential application of the immune response to the detection and management of cancer.

Less publicized, but of great importance to humanity, is the success of immunology in the prevention and virtual elimination of many infectious diseases. Vaccination against infectious diseases has been an effective form of prophylaxis. Immunoprophylaxis against the virus that causes poliomyelitis has reduced this dreadful disease to insignificant importance in many parts of the world. Furthermore, for the first time, a previously widespread disease, smallpox, has been eliminated from the face of the earth. Recent developments in immunology hold the promise of immunoprophylaxis against malaria and several other parasitic diseases that plague many parts of the world and that affect billions of people. Vaccination against diseases of domestic animals promises to increase the production of meat in developing countries. Also, vaccination against various biochemical compounds that play roles in the reproductive processes in mammals offers the exciting possibility of contraception by vaccination of humans and companion animals such as cats and dogs.

During the past twenty years, we have witnessed very rapid advances in the field of immunology. The advances, both conceptual and technical, cover an enormous range of topics and make it difficult for the uninitiated to distinguish "the forest from the trees." This chapter offers an overview of immunology; it is intended to give the highlights of the field, all of which are discussed in more detail in the chapters that follow.

INNATE AND ACQUIRED IMMUNITY

The term ***immunity*** refers to all the mechanisms used by the body as protection against environmental agents that are foreign to the body. These agents may be microorganisms or their product's foods, chemicals, drugs, pollen, and animal hair and dander. Immunity may be innate or acquired. ***Innate immunity*** derives from all those elements with which an individual is born and that are always present and available at very short notice to protect the individual from challenges by "foreign" material. These elements include body surfaces as well as internal components. For example, the skin, the mucous membranes, and the cough reflex present effective barriers to environmental agents. Combined with these physical barriers, chemical influences such as pH, secreted fatty acids and the enzyme lysozyme constitute effective barriers against invasion by many microorganisms.

Numerous internal elements are also features of innate immunity: fever, interferon and other substances released by leukocytes, as well as a variety of serum proteins such as β-lysin, lysozyme, the polyamines, and the kinins, among others. The internal elements of innate immunity also include cells such as granulocytes, macrophages, the microglial cells of the central nervous system, and the cytotrophoblasts of placental villi. These cells all participate in the destruction and elimination of foreign material that has succeeded in penetrating the physical and chemical barriers of the innate immune system.

Acquired immunity is more specialized than innate immunity, and it supplements the protection provided by innate immunity. Acquired immunity came into play relatively late, in evolutionary terms, and is present only in vertebrates.

Although an individual is born with the capacity to mount the defenses provided by acquired immunity, this form of immunity to a foreign agent is not exhibited unless that individual has had prior contact with the same agent. Thus, as the name implies, this form of immunity must be acquired. The initial contact with the foreign agent (immunization) triggers a chain of events that leads to the activation of certain cells ***(lymphocytes)*** and the synthesis of proteins ***(antibodies)*** with specificity against the foreign agent. By this process, the individual acquires the immunity to withstand and resist a subsequent attack by, or exposure to, the same offending agent. Unlike innate immunity, acquired immunity exhibits specificity only against the agent that was used for immunization.

The discovery of acquired immunity predates many of the concepts of modern medicine. It has been recognized for centuries that people who did not die from such life-threatening diseases as bubonic plague or smallpox were subsequently more resistant to the disease than people who had never been exposed to it. The rediscovery of acquired immunity is credited to the English physician, Edward Jenner, who in the late 18th century experimentally induced immunity to smallpox in a young boy. Jenner inoculated the boy with pus from a lesion of a dairy maid who had cowpox, a relatively benign disease that is related to smallpox. Subsequent exposure of the boy to smallpox failed to cause disease. Because of the protective effect of inoculation with cowpox, the process of inducing acquired immunity has been termed ***vaccination,*** from the Latin *vacca,* which means cow.

The concept of vaccination or immunization was expanded by Louis Pasteur and Paul Ehrlich almost 100 years after Jenner's experiment. By the year 1900, it had become apparent that immunity could be induced not only against microorganisms but also their products. We now know that immunity can be induced against thousands of natural and synthetic compounds, which include metals, simple compounds of low molecular weight, carbohydrates, proteins, and nucleotides.

IMMUNOGENS AND ANTIGENS

The ability of a compound to induce an immune response is termed its ***immunogenicity.*** A compound capable of inducing an immune response is called an ***immunogen.***

Another immunologically important property of a compound is its ability to combine with elements of acquired immunity that are specific to that compound. This ability is called ***antigenicity,*** and a compound with this ability is termed an ***antigen.*** While all immunogens are antigens, not all antigens are immunogens, as we will see later.

Immunogenic compounds generally have the following properties: 1) they are ***foreign*** to the immunized individual, 2) they are generally of ***high molecular weight,*** and 3) they have significant ***chemical complexity.*** Thus, foreign substances of high molecular weight, which are chemically complex, are usually immunogenic. Proteins are common examples of such immunogenic compounds. When a protein is used as an immunogen, it induces an immune response, the components of which—cells and antibodies—exhibit a remarkable specificity against that protein.

In many instances an acquired immune response can be induced against relatively simple compounds of low molecular weight, such as dinitrophenol (DNP) or penicillin. These chemicals, when injected alone, are not immunogenic. However, an immune response against them may be induced if they are injected when chemically linked to a substance of high molecular weight, like a protein. The small compound that, by itself, cannot induce an immune response, but against which a response can be induced by immunization with that compound coupled to a substance of high molecular weight, is called a ***hapten.*** A substance with high molecular weight to which the hapten is conjugated for immunogenicity, is called a ***carrier.*** By judicious choice of carriers, an immune response can be induced to thousands of haptenic compounds that are not themselves immunogenic.

CELLS INVOLVED IN ACQUIRED IMMUNITY

There are three types of cells that play major roles in acquired immunity. Their properties are summarized here and are described in more detail in Chapter 9.

B Lymphocytes

B lymphocytes exhibit antigenic specificity. They proliferate in response to a particular antigen and differentiate into nonproliferating but antibody-secreting plasma cells.

T Lymphocytes

T lymphocytes also exhibit antigenic specificity, and they also proliferate and differentiate in the presence of antigen, releasing substances called ***lymphokines,*** which have important biological properties. While ***T cells do not synthesize antibodies,*** they do fulfill many other, immunologically important functions such as ***"helping"*** B cells to synthesize antibodies, ***killing*** microorganisms, and ***regulating*** the immune response.

Macrophages

Macrophages are phagocytic cells that digest antigens and "process" them for presentation to T cells. This processing is a necessary step in the activation of the T cells. Macrophages do not exhibit antigenic specificity; unlike B cells or T cells, a given macrophage can phagocytize and process many different antigens.

In addition to these three types of cells, others, such as polymorphonuclear leukocytes and mast cells, are recruited to participate in acquired immunity. Although their presence is not essential for the inductive phase of acquired immunity, they are important in the later, effector phase of acquired immunity.

HUMORAL AND CELLULAR IMMUNITY

Humoral Immunity

Humoral immunity is mediated by serum ***antibodies.*** Antibodies are a heterogeneous mixture of serum ***globulins,*** all of which share the ability to bind individually to specific antigens. All serum globulins with antibody activity are referred to as ***immunoglobulins (Ig).***

All immunoglobulin molecules have many common structural features, but they differ from one another in that portion of the molecule that binds specifically to the respective antigen. Basically, each immunoglobulin molecule consists of two identical ***light (L) chains*** (molecular weights 25,000 daltons each) and two identical ***heavy (H) chains*** (molecular weights 50,000 daltons each). Each light chain is linked by a disulfide bridge to a heavy chain, and the two H chains are linked to each other by a disulfide bridge. The resultant structure can be represented schematically as shown below:

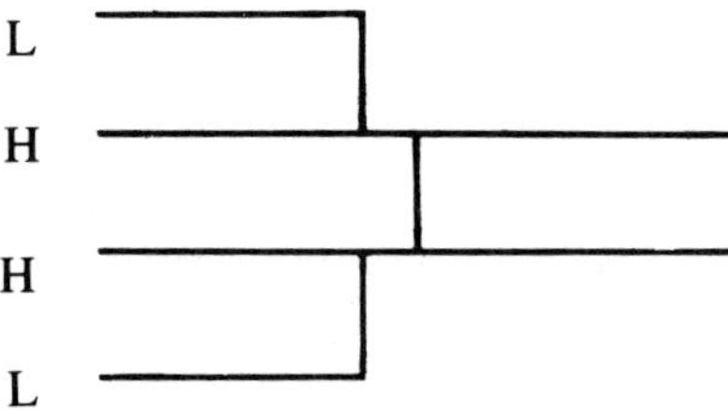

The portion of the molecule that binds antigen consists of the amino-terminal regions of the H and L chains. Thus, each immunoglobulin molecule is symmetrical and is capable of binding two identical haptens or antigenically specific areas (determinants) of a given antigen, whether the two areas are on the same molecule or on two different molecules of that antigen.

In addition to differences in the antigen-binding portion of different immunoglobulin molecules, there are other differences, the most important of which are those in the H chains. There are five different classes of H chains, termed G, M, A, E, and D. Based on the differences in their H chains, immunoglobulin molecules are divided into five major *classes*: ***IgG, IgM, IgA, IgE,*** and ***IgD.*** Each of these five classes of immunoglobulins has several unique biological properties. For example, IgG is the only class of immunoglobulin that crosses the placenta, conferring the mother's immunity on the fetus; IgE binds with high affinity to mast cells and is the major class of immunoglobulin involved in allergy; IgM is a powerful antibody, that can activate other serum components to cause lysis of bacteria and other cells; IgA is the major antibody found in secretions such as tears and saliva; and IgD is found on lymphocytes at certain stages of development. It is important to remember that antibodies in all five classes may possess precisely the same specificity against an antigen, while, at the same time, having different functional properties.

The binding between antigen and antibody does not involve covalent bonds but depends upon many relatively weak forces, such as hydrogen bonds, Van der Waal forces, and hydrophobic interactions. Since these forces are weak, successful binding between antigen and antibody depends upon a very close fit over a sizeable area, much like the contacts between a lock and key.

It has already been mentioned that a single antibody molecule can bind two identical hapten molecules. Similarly, an antibody can bind the two identical determinants that are present on two separate, complex molecules, such as two identical proteins, thereby linking the two molecules. A given protein molecule may have many different antigenic determinants, each of which can give rise to a specific antibody that reacts with the protein. Thus, the reaction of a protein and its antiserum allows the antibodies to cross-link antigen molecules or particles, resulting in large antigen–antibody complexes. As a result, many consequences ensue in vitro that may have deleterious effects in vivo. For example, if the antigen is particulate, like a bacterium, the reaction with antibodies may result in the clumping or ***agglutination*** of the particles or bacteria; if the antigen is soluble, then the reaction with antibodies may produce a ***precipitate*** (see Chapter 7).

Depending on the class of antibody in question, the reaction between antigen and antibodies may activate a humoral system—the ***complement*** system—which, if the antigen is a bacterium, will result in lysis or in enhanced phagocytosis of the bacterium by phagocytic cells. The activation of complement (see Chapter 8) also results in the recruitment of ***polymorphonuclear cells (PMN),*** which constitute part of the innate immune system. When these cells become activated, they release their lysosomal enzymes and destroy the invader. Another type of reaction between antigen and certain antibodies may result in the degranulation of ***mast cells*** and the release of pharmacologically active compounds such as ***histamine.*** Histamine produces an increase in vascular permeability, causing more serum, and therefore more antibodies, to accumulate at the site of the immune reaction.

All these activities are, of course, of great survival value because they maximize the effective response against invading agents.

Cell-Mediated Immunity

While the antigen-specific arm of acquired humoral immunity consists of the immunoglobulins, the antigen-specific arm of ***cell-mediated immunity*** consists of the ***T lymphocytes***. In contrast to an antibody molecule that recognizes two identical antigenic determinants, each T cell has many identical receptors, each directed against the same antigenic determinant. Complex antigens, such as those present on the surface of microorganisms, have many determinants; consequently, many different T cells will be directed against the same antigen.

There are several subpopulations of T cells, each of which may have the same specificity for an antigenic determinant, even though each subpopulation may perform different functions. It is important to reiterate that T cells do not synthesize or secrete antibodies. However, it is well established that, when an antigen is presented to the T cell by an ***antigen-presenting cell,*** such as a macrophage, the result is the activation of the T cell so that it can perform a variety of functions, the exact nature of which depends on the nature of the subpopulation of T cells. The functions of activated T cells include cooperation with B cells to induce production of antibodies by the B cells. Activation of T cells also results in the release of ***lymphokines*** (soluble substances released by lymphocytes), some of which have a profound effect on other T cells. Other lymphokines attract mononuclear cells (mostly macrophages) into the area of the immune response and activate them. Thus, if the invading agent consists of bacteria, cell-mediated immunity may result in the killing of the bacteria by macrophages, which have been recruited into the area and then activated by the T cell lymphokines. Again, as in the case of humoral immunity, cell-mediated immunity consists of some components—the T cells—that specifically recognize the antigen, and of other components—the macrophages—that are elements of innate immunity and do not exhibit antigenic specificity.

It is important to realize that an acquired immune response to such antigens as bacteria usually consists of both a humoral and a cell-mediated immune response, interacting with each other and with components of innate immunity to destroy the invader.

Generally, the immune response is directed against foreign invaders. However, under special circumstances, it may be directed against tumor cells, which have structures on their surfaces that differ from their normal counterparts. These structures (antigens) may be recognized as foreign and will therefore induce an immune response against themselves. Such responses are the subject of an area of intense investigation—tumor immunology (see Chapter 19).

DAMAGING EFFECTS OF THE IMMUNE RESPONSE

The great survival value of acquired immunity is self-evident. Central to acquired immunity is the recognition of the distinction between "self" and "non-self." Acquired immunity is invoked against a foreign invader, with the ultimate goal of eliminating the foreign material. In the process, some tissue damage may occur as a result of the accumulation of components that do not exhibit antigenic specificity. This damage, however, is only temporary. As soon as the invader is eliminated, the situation at that site soon reverts to normal.

Hypersensitivity

There are instances in which the power of the immune response is directed against substances that, although they are foreign, are innocuous to the body. Harmless substances, such as animal hair and dander, pollen, environmental chemicals, food proteins, and the like are recognized as foreign. The acquired immune response, both humoral and cellular, with all its mediators, is mounted against these harmless substances in just the same way as it is mounted against a deadly microorganism or toxin. Exposure to these harmless substances immunizes or ***sensitizes*** the individual, so that when a subsequent exposure or ***challenge*** with the same substance occurs, the sensitized, or ***allergic,*** individual exhibits ***hypersensitivity*** or an allergic reaction (see Chapters 13 and 14). The same mechanisms as those described earlier operate during the reaction of the immune response to the foreign antigen or ***allergen***. If the dose of the challenging antigen or allergen is sufficiently high, or if the antibody response to the allergen is excessive, the reaction may result in severe pathological consequences, and even death. Continuous exposure of an allergic (sensitized) individual to a particular allergen results in chronic allergy (hypersensitivity), the effects of which range from mild to incapacitating.

One or both aspects of acquired immunity (humoral or cell mediated) may be involved in hypersensitivity. When an allergic person is ***challenged*** with an allergen, for example in a skin test, one type of allergic reaction may appear within minutes; another, an hour or so later. Because of the short time between the challenge and the appearance of the allergic reaction, these reactions are called ***immediate hypersensitivity reactions.*** Alternatively, the reaction may appear 18–48 hours after the challenge, and such a reaction is called a ***delayed hypersensitivity reaction.*** Often a challenge can elicit both an immediate reaction, which may or may not subside within a few hours, and a delayed reaction, which may last a few days (or occasionally even a few weeks).

Immediate and delayed hypersensitivity reactions are differentiated, not only by the time between the challenge and the appearance of the reaction but also, and more importantly, by the components that mediate the reactions. Consideration of these mediators is important in the treatment of hypersensitivity reactions.

IMMEDIATE HYPERSENSITIVITY. Immediate hypersensitivity is mediated by antibodies, either IgE or IgG and IgM. A central event in the immediate hypersensitivity reaction due to IgE antibody is the release of histamine from mast cells. This release is achieved when the allergen combines with specific IgE antibodies that are attached to the outer membrane of the mast cells. The binding triggers the degranulation of the mast cells and the release of pharmacologically active compounds, most notably histamine. In hypersensitivity reactions due to IgG and IgM, the activation of the components of serum complement, when they are bound to antigen, may also bring about the release of histamine, but the major outcome of the activation of complement results in the release of factors that recruit polymorphonuclear cells into the area of the immune reaction. These cells become activated and release their ***lysosomal enzymes,*** causing damage to surrounding tissue. Thus, immediate hypersensitivity, which is mediated by antibodies, results from the release of chemical mediators such as histamine and/or damage to tissue by lysosomal enzymes.

DELAYED HYPERSENSITIVITY. Delayed hypersensitivity is mediated by T cells. Antigen-presenting cells, such as macrophages, present the antigen or allergen to T cells. In response, the T cells become activated and release lymphokines. These lymphokines activate macrophages and cause them to become voracious killers of foreign invaders, or even of normal tissue. Delayed hypersensitivity reactions do not have an antibody component, they are strictly cellular reactions that involve T cells and macrophages.

Autoimmunity

While normally acquired immunity is carefully regulated so that it is not induced against components of "self," for various reasons, when this regulation is defective, an immune response against "self" is mounted. This type of immune response is termed ***autoimmunity.*** Some of the diseases that are the most difficult to treat are the autoimmune diseases, and they often lead to premature death (see Chapter 16).

Transplantation and Transfusion Reactions

In many cases, exposure to foreign substances results from clinical situations in which tissue is transplanted or blood is transfused from one person to another. Unless the donor and recipient are identical twins, the transplanted tissue or transfused blood contains antigens that are foreign to the recipient, and an immune response will be mounted that results in rejection of the transplanted tissue or transfused blood (see Chapters 17 and 18). Rejection of the transplant or transfusion is not a manifestation of some force of nature designed to frustrate the physician and the patient. Rather, such rejection occurs because of the central tenet of acquired immunity— recognition and elimination of "non-self."

REGULATION OF THE IMMUNE RESPONSE

The immune response is complex and may exert deleterious effects on the body. We would therefore expect that its evolution was accompanied by the development of highly sophisticated and very precise mechanisms for the regulation of the nature and extent of the response. Indeed, mechanisms exist that have the ability either to heighten or to reduce the response (see Chapters 12 and 15). Disturbances in these regulatory mechanisms may be caused by conditions such as congenital defect, infection, or hormonal imbalance, any of which may have disastrous consequences. The acquired immune deficiency syndrome (AIDS) is a defect in the regulation of the immune response and the subject of much current research. As a result of infection with the human AIDS virus, there is a decrease in one subpopulation of T cells (the helper T cells) that leads to immunological deficiency, which renders the patient susceptible to infectious microorganisms that are normally benign, and to malignancies, the most common of which is Kaposi's sarcoma.

TRANSFER OF IMMUNITY

Acquired immunity, with specificity directed against a particular antigen, can be transferred from one individual to another by the transfer of serum or of cells. The term ***active immunization*** refers to immunization of an individual by administration of an antigen. ***Passive immunization*** refers to immunization by the transfer of specific antibodies in serum. ***Adoptive transfer (immunization)*** refers to the transfer of immunity by the transfer of immune cells. It should be noted that, although passive immunization is not generally associated with significant risk, the success of adoptive immunization depends upon the careful matching of donor tissue to the recipient; if the recipient recognizes the donor's lymphocytes as foreign, they will be rejected.

CURRENT ADVANCES IN IMMUNOLOGY

The past twenty years have witnessed great advances in immunology. Research during this period was generally directed toward two major goals: 1) an understanding of the mechanisms that operate in acquired immunity and 2) the manipulation of the immune response for improvement of public health and the conquest of disease.

Many of the most exciting recent advances have resulted from the juxtaposition of the techniques of modern molecular biology and the use of cells from the immune system, which together provide one of the best systems for the productive application of these techniques. This research has produced an expanding body of knowledge about the genetic basis of antibody specificity. It has been demonstrated that immunoglobulin genes are representative of a new type of genetic organization in which the final protein product results from rearrangement of a series of genes, each of which encodes a portion of the final molecule. Elucidation of the mechanisms of ***gene rearrangement*** and ***splicing*** has provided a detailed understanding of how antibodies of many different specificities are made from a relatively small number of genes. The process involves rearrangement of several gene segments that make up an antibody's ***combining site.*** In addition, the ease and rapidity with which the nucleotide sequences of long segments of DNA can be obtained have allowed scientists to determine the structures of antibodies of different specificities much more rapidly than is possible by sequencing their constituent amino acids. Elucidation of the detailed structures of antibodies has, in turn, provided insight into how antibody-combining sites function and how they may be altered to generate a site of higher affinity for the antigen. It is already conceivable that, by use of gene-splicing techniques, antibodies may be synthesized to order, and for specific purposes. For example, the genes for a specific combining site may be spliced to the gene for a toxin molecule to produce a ***hybrid antibody*** capable of binding to a specific target, such as a tumor cell, and killing it.

In another area of investigation of the nature of ***T cell receptors,*** the methods of molecular biology have proved to be invaluable. After many years of failure of classical techniques to detect, much less to characterize, the receptors on T cells that give them their functional specificity, application of the techniques of molecular genetics has demonstrated that T cell receptors share many properties with the immunoglobulin receptors of B cells, in having a limited number of genes that rearrange to form a two chain receptor molecule with many specificities. In addition, however, the greater complexity of the T cell receptors has been demonstrated by the discovery of additional polypeptide chains and their genes, which are coexpressed and required for the complete activation of T cells.

Elucidation of the genetic mechanisms for the synthesis and expression of antigen-specific receptors on B and T cells is one of the triumphs of the marriage of molecular biology and immunology. The practical results of such remarkable progress are already visible on the horizon, in the form of a greater understanding of the normal ontogeny of B and T cells, and as insights into the causes of malignancies in these cell lines. The latter insights may eventually lead to the development of more rational approaches to the treatment of such malignancies.

In addition to providing the basis for the synthesis of receptors of known specificity by genetic manipulations, these techniques have provided a powerful impetus to the development of novel vaccines. Instead of a laborious, empirical search for an attenuated virus or bacterium for use in immunization, new approaches are being employed. For example, it is now possible to obtain the nucleotide sequence of the DNA that encodes a viral coat protein, or of the DNA that encodes a surface component of an organism as complex as the malarial parasite. By examination of such sequences, educated guesses can be made about which segments of the proteins are most likely to be antigenic determinants. Such segments can then be readily synthesized and tested for use as a vaccine. Many applications of this technique are already underway, and there is considerable optimism toward their potential success.

Another area of great promise is the characterization and synthesis of ***immune modulators.*** Again, the techniques of gene isolation, clonal reproduction and biosynthesis have contributed to rapid progress. Powerful and important modulators, such as ***interleukin-1*** and ***-2*** and ***interferons*** have been synthesized by the methods of recombinant DNA technology and are being tested for their therapeutic efficacy in a variety of diseases that includes many different cancers. Thus, our burgeoning understanding of the functioning of the immune system, combined with the recently acquired ability to alter and manipulate its components, carries enormous implications for the future of mankind.

CHAPTER

2

ELEMENTS OF IMMUNITY

INTRODUCTION

Every living organism is confronted by continual assaults from its environment. To survive, every organism has therefore had to develop defenses that render it resistant, or immune, to such assaults. These defenses range from physical barriers, such as a cell wall, to highly sophisticated systems, such as the acquired immune response. This chapter describes the defense systems: the elements that constitute the defense, the participating cells and organs, and the action of the participants in the immune response to foreign substances that invade the body.

In vertebrates, immunity against microorganisms and their products is divided into two major categories: ***innate or natural immunity,*** and ***acquired immunity*** (Fig. 2.1). These two types of immunity, their origins, and their components are discussed in the paragraphs that follow.

INNATE OR NATURAL IMMUNITY

Innate (natural) immunity is present from birth and consists of many factors that are relatively nonspecific; i.e. they operate against almost any substance that threatens the body. Some of the important non-antigen-specific factors that are part of innate immunity are given below.

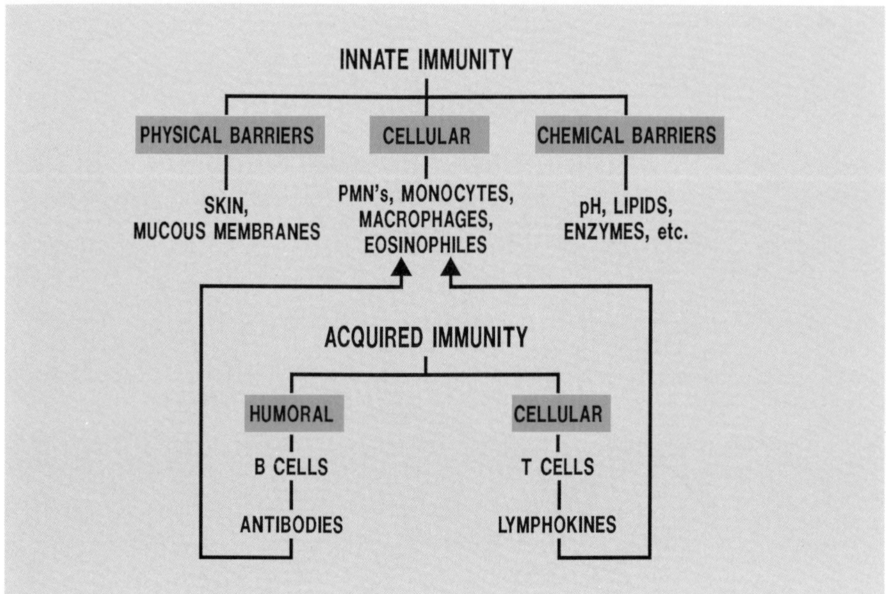

Figure 2.1.
The relationship between innate and acquired immunity.

Physiologic Barriers (Skin and Mucous Membranes)

Most organisms cannot penetrate intact skin, although they can enter the body if the skin is cut. Some microorganisms can enter the body through sebaceous glands and hair follicles. However, the ***acid pH*** of sweat and sebaceous secretions, the presence of various ***fatty acids*** and of ***enzymes*** (e.g. lysozyme), all of which have some antimicrobial effect, minimize the importance of this route of infection.

Mucus covers the surface of many areas in the body, such as the respiratory and the gastrointestinal tracts. In the respiratory tract, the mucus and any microorganisms trapped in it are constantly being driven upward by ciliated cells, toward the external openings. Also, the hairs in the nostrils and the cough reflex are helpful in preventing organisms from infecting the respiratory tract. Alcohol, cigarette smoke, and narcotics suppress this entire defense system.

The elimination of microorganisms from the respiratory tract is aided by pulmonary or alveolar macrophages, which are phagocytic cells able to destroy some microorganisms. Other microorganisms that have penetrated the mucous membrane can be picked up by macrophages or otherwise transported to lymph nodes, where many are destroyed.

The environment of the gastrointestinal tract is hostile to many microorganisms: the ***hydrolytic enzymes in saliva***, the ***low pH of the stomach***, and the ***proteolytic enzymes and bile in the small intestine***, all contribute to an unfavorable environment for many (but not all) microorganisms. Similarly, the ***low pH of the vagina*** inhibits growth of some organisms.

Phagocytosis

Phagocytosis is the ingestion and destruction by individual cells of invading foreign particles, such as bacteria. Many microorganisms release substances that attract phagocytic cells. Phagocytosis may be enhanced by a variety of factors that make the foreign particle an easier target. These factors, collectively referred to as ***opsonins,*** consist of antibodies and of various serum components of complement (see Chapter 8). After ingestion, the foreign particle is entrapped in a ***phagocytic vacuole*** into which ***lysosomes*** release their enzymes, which then digest the particle.

The phagocytic cells consist of polymorphonuclear leukocytes; phagocytic monocytes, i.e. macrophages; and fixed macrophages of the reticuloendothelial system.

1) ***Polymorphonuclear leukocytes (PMN),*** also referred to as ***granulocytes,*** are short-lived, phagocytic cells that contain granules filled with hydrolytic enzymes. Some granules also contain proteins such as lactoferrin, which are bactericidal. The PMN play a major role in protection against infection. Defects in PMN function are accompanied by chronic or recurrent infection.

2) ***Macrophages*** are circulating ***phagocytic monocytes*** that are relatively long-lived (compared to granulocytes) and that have relatively few granules, unless they become activated through a variety of mechanisms (in particular, by substances released from T lymphocytes; see Chapter 14). Activated macrophages contain many lysosomes, and activation leads to increased phagocytosis and intracellular killing of ingested bacteria. In addition, macrophages play an important role in the "processing" of antigen and its "presentation" to T lymphocytes (see Chapters 10 and 11).

3) ***Fixed macrophages of the reticuloendothelial (RE) system*** are the phagocytic macrophages that are present in lymphoid tissue, such as the spleen and lymph nodes, in the liver (Kupffer cells), in lungs (alveolar macrophages),

in connective tissue, and along the lining of the blood and lymph sinuses. The function of the RE system is to trap microorganisms and foreign substances that are in the bloodstream and in various tissues, and to expose them to phagocytosis by the macrophages. The RE system also functions in the destruction of aged and imperfect cells of the host, such as erythrocytes.

Phagocytosis constitutes an important component of ***inflammation.*** Inflammation is initiated by injury to tissue, which includes injury as a result of infection by microorganisms. The process of inflammation involves enhanced capillary permeability that results in the accumulation of fluid ***(edema)*** and leukocytes present in the blood or lymph. PMN, which are attracted to the area, can phagocytose foreign particles or even damaged host cells, contributing to their destruction by intracellular digestion as well as by the action of their lysosomal enzymes. In the process, many leukocytes are lysed. Mononuclear macrophages subsequently infiltrate the area and phagocytize the debris; then the inflammation subsides.

Fever

Although fever is one of the most common manifestations of infection and inflammation, there is limited information about the significance of fever in the course of infection in mammals. Fever is caused by many bacterial products, most notably the endotoxins of gram-negative bacteria, generally as the result of the release of endogenous ***pyrogens*** that derive from monocytes and macrophages and that include ***interleukins*** and ***interferons*** (see Chapter 14).

Biologically Active Substances

Many tissues synthesize substances that are harmful to microorganisms. Some examples of these harmful substances are ***degradative enzymes, toxic free radicals, acids***, and ***inhibitors of growth***. Thus, depending on their ability to synthesize these substances, certain tissues may have a heightened resistance to infection by some microorganisms.

Innate or natural immunity is related to many attributes of the individual that are determined genetically. Differences in innate immunity between various people may, in addition, be attributed to age, race, and to the hormonal and metabolic conditions of the individual.

ACQUIRED IMMUNITY

In contrast to innate immunity, which is an attribute of every living organism, acquired immunity is a more specialized form. It has developed late in evolution and is found only in vertebrates. The various elements that participate in innate immunity do not exhibit specificity against the foreign agent that they encounter, while acquired immunity always exhibits such specificity. As its name implies, acquired immunity is a consequence of an encounter with a foreign substance. The first encounter with a foreign substance that has penetrated the body triggers a chain of events that induce an immune response with specificity against this foreign substance.

Although an individual is genetically endowed with the capacity to mount an immune response against a certain substance, acquired immunity is usually exhibited only after an initial encounter with this substance. Thus, acquired immunity develops only after exposure to, or ***immunization*** with, a given substance. As mentioned above, ***unlike innate immunity, acquired immunity exhibits specificity:*** it develops only against that substance which was used for immunization.

There are three major types of cells that participate in acquired immunity: ***B lymphocytes, T lymphocytes***, and ***macrophages***. B lymphocytes and T lymphocytes are responsible for the specificity exhibited by the acquired immune response. Macrophages, which do not exhibit specificity against a given substance, are involved in the processing and presentation of foreign substances to T lymphocytes (see Chapters 10 and 11). B lymphocytes synthesize and secrete antibodies with specificity against the foreign substance. The T lymphocytes, which also exhibit specificity against the foreign substance, do not make antibodies, but they are of prime importance in many aspects of acquired immunity. For example, T lymphocytes interact with B cells and "help" the latter make antibodies, they activate macrophages, and they have a central role in the regulation of acquired immunity (see Chapter 15).

There are two major components of acquired immunity: ***humoral immunity,*** which is mediated by specific antibodies present in the serum; and ***cellular immunity,*** which is mediated by cells, with the T cells being the antigen-specific elements of cellular immunity.

Lymphatic Organs

The ***lymphatic organs*** are those organs in which maturation, differentiation, and proliferation of lymphocytes take place. ***Lymphocytes*** are derived from the pluripotential ***hematopoietic bone marrow stem cells,*** which give rise to all blood cells. The ***erythroid*** and ***myeloid*** cells, which differentiate into erythrocytes and granulocytes, are derived from these stem cell progenitors. Other progenitor cells differentiate into lymphocytes.

The ***primary, or central, lymphoid organs*** are those organs in which the maturation of T and B lymphocytes into antigen-recognizing lymphocytes takes place. The ***secondary lymphoid organs*** are those organs in which antigen-driven proliferation and differentiation take place.

PRIMARY LYMPHOID ORGANS. There are two major, primary lymphoid organs, one in which the T cells develop, and the other in which the B cells develop.

The Thymus Gland. Progenitor cells from the bone marrow migrate to the ***thymus gland***, where they differentiate into ***T lymphocytes***. The thymus gland (Fig. 2.2) is a bilobed structure, derived from the endoderm of the third and fourth pharyngeal pouches. During fetal development, the size of the thymus increases and reaches its maximum at birth. After birth, the thymus begins to decrease in size and undergoes atrophy with aging. The thymus is a ***lymphoepithelial*** organ and consists of lymphoid cells (thymocytes) and epithelial cells organized into cortical and medullary areas. The ***cortex*** contains epithelial cells and is densely populated with lymphocytes of various sizes, most of which are immature. T lymphocytes mature in the cortex and migrate to the ***medulla***, which they then leave to enter the peripheral blood circulation,

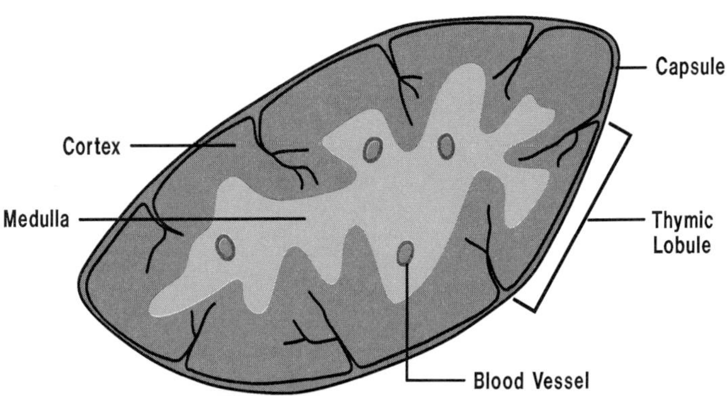

Figure 2.2
A diagramatic representation of a section of the thymus gland.

through which they are transported to the ***secondary lymphoid organs*** (see below). It is in these secondary lymphoid organs that the T cells encounter and respond to foreign antigens, and while T cells do not, themselves, make antibodies they help B cells to do so. By release of soluble mediators called ***lymphokines,*** T cells participate in cell-mediated immunity and in a variety of regulatory functions.

Maturation of the T lymphocyte involves the commitment of a given T cell to recognize and respond to a given determinant or ***epitope*** of a foreign antigen. This recognition is achieved by a specific receptor on the T cell (see Chapters 9 and 11). Mature T lymphocytes in the medulla are capable of responding to foreign antigens in the same way that they would respond in the secondary lymphoid organs. Thus, although the thymus is considered to be a primary lymphoid organ, antigen-driven proliferation and differentiation (events that generally take place in secondary lymphoid organs, as described below) may occur in the thymus.

The thymus gland is the organ in which T cells mature and become committed to respond to a single antigenic determinant. This commitment occurs only during fetal development and for a short time after birth. In fact, removal of the thymus from an adult generally has little effect on the quantity and quality of the T lymphocytes, which have already matured and populated the secondary lymphoid organs. However, adult thymectomy could, in time, result in a deficiency in T cells after the eventual death of the T cells that originally populated the secondary lymphoid organs. Without the thymus there would be no mechanism for repopulation of the secondary organs with new T lymphocytes. In contrast, removal of the thymus gland from a neonate results in an immediate severe reduction in the quantity and quality of T lymphocytes and produces a potentially lethal wasting disease.

Only 5–10% of maturing lymphocytes survive and eventually leave the thymus; 90–95% of all thymocytes die in the thymus. It is believed that the lymphocytes that die have developed specificity to "self" structures or have failed to make functional receptors and therefore, by some unexplained mechanism, they are eliminated. The lymphocytes that survive develop specificity against foreign antigens.

Bursa of Fabricius or Its Equivalent. A primary lymphoid organ in birds, in which B cells undergo maturation, is the ***bursa of Fabricius.*** This organ, situated near the cloaca, consists of lymphoid centers that contain epithelial cells and lymphocytes. Unlike the lymphocytes in the thymus, these lymphocytes consist solely of antibody-producing ***B cells*** (see Chapter 9). Like the thymus, the bursa is largest at hatching and undergoes atrophy with maturation.

Mammals do not have a bursa of Fabricius. In consequence, much work has been directed toward the identification of a mammalian equivalent of the primary lymphoid organ in which development and maturation of B cells occur. A structure with functions equivalent to that of the avian bursa, may be the ***bone marrow.***

Mature B lymphocytes, each with antigen-specific receptors that have a structure and specificity identical to that of the antibody synthesized by the B cell, are transported from the bursa or equivalent structure, by the circulating blood, to the secondary lymphoid organs, where they encounter and respond to antigens.

SECONDARY LYMPHOID ORGANS. The secondary lymphoid organs consist of certain structures in which mature, antigen-committed lymphocytes are stimulated by antigen to undergo further division and differentiation. The major secondary lymphoid organs are the ***spleen*** and the ***lymph nodes.*** In addition, clusters of lymphocytes (***Peyer's patches***), which are spread throughout the lining of the intestinal wall, tonsils and appendix constitute secondary lymphoid organs where mature lymphocytes interact with antigens and differentiate to synthesize specific antibodies.

The secondary lymphoid organs have two major functions: they are highly effective in trapping and concentrating foreign substances, and they are the main sites of production of antibodies and the generation of antigen-specific T lymphocytes.

The Spleen. The spleen (Fig. 2.3) is the largest of the secondary lymphoid organs. It is a highly efficient organ that traps and concentrates foreign substances carried in the blood. It is the major organ in the body in which antibodies are synthesized and from which they are released into the circulation. The spleen is composed of ***white pulp***, rich in lymphoid cells, and ***red pulp***, which contains many sinuses, as well as large quantities of erythrocytes and macrophages, some lymphocytes, and a few other cells.

The areas of white pulp are located mainly around small arterioles, the peripheral regions of which are rich in T cells, with more central regions that are rich in B lymphocytes. Approximately 50% of spleen cells are B lymphocytes; 30–40% are T lymphocytes. After antigenic stimulation, ***germinal centers*** containing large numbers of B cells and ***plasma cells*** appear in the periarteriolar areas and almost completely replace the T cells. These cells synthesize and release antibodies.

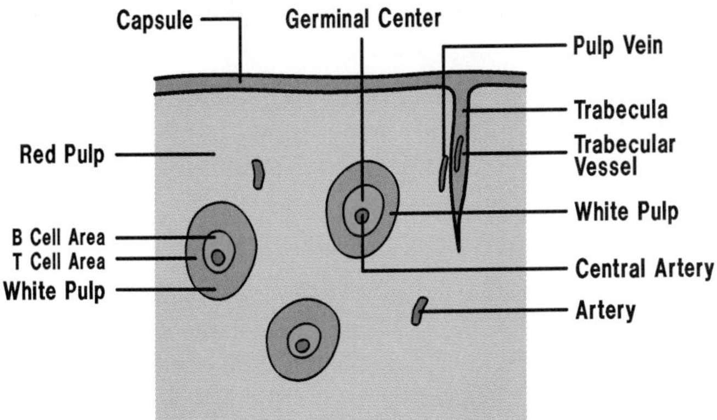

Figure 2.3.
A diagramatic representation of a section of the spleen.

Lymph Nodes. Lymph nodes are small ovoid structures (normally less than 1 cm in diameter) found in various regions throughout the body (Fig. 2.4). They are close to major junctions of the ***lymphatic channels,*** which are connected to the ***thoracic duct.*** The thoracic duct transports lymph and lymphocytes to the ***vena cava,*** the vessel that carries blood to the right side of the heart.

Lymph nodes are composed of a ***medulla*** with many sinuses, and a ***cortex***, which is surrounded by a capsule of connective tissue. The cortical region contains ***primary lymphoid follicles***. Upon antigenic stimulation, these

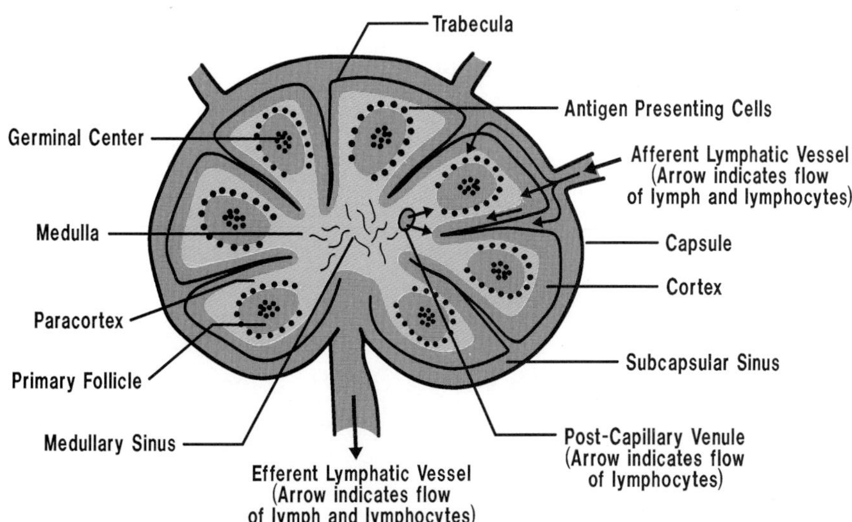

Figure 2.4.
A diagramatic representation of a section of a lymph node.

structures form ***germinal centers*** that contain dense populations of lymphocytes—mostly B cells—that are undergoing mitosis. The deep cortical area or paracortical region contains T cells and macrophages. The macrophages trap, process, and present the antigen to the T cells that have specificity against that antigen, events that result in activation of the T cells. The medullary area of the lymph node contains antibody-secreting plasma cells that have traveled from the cortex to the medulla via the lymphatic vessels.

The lymph node is highly efficient in trapping antigen. Antigen enters the node through the ***afferent lymphatic vessels.*** In the node, the antigen interacts with macrophages, T cells, and B cells, and that interaction brings about an immune response, manifested by the generation of antibodies and antigen-specific T cells. Lymph, antibodies, and cells leave the lymph node through the ***efferent lymphatic vessel,*** which is just below the medullary region.

CIRCULATION OF LYMPHOCYTES

Blood lymphocytes enter the lymph nodes through ***post-capillary venules*** and leave the lymph nodes through efferent lymphatic vessels. The vessels from numerous lymph nodes throughout the body converge in the thoracic duct, which empties into the ***vena cava***, the vessel that returns the blood to the heart. Lymph and lymphocytes also enter the lymph nodes through numerous afferent lymphatic vessels.

The spleen functions in a similar manner. Arterial blood lymphocytes enter the spleen through the ***hilus*** and pass into the ***trabecular artery***, which along its course becomes narrow and branched. At the farthest branches of the trabecular artery, capillaries lead to lymphoid nodules. Ultimately, the lymphocytes return to the venous circulation through the ***trabecular vein***, but it is unclear how the cells pass from the capillaries to the trabecular vein. Like lymph nodes, the spleen contains efferent lymphatic vessels through which lymph empties into the lymphatics from which the cells continue their recirculation through the body and back to the afferent vessels.

THE FATE OF ANTIGEN AFTER PENETRATION

The reticuloendothelial system is designed to trap foreign antigens that have penetrated the body and to subject them to phagocytosis—by the phagocytic cells of the system. Also, there is constant movement of lymphocytes throughout the body, and this movement permits deposition of lymphocytes in strategic places along the lymphatic vessels. The system not only traps antigens but also provides loci (the secondary lymphoid organs) where antigen, macrophages, T cells and B cells can interact in a very small area to initiate an immune response.

The fate of an antigen that has penetrated the physical barriers, and the cellular and antibody components of the ensuing immune response are shown in Figure 2.5. As illustrated, there are three major routes that may be followed by an antigen after it has penetrated the interior of the body.

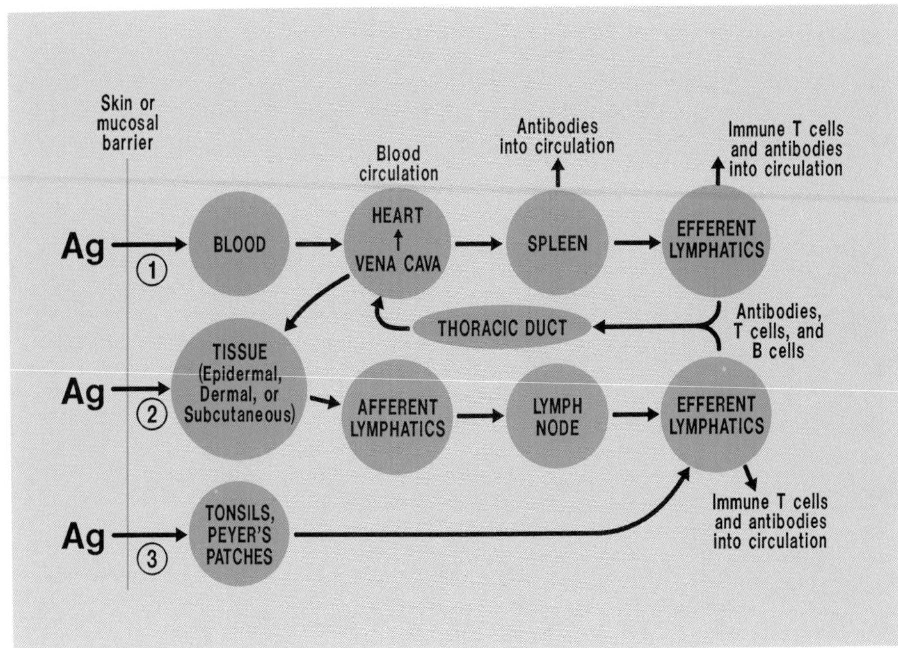

Figure 2.5.
Circulation of lymph and fate of antigen following penetration through 1) the bloodstream, 2) the skin, and 3) the gastrointestinal or respiratory tract.

1. The antigen may enter the body through the ***bloodstream***. In this case, it is carried to the ***spleen***, where it interacts with macrophages, T cells, and B cells to generate an antigen-specific immune response. The spleen then releases

the antibodies directly into the circulation. Lymphocytes also leave the spleen through the efferent lymphatics, to re-enter the circulation via the thoracic duct.

2. The antigen may lodge in the ***epidermal, dermal***, or ***subcutaneous tissue***, where it may cause an inflammatory response. From these tissues the antigen, either free or trapped by macrophages, is transported through the afferent lymphatic channels into the regional, ***draining lymph node***. In the lymph node, the antigen, macrophages, T cells, and B cells interact to generate the immune response. Eventually, antigen-specific T cells and antibodies, which have been synthesized in the lymph node, enter the circulation and are transported to the various tissues. Antigen-specific T cells, B cells, and antibodies also enter the circulation via the thoracic duct.

3. The antigen may enter the ***gastrointestinal*** or ***respiratory tract,*** where it lodges in lymphoid organs such as ***Peyer's patches*** or the ***tonsils.*** There, it will interact with macrophages and lymphocytes. Antibodies synthesized in these organs are deposited in the local tissue. In addition, lymphocytes entering the efferent lymphatics are carried through the ***thoracic duct*** to the circulation and are thereby redistributed to various tissues.

The induction of an acquired immune response necessitates the interaction of the foreign antigen with lymphocytes that recognize that specific antigen. It has been estimated that in a ***naive (nonimmunized)*** animal, only one in every 10^3–10^5 lymphocytes is capable of recognizing a typical antigen. Therefore, the probability that an antigen will encounter such cells is very low. The problem is compounded by the fact that, for synthesis of antibody to ensue, two different kinds of lymphocyte—the T lymphocyte and the B lymphocyte—each with specificity against this particular antigen, must interact. Moreover, for the activation of most subpopulations of T cells, the antigen has to be presented on the surface of a macrophage. Statistically, the chances for the interaction of specific lymphocytes with their particular antigen, and then for their interaction with B cells specific for the same antigen, are very low. However, a mechanism exists for bringing all these cells into contact with antigen. The antigen is carried, via the draining lymph nodes, to the secondary lymphoid organs. In these organs, the antigen is exposed on the surface of fixed macrophages. Because both T and B lymphocytes circulate at a rather rapid rate, making the rounds every several days, some circulating lymphocytes with specificity for the particular antigen should pass by the fixed antigen within a relatively short time. When these lymphocytes recognize the antigen, a specific interaction takes place: the lymphocytes become activated and the acquired immune response, with specificity against this antigen, is triggered.

SUMMARY

1. There are two forms of immunity: 1) innate, or natural, and 2) acquired.

2. Three major types of cell participate in acquired immunity: 1) the B lymphocyte; 2) the T lymphocyte; and 3) the macrophage.

3. B and T lymphocytes have receptors that are specific for particular antigens and, thus, constitute the components of acquired immunity that are responsible for antigenic specificity.

4. B lymphocytes and T lymphocytes develop in primary lymphoid organs. Their development and maturation is independent of antigen.

5. B and T lymphocytes differentiate and proliferate in response to antigenic stimulation. These events generally take place in secondary lymphoid organs.

6. B lymphocytes synthesize and secrete antibodies; T lymphocytes do not make antibodies. However, T lymphocytes participate in cell-mediated immunity; they "help" B cells make antibodies; they also participate in various regulatory aspects of the immune response through soluble factors (lymphokines), which they release.

7. Macrophages constitute an essential part of the reticuloendothelial system and function to trap, process, and present antigen to T lymphocytes.

REFERENCES

Butcher EC, Weissman IL (1984). In Paul WE (ed): Fundamental Immunology. New York: Raven Press.

Cline MJ (ed) (1975): The White Cell. Cambridge, Massachusetts: Harvard University Press.

Van Furth R (ed) (1985): Mononuclear phagocytes—characteristics, physiology and function. Boston: Martinus Nijhoff.

Weiss L (1972): The Cells and Tissues of the Immune System: Structure, Functions, Interactions. Englewood Cliffs, New Jersey: Prentice-Hall.

(Continued on next page)

REVIEW QUESTIONS

For each of the incomplete statements below, ONE or MORE of the completions given is correct. Choose the appropriate answer:
A) if only *1, 2, 3* are correct
B) if only *1 and 3* are correct
C) if only *2 and 4* are correct
D) if only *4* is correct
E) if *all* are correct

1. Which of the following apply to *both* primary and secondary lymphoid organs:
   1) cellular proliferation.
   2) differentiation of lymphocytes.
   3) cellular interaction.
   4) antigen-dependent response.

2. Which of the following apply uniquely to secondary lymphoid organs:
   1) antigen-dependent response.
   2) circulation of lymphocytes.
   3) terminal differentiation.
   4) cellular proliferation.

3. Which of the following apply to "innate" immune mechanisms:
   1) absence of specificity.
   2) activation by a stimulus.
   3) involvement of multiple cell types.
   4) a memory component.

4. Which of the following is the major function of the lymphoid system:
   1) innate immunity.
   2) inflammation.
   3) phagocytosis.
   4) acquired immunity.

5. Removal of the bursa of Fabricius from a chicken results in
   1) a markedly decreased number of circulating lymphocytes.
   2) anemia.
   3) delayed rejection of skin graft.
   4) low levels of antibodies in serum.

ANSWERS TO REVIEW QUESTIONS

1. ***A*** Cellular proliferation, differentiation of lymphocytes, and cellular interactions can take place in primary lymphoid organs (bursa of Fabricius or equivalent, thymus gland). However, antigen-dependent responses occur in the secondary lymphoid organs, such as spleen and lymph nodes.

2. ***B*** Antigen-dependent responses of proliferation and differentiation (as well as terminal differentiation of B cells into plasma cells) occur only in secondary lymphoid organs, such as spleen and lymph nodes. However, circulation of lymphocytes and cellular proliferation (but not antigen-dependent responses of terminal differentiation) take place in the primary lymphoid organs, such as the bursa of Fabricius or its equivalent, or the thymus.

3. ***A*** Innate immunity has none of the antigenic specificity exhibited by acquired immunity. It is activated by such stimuli as the invasion of foreign particles into the body. Innate immunity involves multiple cell types, such as those of the monocytic series (macrophages) and those of the granulocytic series (neutrophils, eosinophils, etc.).

4. ***D*** The major function of the lymphoid system is the recognition of foreign antigen by lymphocytes, which leads to the acquired immune response. Functions such as phagocytosis and inflammation do not necessarily require the lymphoid system, and they constitute part of innate immunity.

5. ***D*** Removal of the bursa of Fabricius from a chicken results in low levels of antibodies in serum, since this organ serves as a primary lymphoid organ in which B lymphocytes (which eventually synthesize and secrete antibodies) undergo maturation. The removal of the organ will not result in a marked decrease in the number of circulating lymphocytes, nor will it result in anemia, characterized by a marked decrease in erythrocyte count, since erythrocytes undergo maturation outside the bursa. The question has no relevance to delayed rejection of skin grafts.

CHAPTER

3

IMMUNOGENS AND ANTIGENS

INTRODUCTION

Immune responses arise as a result of exposure to foreign stimuli. The compound that evokes the response is referred to either as "antigen" or as "immunogen." The distinction between these terms is functional. An ***immunogen*** is any agent capable of inducing an immune response. In contrast, an ***antigen*** is any agent capable of binding specifically to components of the immune response, such as lymphocytes and antibodies. The distinction between the terms is necessary because there are many compounds that are incapable of inducing an immune response, yet they are capable of binding with components of the immune system that have been induced specifically against them. Thus, all immunogens are antigens, but not all antigens are immunogens, although many are. This difference becomes obvious in the case of low molecular weight compounds, a group of substances that includes many antibiotics and drugs. By themselves, these compounds are incapable of inducing an immune response, but when they are coupled with much larger entities, such as proteins, the resultant conjugate induces an immune response that is directed against various parts of the conjugate, including the low molecular weight compound. When manipulated in this manner, the low molecular weight compound is referred to as a ***hapten*** (from the Greek *hapten,* which means to grasp); the high molecular weight compound to which the hapten is conjugated is referred to as a ***carrier***. Thus, a hapten is a compound that, by itself, is incapable of inducing an immune response, but against which an immune response can be induced by immunization with the hapten conjugated to a carrier.

In the present chapter we shall deal with some attributes of compounds which render them immunogenic and antigenic.

REQUIREMENTS FOR IMMUNOGENICITY

There are three characteristics that a compound must possess to be immunogenic. They are ***foreignness, high molecular weight,*** and ***chemical complexity.***

Foreignness

Animals normally do not respond defensively to "***self***." Thus, for example, if a rabbit is injected with its own serum albumin, the rabbit will not mount an immune response; it recognizes the albumin as self. In contrast, if rabbit serum albumin is injected into a guinea pig, the guinea pig, recognizing the rabbit serum albumin as "***foreign***," mounts an immune response against it. To prove that the rabbit, which did not respond to its own serum albumin, is immunologically competent, it can be injected with guinea pig albumin. The competent rabbit will mount an immune response to guinea pig serum albumin because it recognizes the substance as foreign. Thus, the first requirement for a compound to be immunogenic is foreignness.

Normally, compounds that are part of self are not immunogenic to the individual. However, there are exceptional cases in which an individual mounts an immune response against components of self. This pathological condition is termed ***autoimmunity*** or ***autoallergy*** (see Chapter 16).

High Molecular Weight

The second requirement that determines whether a compound is immunogenic is that it must have a certain minimal molecular weight. Low molecular weight chemicals are usually not immunogenic, whereas high molecular weight chemicals are. In general, compounds that have a molecular weight of less than 1,000 daltons (e.g. penicillin, progesterone, aspirin) are not immunogenic; those of molecular weight between 1,000 and 6,000 daltons (e.g. insulin, adrenocorticotropic hormone, ACTH) may or may not be immunogenic; and those of molecular weight ***greater than 6,000 daltons*** (e.g. albumin, tetanus toxin) ***are generally immunogenic.***

Chemical Complexity

The third characteristic necessary for a compound to be immunogenic is a certain degree of physicochemical complexity. Thus, for example, various homopolymers of amino acids, such as a polymer of lysine of molecular weight 30,000 daltons, are usually not good immunogens. Similarly, a homopolymer of poly-gamma-D-glutamic acid (the capsular material of *Bacillus anthracis*), of molecular weight 50,000 daltons, is not immunogenic. This absence of immunogenicity is because these compounds, although of high molecular weight, are not chemically complex enough to be immunogenic. However, if various moieties, such as dinitrophenol or other low molecular weight compounds, which by themselves are not immunogenic, are attached to the epsilon amino groups of poly-lysine, the entire macromolecule becomes immunogenic. The resulting immune response is directed not only against the small haptens but also against the high molecular weight homopolymer. In general, an increase in the chemical complexity of a compound is accompanied by an increase in its immunogenicity. Thus polymers of several amino acids such as poly-glutamic, alanine, and lysine (poly-GAT) are highly immunogenic.

HAPTENS

Haptens are low molecular weight compounds that are not immunogenic but that become immunogenic if they are ***conjugated*** to high molecular weight ***carriers.*** Thus, an immune response can be evoked to thousands of chemical compounds—those of high molecular weight and those of low molecular weight. Immune responses have been demonstrated against all the known biochemical families of compounds: carbohydrates, lipids, proteins, and nucleic acids. Moreover, immune responses to thousands of low molecular weight compounds have been reported, examples of which include drugs, antibiotics, food additives, cosmetics, and many small synthetic peptides. Immunogenicity, in every case, is conferred by fulfillment of the three criteria: foreignness, high molecular weight, and chemical complexity. If these critera are not met, immunogenicity can be achieved by conjugating a compound covalently to any of various carriers, thus increasing the molecular weight and the degree of chemical complexity.

THYMUS-DEPENDENT AND THYMUS-INDEPENDENT ANTIGENS

It is well established that both T and B lymphocytes participate in the immune response (see Chapters 9 and 10 for a detailed discussion). Generally, the B cell, which is the antibody-producing cell, requires the cooperation of a T cell for the production of antibodies and, in particular, for the production of antibodies of the IgG class.

Most immunogenic molecules, such as proteins, which induce an immune response and the production of antibodies, require both T and B lymphocytes. Because T lymphocytes mature in the thymus these immunogens are referred to as ***thymus-dependent antigens.*** There are, however, certain types of molecules that can induce the production of antibodies without the apparent participation of T lymphocytes. Such molecules are referred to as ***thymus-independent antigens,*** and are generally substances of high molecular weight with repeating structures, such as bacterial polysaccharides and polymerized proteins. Immunization with thymus-independent antigens (or more correctly, immunogens) leads to the production of antibodies exclusively of the IgM class and generates little or no immunological memory (see Chapter 10). However, IgG antibodies against such immunogens may be induced by immunization with the thymus-independent antigen conjugated to thymus-dependent antigens.

ANTIGENICITY

An immune response induced by an antigen generates immune components, some of which react specifically with the antigen. The specificity of this interaction is analogous to the interaction of an enzyme with its substrate. The antigen-binding site of an antibody or of a receptor on a lymphocyte has a unique structure that allows a complementary "fit" to some structural aspect of the specific antigen. The portion of the antigen that binds specifically with the binding site of an antibody or a receptor on a lymphocyte is termed an ***antigenic determinant*** or ***epitope.***

Various studies on the size of antigenic determinants indicate a size approximately equivalent to 5–7 amino acids or, roughly 7 × 12 × 35 Å. These dimensions were calculated from experiments that involved the binding of antibodies to polysaccharides, as well as to peptide determinants. These dimensions would also be expected to correspond roughly to the size of the antibody-combining site, and indeed this expectation has been confirmed by X-ray crystallography. Thus, in current immunologic terminology, the size of an epitope is approximately 7 × 12 × 35 Å, and the size of the complementary site on the antibody, or the ***paratope,*** has approximately the same dimensions.

With respect to their epitopes, antigens may have the following characteristics (shown schematically in Figure 3.1).

1. The antigen may have only a single epitope of a given specificity on its surface, which is capable of binding to antibodies. Such a compound is called a ***unideterminant, univalent antigen;*** i.e. there is only one determinant or one epitope on the molecule.

2. The antigen may have two or more determinants of the same kind on the molecule. Such an antigen is called a ***unideterminant, multivalent antigen,*** since it has only one kind of determinant, but many such determinants on each molecule.

3. Some antigens, including most proteins, are ***multideterminant and univalent***. Such molecules have many epitopes of different kinds, but only ***one of each kind***.

4. High molecular weight, chemically complex compounds or polymerized proteins are usually ***multideterminant, multivalent antigens,*** having ***many kinds of determinants*** and many determinants of each kind on each molecule.

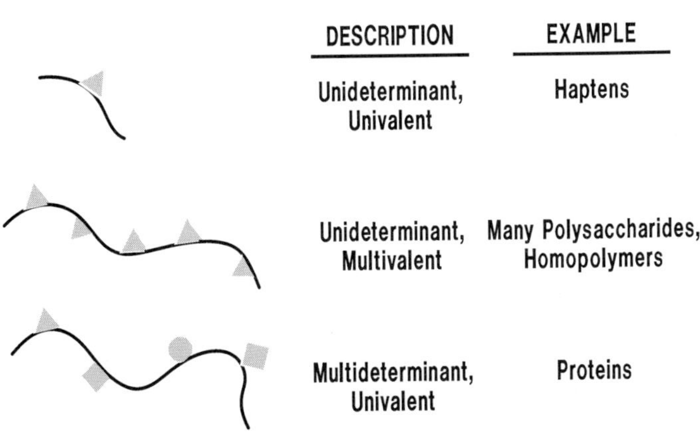

DESCRIPTION
EXAMPLE
Unideterminant, Univalent
Haptens
Unideterminant, Multivalent
Many Polysaccharides, Homopolymers
Multideterminant, Univalent
Proteins

Figure 3.1
Representation of various possible antigenic structures.

MAJOR CLASSES OF ANTIGENS

The following major chemical families may be antigenic:

1. ***Carbohydrates (polysaccharides).*** Polysaccharides are potentially, but not always, immunogenic. Normally, polysaccharides, which form part of more complex molecules such as cell surface ***glycoproteins***, elicit an immune response directed specifically against the polysaccharide moiety of the molecule. An immune response, consisting primarily of humoral antibodies, can be induced against many kinds of polysaccharide molecules such as components of microorganisms and eukaryotic cells. An excellent example of this antigenicity is the immune response associated with the ***ABO blood groups,*** which derive their antigenicity and immunological specificity from polysaccharides on the surface of the red blood cells.

2. ***Lipids.*** Lipids are usually not immunogenic, but an immune response to lipids may be induced if the lipids are conjugated to protein carriers. Thus, in a sense, lipids may be regarded as haptens. Immune responses to ***sphingolipids*** have also been reported.

3. ***Nucleic acids.*** Nucleic acids are poor immunogens by themselves, but they become immunogenic when they are conjugated to protein carriers. DNA, in its native helical state, is usually nonimmunogenic in normal animals. However, immune responses to nucleic acids have been reported in many instances. One important example in clinical medicine is the appearance of anti-DNA antibodies in patients with ***systemic lupus erythematosus***.

4. ***Proteins.*** Virtually all proteins are immunogenic in an appropriate individual. Thus, the most common immune responses are those to proteins. Furthermore, the greater the degree of complexity of the protein, the more vigorous will be the immune response to that protein. In general, proteins are multideterminant univalent antigens with immune responses directed against many, or all, of the determinants.

The immune response recognizes many structural features and physicochemical properties of compounds. For example, antibodies can recognize various structural features of a protein, such as its ***primary structure*** (the amino acid sequence); ***secondary structures*** (the structure of the backbone of the polypeptide chain, such as an α-helix or β-pleated sheet); ***tertiary structures*** (formed by the three-dimensional configuration of the protein, which is conferred by the folding of the polypeptide chain and held together by disulfide bridges, hydrogen bonds, hydrophobic interactions, etc.); and ***quaternary***

structures (formed by the juxtaposition of separate parts if the molecule is composed of more than one protein subunit). Antibodies are also capable of recognizing and distinguishing differences as subtle as the various positions of substituents on a benzene ring (ortho, meta, or para positions), as well as various optical isomers of a compound. In general, it can be said that antibodies are exquisitely specific reagents for the detection of numerous physicochemical characteristics or structures of compounds.

BINDING OF ANTIGEN WITH ANTIBODIES OR IMMUNOLOGICALLY COMPETENT CELLS

The binding between antigen and various immune components is discussed in detail in Chapter 7. At this point, it is important to mention only that the binding of antigen with antibodies or immunocompetent cells does not involve covalent bonds. The binding may involve ***electrostatic interactions, hydrophobic interactions, hydrogen bonds,*** and ***Van der Waal forces.*** Since these interactive forces are relatively weak, the "fit" between antigen and its complementary site on the antibody must occur over an area large enough to allow the summation of all the possible available interactions. This requirement is the basis for the exquisite specificity observed in antigen–antibody interactions.

CROSS-REACTIVITY

Since macromolecular antigens contain several distinct antigenic determinants, some of these structures can be altered without totally changing the immunogenic and antigenic structure of the entire molecule. This concept is important in relation to immunization against highly pathogenic microorganisms or highly toxic compounds, when the microorganism or the toxin is used for immunization. For example, a lethal dose of tetanus toxin for mice is measured in picograms (10^{-12} gm), while a dose required for immunization is measured in micrograms (10^{-6} gm). Obviously, immunization with the toxin would be unwise. However, it is possible to destroy the biological activity of this and a broad variety of other toxins (e.g., bacterial toxins and snake venoms) without appreciably affecting their antigenicity or immunogenicity. A toxin that has been modified to the extent that it is no longer toxic but still maintains some of its immunochemical characteristics is called a ***toxoid***. A toxoid is a molecule that ***cross-reacts*** immunologically with the toxin. Thus, it is possible to immunize individuals with the toxoid and thereby induce immune responses to some of the antigenic determinants that the toxoid still shares with the native toxin, because these determinants have not been destroyed by the modification. Although the molecules of toxin and toxoid differ in many physicochemical and biological respects, they nevertheless share enough antigenic determinants to allow the immune response to the toxoid to mount an effective defense against the toxin itself.

An immunologic reaction in which the immune components, either cells or antibodies, react with two molecules that share antigenic determinants, but that are otherwise dissimilar, is called a ***cross-reaction.*** When two compounds cross-react immunologically, it means that the compounds have one or more antigenic determinants in common, and that the immune response to one of the compounds recognizes one or more of the same antigenic determinant(s) on the other compound, and reacts with it. Another form of cross-reactivity is seen when antibodies to one determinant bind, usually more weakly, to another determinant that is not quite identical but that has a structural resemblance to the first determinant.

To denote that the antigen used for immunization is different from the one with which the induced immune components are then allowed to react, the terms homologous and heterologous are used. ***Homologous*** denotes that the antigen and the immunogen are the same; ***heterologous*** denotes that the compound used to induce the immune response is different from the compound that is then allowed to react with the products of induced response. In the latter case, the heterologous antigen may or may not react with the immune components. If reaction takes place, it may be concluded that the heterologous and homologous antigens exhibit ***immunologic cross-reactivity.***

Although the hallmark of immunology is specificity, immunologic cross-reactivity has been observed on many levels. Such observations do not mean that the immunologic specificity has been diminished, but rather that the compounds that cross-react share antigenic determinants. In cases of cross-reactivity, the antigenic determinants of the cross-reacting substances may have identical chemical structures, or they may be composed of similar but not identical physicochemical configurations. In the example given above, a toxin and its corresponding toxoid represent two molecules, the toxin being the ***native*** molecule, and the toxoid being a ***modified*** molecule that cross-reacts with the native molecule.

There are other examples of immunological cross-reactivity, wherein the two cross-reacting substances are unrelated to each other except insofar as they have one or more antigenic determinants in common. Common antigenic determinants that are found on unrelated substances are referred to as ***heterophile antigens.*** For example, human blood group A antigen reacts with antiserum raised against pneumococcal capsular polysaccharide (type XIV). Similarly, human blood group B antigen reacts with antibodies to certain strains of *Escherichia coli.* In these examples of cross-reactivity, the antigens of the microorganisms are referred to as the heterophile antigens (with respect to the blood group antigen).

IMMUNOLOGIC ADJUVANTS

To enhance the immune response to a given immunogen, immunologic adjuvants are often used. An ***adjuvant*** is a substance which, when mixed with an immunogen, enhances the immune response against the immunogen. It is important to distinguish between a carrier for a hapten and an adjuvant. A hapten will become immunogenic when conjugated covalently to a carrier; it will not become immunogenic if mixed with an adjuvant. Thus, an adjuvant enhances the immune response to immunogens but does not confer immunogenicity to haptens.

There are various adjuvants that are widely used to enhance the immune response. One such adjuvant is ***Freund's complete adjuvant (CFA)***, which consists of a water-in-oil emulsion, and killed *Mycobacterium tuberculosis* or *butyricum.* The antigen is contained in the water phase. Other microorganisms used as adjuvants are ***BCG*** (bacillus Calmette-Guérin, an attenuated *Mycobacterium*), *Corynebacterium parvum,* and *Bordetella pertussis.* These adjuvants are presumed to release antigen slowly but continuously and to stimulate certain subpopulations of lymphocytes (T cells) and macrophages. Other adjuvants are toxins and polysaccharides such as ***lipopolysaccharide*** (endotoxin or LPS), and still others contain a synthetic ***muramyldipeptide*** (N-acetyl-muramyl-L-alanyl-D-isoglutamine [MDP]). LPS enhances the antibody response by stimulating a subpopulation of lymphocytes (B cells) while muramyldipeptide, the effective constituent of mycobacterial cell walls, stimulates T cells.

The most widely used adjuvant in humans is ***alum precipitate,*** a suspension of aluminum hydroxide on which the antigen is adsorbed. This adjuvant allows continuous release of antigen and, in addition, the adjuvant has a slight irritant effect which enhances the ingestion and processing of antigen by macrophages (see Chapter 10).

SUMMARY

1. Immunologically, a compound may have one or both of the following two major attributes:

a) *Immunogenicity*—the capacity to induce an immune response. Immunogenicity requires that a compound i) is foreign to the immunized individual, ii) possesses a certain minimal molecular weight, and iii) possesses a certain degree of chemical complexity. Compounds that are of high molecular weight but that are not chemically complex are usually not good immunogens.

b) *Antigenicity*—the ability to bind with antibodies or with cells of the immune system. This binding is highly specific; the immune components are capable of recognizing various physicochemical aspects of the compound. The binding between antigen and immune components involves Van der Waal forces, electrostatic interactions, hydrophobic interactions, and hydrogen bonds, it does not involve covalent bonds.

2. The smallest unit of an antigen that is capable of binding with antibodies is called an *antigenic determinant* or *epitope*. Compounds may have one or more epitopes capable of reacting with immune components. The immune response against these compounds involves the production of antibodies or the generation of cells with specificities directed against most or all of the epitopes.

3. Immunologic cross-reactivity denotes a situation in which two or more compounds, that may have various degrees of dissimilarity, share antigenic determinants and would, therefore, react with immune components induced against any one of these compounds. Thus, a toxoid, which is a modified form of a toxin, may have one or more antigenic determinants in common with the toxin. Immunization with the toxoid leads to an immune response capable of reacting not only with the toxoid but also with the native toxin.

4. Most antigens are thymus-dependent; they require both T and B lymphocytes for induction of the immune response. However, some antigens are thymus-independent and appear not to require T lymphocytes for production of antibodies by the B lymphocytes. Thymus-independent antigens induce primarily antibodies of the IgM class and do not induce immunologic memory.

REFERENCES

Atassi MZ (ed) (1977): Immunochemistry of Proteins, Vols 1 and 2. New York: Plenum.

Goodman JW (1984): Immunogenicity and antigenic specificity. In Stites DP, Stobo JD, Fudenberg HH, Wells JV (eds): Basic and Clinical Immunology, Ed 5. Los Altos, California: Lange Medical Publications.

Landsteiner K (1962): The Specificity of Serologic Reactions, Rev Ed. New York: Dover Press. (original: Harvard University Press, 1945).
Sela M (1973): The Antigens, Vols 1–5. New York: Academic Press.
Young CR (1984): Structural requirements for immunogenicity and antigenicity. In Atassi MZ, Van Oss CJ, Absolom DR (eds): Molecular Immunology. New York: Marcel Dekker.

REVIEW QUESTIONS

Each of the questions below (questions 1–3) is followed by several suggested answers or completions. Select ONE that is BEST in each case.

1. The following properties render a substance immunogenic
   a) high molecular weight.
   b) chemical complexity.
   c) sufficient stability and persistence after injection.
   d) all of the above.
   e) all of the above are essential but not sufficient.

2. The protection against smallpox afforded by prior infection with cowpox represents
   a) antigenic specificity.
   b) antigenic cross-reactivity.
   c) viral superinfection.
   d) innate immunity.
   e) passive protection.

3. Converting a toxin to a toxoid
   a) makes the toxin more immunogenic.
   b) reduces the pharmacologic activity of the toxin.
   c) enhances binding with antitoxin.
   d) induces only innate immunity.
   e) increases phagocytosis.

For the incomplete statement below (question 4), ONE or MORE of the completions given is correct. Choose the appropriate answer:
A) if only *1, 2, 3* are correct
B) if only *1 and 3* are correct
C) if only *2 and 4* are correct
D) if only *4* is correct
E) if *all* are correct

4. Haptens
   1) require carrier molecules in order to be immunogenic.
   2) will not react with specific antibodies in vitro unless homologous carriers are employed.
   3) interact with specific antibody even if the hapten is monovalent.
   4) can stimulate secondary antibody responses without carriers.

(*Continued on next page*)

ANSWERS TO REVIEW QUESTIONS

1. ***e*** All of the properties are essential but not sufficient, since for immunogenicity the substance must be foreign to the immunized individual.

2. ***b*** The protection against smallpox provided by prior infection with cowpox is an example of antigenic cross-reactivity. Immunization with cowpox leads to the production of antibodies capable of reacting with smallpox because the two viruses share several identical, or structurally similar, determinants.

3. ***b*** Conversion of a toxin to a toxoid is performed in order to reduce the pharmacologic activity of the toxin, so that sufficient toxoid can be injected to induce an immune response.

4. ***B*** Haptens are substances, usually of low molecular weight and univalent, that by themselves, cannot induce an immune response, but that can do so if conjugated to high molecular weight carriers. The haptens can and do interact with the induced antibodies, without it being necessary that they be conjugated to the carrier.

CHAPTER

4

ANTIBODY STRUCTURE

INTRODUCTION

One of the major functions of the immune system is the production of soluble proteins that circulate freely and exhibit a variety of properties, all of which contribute, in some way, to immunity and protection against foreign material. These soluble proteins are the ***antibodies***, and they belong to the class of proteins called ***globulins*** because of their globular structure. Initially, because of their migratory properties in an electrophoretic field they were called γ-***globulins*** (in relation to albumin, α-globulin and β-globulin); today they are known collectively as ***immunoglobulins (Ig)***.

The structure of immunoglobulins must incorporate several features essential for their participation in the immune response. The two most important of these features are ***specificity*** and ***biologic activity***. Specificity requires a mechanism that restricts the molecules with which the antibody can combine to those that contain one, particular antigenic structure. The existence of a vast array of potential antigenic determinants (see Chapter 3) has necessitated the evolution of a system for producing a repertoire of molecules, each of which is capable of combining with a single antigenic structure. Thus, antibodies exhibit not only great diversity, in terms of the types of molecular structure with which they are capable of reacting, but also a high degree of specificity, since each is able to react with only one antigenic determinant. Despite the large numbers of antibodies capable of reacting with many different structural entities, the biologic effects of such a combination are rather few in number (e.g. complement fixation, crossing of the placenta, activation of mast cells). Therefore, while one part of the molecule is adapted to allow tremendous variation in the determinants that can be recognized, another part must be adapted to allow the antibody to participate in biological functions common to all antibodies. This chapter deals with the ways in which the antibody molecule fulfills these two functions.

ISOLATION AND CHARACTERIZATION

Serum is the residue that is left when blood has clotted and the clot, which contains cells and clotting factors, is removed. When serum is subjected to ***electrophoresis*** (separation in an electrical field) at slightly alkaline pH (8.2), five major components can normally be visualized (see Fig. 4.1). The slowest, in terms of migration toward the anode is called ***γ-globulin,*** and was shown by Kabat and Tiselius in 1939 to contain antibody. This demonstration entailed the simple comparison of the electrophoretic pattern of antiserum from a hyperimmune rabbit before and after the specific antibody had been removed by precipitation with the antigen. Only the size of the γ-globulin fraction was

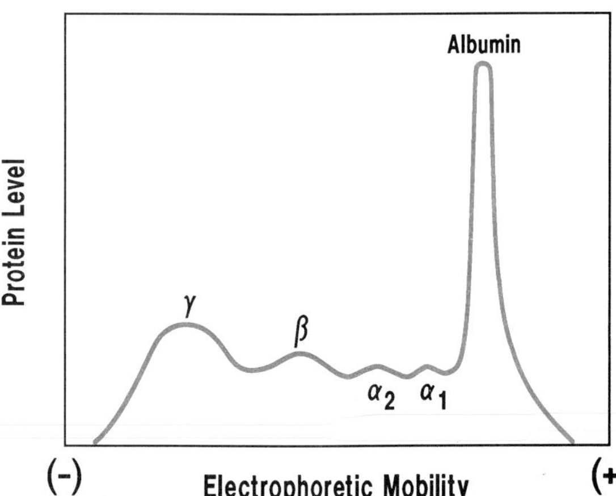

Figure 4.1.
Electrophoretic mobility of serum proteins.

diminished by this procedure. Subsequent analysis showed that, when this fraction was collected separately, all measureable antibodies were contained within it.

From the broad electrophoretic peak of this fraction, it is clear that a ***heterogeneous*** collection of molecules with different charges (generically known as ***immunoglobulins***) is present. This heterogeneity was one of the early obstacles in attempts to determine the structure of antibodies, since analytical chemistry requires homogeneous, crystallizable compounds as starting material. This problem was solved, in part, by the discovery of ***myeloma proteins,*** which are homogeneous immunoglobulins produced by the progeny of a single plasma cell that has become neoplastic and reproduced itself endlessly in the disease called ***multiple myeloma***. When it became clear that some myeloma proteins bind antigen, it also became apparent that they could be dealt with as typical immunoglobulin molecules. Another aid to structural studies of antibodies was the discovery of ***Bence-Jones proteins*** in the urine. These homogeneous proteins, produced in large quantities by some patients with multiple myeloma, are ***dimers of antibody light chains***. They were very useful in the determination of the structure of this portion of the immunoglobulin molecule. Today, the powerful technique of cell–cell hybridization permits the production of large quantities of homogeneous preparations of monoclonal antibody of virtually any specificity (see Chapter 8).

STRUCTURE OF LIGHT AND HEAVY CHAINS

The analysis of the structure of antibody molecules really began in 1959 with two discoveries which, for the first time, revealed that the molecule could be separated into analyzable parts suitable for further study. Porter found that proteolytic treatment with the enzyme papain split the molecule (molecular weight 150,000 daltons) into three fragments of about equal size (45,000 daltons) (see Fig. 4.2). Two of these fragments were found to retain the antibody's ability to bind antigen specifically, although they could no longer precipitate the antigen from solution. These two fragments are referred to as ***Fab*** (fragment antigen binding) fragments and were considered to be univalent, possessing one binding site each and being in every way identical to each other. The third fragment could be crystallized out of solution, a property indicative of its apparent homogeneity. This fragment is called ***Fc*** (fragment crystallizable). It cannot bind antigen, but, as was subsequently shown, it is responsible for the biological functions of the molecule after antigen has been bound to the Fab part of the intact molecule.

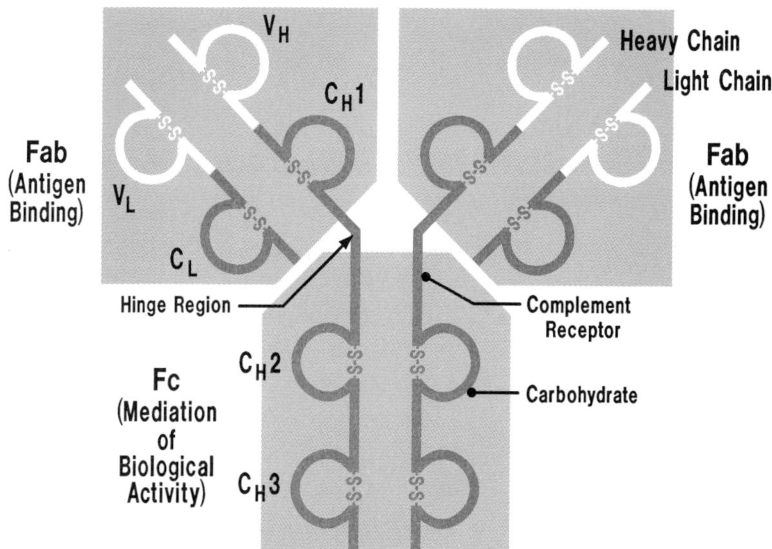

Figure 4.2.
Schematic representation of an immunoglobulin molecule.

At about the same time, Edelman discovered that when γ-globulin was extensively reduced by treatment with ***mercaptoethanol*** (a reagent that breaks S–S bonds) the molecule fell apart into four chains: two identical chains with molecular weight of about 53,000 daltons each, and two others of about 22,000 daltons each. The larger chains were designated ***heavy (H)*** and the smaller ones ***light (L).*** Based on these results, the structure of immunoglobulin molecules, as depicted in Figure 4.2, was proposed. This model was subsequently shown to be essentially correct; Porter and Edelman shared the Nobel prize for the elucidation of antibody structure. Thus, all immunoglobulin molecules consist of a basic unit of 4 polypeptide chains, ***2 identical H chains*** and ***2 identical L chains,*** held together by a number of ***disulfide bonds.***

As in the case of any other protein, immunoglobulins of one species are immunogenic in another species. The use of immunoglobulins as antigens allowed the production of a variety of antisera that could distinguish between features of different immunoglobulin chains. By a combination of biochemical and serologic (utilizing serum antibodies) techniques, it was shown that almost all species studied have two major classes of L chains, called κ and λ. Any one individual of a species produces both types of L chain, but the ratio of κ-chains to λ-chains varies with the species (mouse: 95% κ; human: 60% κ). However, in any one immunoglobulin molecule, the L chains are always either both κ or both λ, not one of each.

By physicochemical and immunochemical techniques, the immunoglobulins of virtually all species have been shown to consist of five different ***isotypes (classes).*** These isotypes differ not only in antigenic reactivity (serologically) and carbohydrate content but also in size and biological function. The H chains, derived from the various immunoglobulin isotypes, are designated with Greek letters, as follows:

Immunoglobulin isotype (class)	Heavy chains
IgM	μ
IgG	γ
IgA	α
IgD	δ
IgE	ϵ

Again, any individual of a species makes all classes of H chains, in proportions characteristic of the species, but in any one antibody molecule both H chains are identical (i.e. 2 γ or 2 ϵ, etc.). Thus, an antibody molecule of the IgG class could have the structure $\kappa2\gamma2$ or $\lambda2\gamma2$, while an antibody of the IgE class could have the structure $\kappa2\epsilon2$ or $\lambda2\epsilon2$. In each case, it is the nature of the H chains that confers on the molecule its unique biologic properties, such as its half-life in the circulation, its ability to bind to certain receptors, or its ability to activate enzymes (see Chapter 8).

Further characterization of these isotypes by specific antisera has led to the designation of several ***subclasses*** (also referred to as ***isotypes***) which have more subtle differences among themselves. Thus, the major class, IgG, can be subdivided into IgG_1, IgG_2, IgG_3, and IgG_4 in humans; IgG_1, IgG_{2a}, IgG_{2b}, and IgG_3 in mice. IgA has been divided similarly into two subclasses, IgA_1 and IgA_2. The subclasses differ from one another in numbers and arrangement of interchain disulfide bonds, as well as by alterations in other structural features. These alterations, in turn, produce some changes in functional properties that will be discussed later.

DOMAINS

Early in the study of the structure of immunoglobulins, it became apparent that, in addition to INTERchain disulfide bonds that hold L and H chains, as well as H and H chains, together, INTRAchain disulfide bonds exist that form loops in the chain. The globular structure of immunoglobulins, and the ability of enzymes to cleave these molecules at very restricted positions into large entities, instead of degrading them to oligopeptides and amino acids, is indicative of a very compact structure. Furthermore, the presence of intrachain disulfide bonds at regular, approximately equal intervals of about 100–110 amino acids each, leads to the prediction that each loop in the peptide chains should form a compactly folded globular ***domain.*** In fact, L chains have two domains each, and H chains have four or five domains, separated by a short unfolded stretch. These configurations have been confirmed by direct observation and by genetic analysis (see Chapter 6). We now know that immunoglobulin molecules are assemblies of separate domains, each centered on a disulfide bond, and each having so much homology with the others as to suggest that they evolved from a single, ancestral gene, which duplicated itself several times and then changed its amino acid sequence to enable the resultant different proteins to fulfill different functions. Each domain is designated by a letter that indicates whether it is on an L chain or an H chain and a number that indicates its position. As we shall soon discuss in more detail, the first domain on L and H chains is highly variable, in terms of amino acid sequence, from one antibody to the next, and it is designated $\boldsymbol{V_L}$ or $\boldsymbol{V_H}$ accordingly (see Fig. 4.2). The second and subsequent domains on both chains are much more constant in amino acid sequence and are designated $\boldsymbol{C_L}$ or $\boldsymbol{C_H1}$, $\boldsymbol{C_H2}$ and $\boldsymbol{C_H3}$ (Fig. 4.2). In addition to their interchain disulfide bonding, the globular domains bind to each other in homologous pairs, largely by hydrophobic interactions, as follows: V_H and V_L; C_H1 and C_L; C_H2 and C_H2; C_H3 and C_H3.

HINGE REGION

In the immunoglobulins (with the possible exception of IgM and IgE), a short additional segment of amino acids is found between the C_H1 and C_H2 regions of the H chains (see Fig. 4.2). This segment is made up predominantly of ***cysteine and proline residues***. The cysteines are involved in formation of interchain disulfide bonds and the proline residues prevent folding into a globular structure. This region of the H chain provides an important characteristic of immunoglobulins. It permits ***flexibility*** between the two Fab arms of the Y-shaped antibody molecule and is called the ***hinge region***. It allows the two Fab arms to open and close to accommodate binding to two antigenic determinants, separated by a fixed distance, as might be found on the surface of a bacterium. Additionally, since this stretch of amino acids is open and as accessible as any other nonfolded peptide, it can be cleaved by proteases, such as papain or pepsin, to generate the Fab and Fc fragments described above.

VARIABLE REGION

The biological functions of the antibody molecule derive from the properties of a ***constant*** region, which is identical for antibodies of all specificities within a particular class. A major problem for immunologists was to determine how so many individual specificities, which are required to meet the enormous variety of antigenic challenges, could be generated.

When the amino acid sequences of proteins of sufficient homogeneity (e.g. myeloma proteins, monoclonal antibodies, Bence-Jones proteins) were determined, it was found that the greatest variability in sequence existed in the first 110 amino acids of both the L and the H chains. Kabat and Wu compared the amino acid sequences of many different V_L and V_H regions. They plotted the variability in the amino acids at each position in the chain and showed that the greatest amount of variability (defined as the ratio of the number of different amino acids at a given position to the frequency of the most common amino acid at that position) occurred in three ***complementarity-determining regions (CDR)*** of the L and the H chain: CDR1, CDR2, and CDR3 (see Fig. 4.3). These regions are called ***hypervariable regions***; the less variable stretches, which occur between these hypervariable regions, are called ***framework regions***.

The hypervariable regions, although separated in the linear, two-dimensional model of the peptide chains, are actually brought together in the folded form of the intact antibody molecule and, together, these hypervariable regions

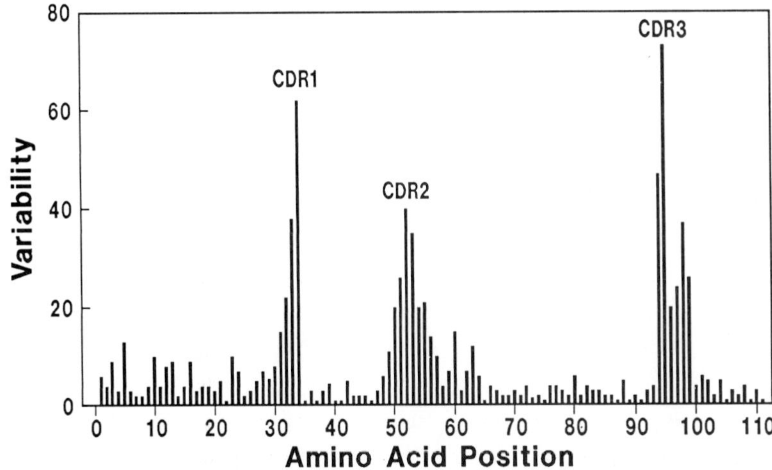

Figure 4.3. Variability of amino acids representing the N-terminal 110 residues of an immunoglobulin chain.

constitute the ***combining site,*** which is complementary to the epitope (Fig. 4.4). The variability in these CDR provides the diversity in the shape of the combining site that is required for the function of antibodies of different specificities. All of the known, weak, non-covalent forces of molecular interactions (e.g. ionic, hydrogen-bonding, and hydrophobic interactions) are involved in antigen–antibody interactions (see Chapter 7). It is therefore necessary that there be a close fit between antigen and antibody over a large enough region to allow a total binding force that is adequate for stable interaction. Contributions to this binding interaction by both H and L chains are involved in the overall association constant between antigen and antibody.

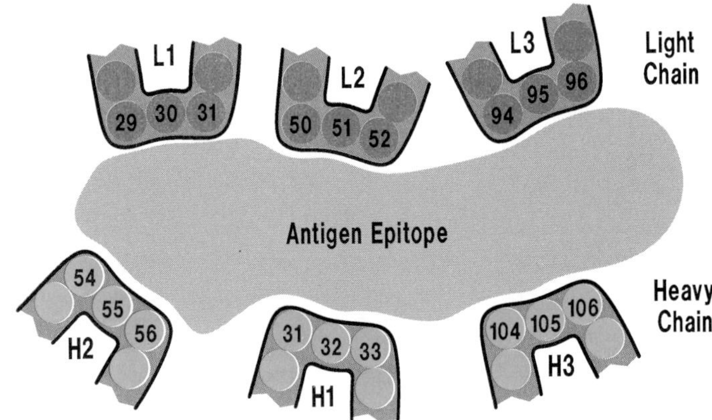

Figure 4.4.
A schematic representation of the complimentarity between an epitope and the antibody combining site consisting of the hypervariable areas of the L and H chains. (Numbered letters denote CDR of H and L chains; circled numbers denote the number of the amino acid residue in the CDRs.)

It should now be apparent that two antibody molecules with different antigenic specificities must have different amino acid sequences in their hypervariable regions, and that those with similar sequences will generally have the same specificity. However, it is possible for two antibodies with different amino acid sequences to have the same specificity. In this case, the binding affinities of the antibodies for the epitope will probably be different because there will be differences in the number and types of binding forces available to bind identical antigens to the different binding sites of the two antibodies.

An additional source of variability involves the size of the antibody-combining site on the antibody, which is usually (but not always) considered to take the form of a depression or cleft. In some instances, especially when small, hydrophobic haptens are involved, antigens do not occupy the entire combining site, yet they achieve sufficient affinity of binding. It has been shown that antibodies specific for such a small hapten may, in fact, react with other antigens that have no obvious similarity to the hapten (e.g. dinitrophenol and sheep red cells). These large, dissimilar antigens bind either to a larger area or to a different area of the combining site on the antibody (see Fig. 4.5). Thus, a particular antibody-combining site on an antibody may have the ability to combine with two (or more) apparently diverse, antigenic determinants, a property called ***redundancy.*** The ability of a single antibody molecule to cross-react with an unknown number of antigenic determinants may limit the number of different antibodies needed to defend an individual against the range of antigenic challenges.

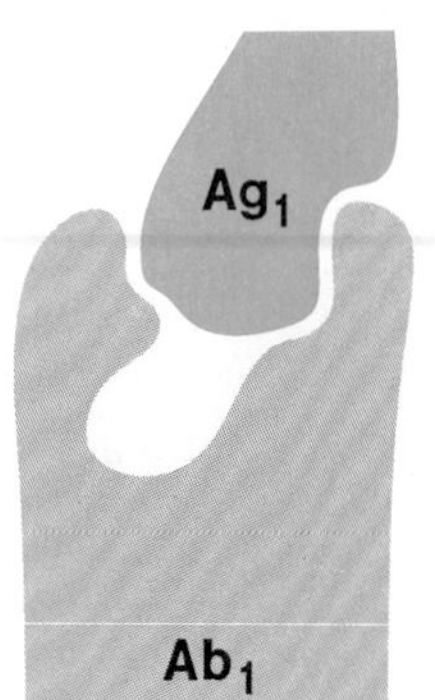

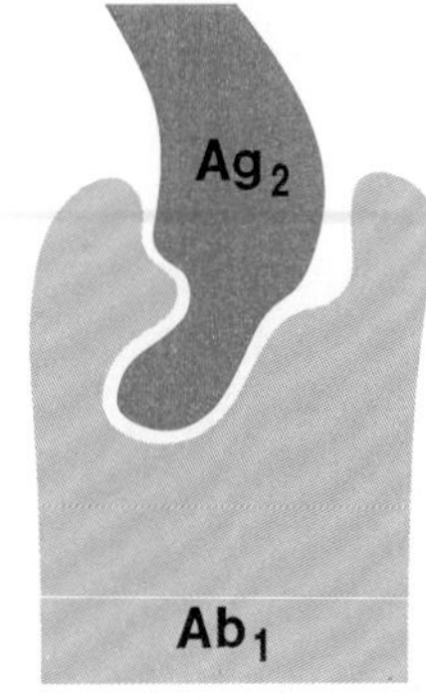

Figure 4.5.
A representation of how an antibody of a given specificity (Ab_1) can exhibit binding with two different epitopes Ag_1 and Ag_2.

IMMUNOGLOBULIN VARIANTS

Classes of Immunoglobulins

Thus far we have described the features common to all immunoglobulin molecules, such as the four-chain unit and the structural domains. In its defense against invading pathogens, the body has evolved a variety of mechanisms, each dependent on a somewhat different property or function of an immunoglobulin molecule. Thus, when a specific antibody molecule combines with a specific antigen or a pathogen, several different effector mechanisms may be available. These different mechanisms derive from the development of different classes of immunoglobulin ***(isotypes),*** each of which may combine with the same epitope but each of which triggers a different response. These differences result from structural variations in H chains, which have generated domains that mediate a variety of functions. ***The biological properties of each class are fully described in Chapter 5. The structural features are discussed here.*** A summary of the properties of the immunoglobulin classes is given in Tables 5.1 and 5.2.

STRUCTURAL FEATURES OF IgG. IgG is the predominant immunoglobulin of internal components such as blood, cerebrospinal fluid and peritoneal fluid. The IgG molecule consists of two γ H chains of molecular weight ~ 50,000 daltons each and two L chains (either κ or λ) of molecular weight ~ 25,000 daltons each, held together by disulfide bonds, to give a total molecular weight of approximately 150,000 daltons and a sedimentation coefficient of 7S. Electrophoretically, the IgG molecule is the ***least acidic*** of all serum proteins, and it migrates to the γ range of serum globulins; hence its designation as γ ***globulin*** or ***7S immunoglobulin.***

The IgG class of immunoglobulins in humans contains four subclasses designated IgG_1, IgG_2, IgG_3, and IgG_4. In the mouse there are four comparable subclasses (IgG_1, IgG_{2a}, IgG_{2b}, and IgG_3), but none has yet been found in the rabbit. All the immunoglobulins have about 90% homology in their amino acid sequences within a class, but only 60% homology between subclasses. This degree of homology means that an antiserum may be raised against a determinant that is common to, and specific for, all members of a class (e.g. all members of the IgG class) while other antisera are specific for determinants found in only one of the subclasses (e.g. in IgG_2). This variation was first detected antigenically by the use of antibodies against various γ chains. The IgG subclasses differ in their chemical and biological properties; the most important of these differences are discussed in Chapter 5.

STRUCTURAL FEATURES OF IgM. IgM is the first immunoglobulin produced in an immune response. Its name derives from its initial description as a ***macroglobulin (M)*** of high molecular weight (900,000 daltons). It has a sedimentation coefficient of 19S. In contrast to the IgG molecule, which has a four-chain structure, five such structures, each of which consists of two L and two μ chains, are joined together by additional disulfide bonds between their Fc portions and by a polypeptide chain termed the ***J chain*** (see Fig. 4.6). The J chain has a molecular weight of 15,000 daltons. This pentameric ensemble

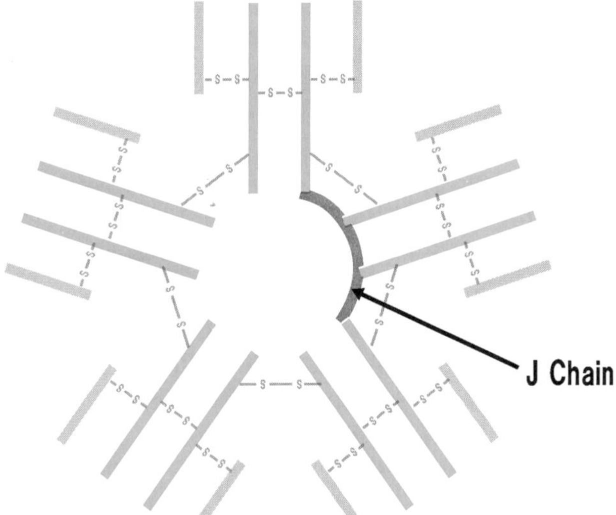

Figure 4.6.
A schematic representation of IgM pentameter.

of IgM, which is held together by disulfide bonds, comes apart after mild treatment with reducing agents such as mercaptoethanol, at which point the binding efficiency with antigen is significantly reduced. Surprisingly, each pentameric IgM molecule has a valence of 5, instead of the expected valence of 10 predicted by the 10 Fab segments contained in the pentamer. This reduction in valence is probably the result of conformational constraints imposed by the polymerization. It is known that pentameric IgM has a planar configuration, such that each of its 10 Fab portions cannot open fully with respect to the "adjacent" Fab, when it combines with antigen, as is possible in the case of IgG. Thus, any large antigen bound to one Fab may block a neighboring site from binding with antigen, making the molecule appear pentavalent (or of even lesser valence).

STRUCTURAL FEATURES OF IgA. IgA is an immunoglobulin whose importance has not been fully appreciated until recently, largely because of the misplaced attention to its function in serum. IgA is the major immunoglobulin in ***external secretions*** such as saliva, mucus, sweat, gastric fluid, and tears. It is, moreover, the major immunoglobulin of colostrum and milk, and it may provide the neonate with a major source of intestinal protection against pathogens.

The IgA molecule consists of either two κ or two λ L chains and two H α chains. The α-chain is somewhat larger than the γ-chain. The molecular weight of monomeric IgA is approximately 165,000 daltons, and its sedimentation coefficient is 7S. Electrophoretically it migrates to the slow β or fast γ region of serum globulins.

IgA, present in ***mucous secretions***, exists as a ***dimer*** consisting of two four-chain units linked by the same ***joining (J) chain*** found in IgM molecules (see Fig. 4.7). In addition IgA has another protein, the ***secretory component,*** or ***S piece*** (molecular weight 70,000 daltons), which is attached. Plasma cells make only the basic IgA molecules and the J chains, which form the dimers. When these dimeric molecules are released from plasma cells, they are bound to the basal membranes of adjacent epithelial cells by a receptor on these cells, which is the secretory component itself. This receptor transports the molecules through the epithelial cells and releases them into extracellular fluids in fully assembled form as dimeric IgA, with the secretory piece attached.

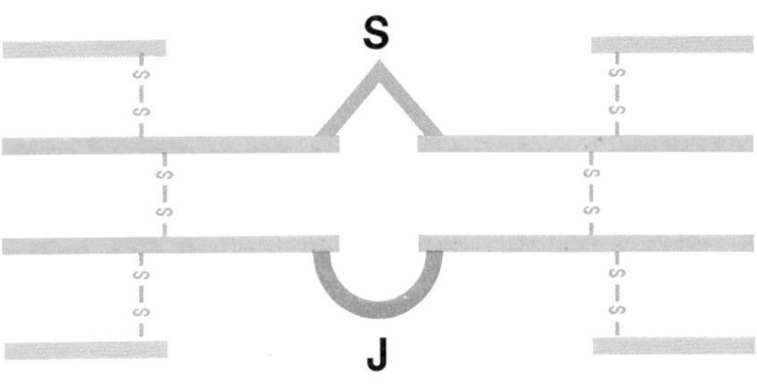

Figure 4.7.
A schematic representation of IgA dimer.

The IgA present in ***serum*** is predominantly ***monomeric*** (one four-chain unit), and has presumably been released before dimerization so that it fails to bind to the secretory component. Secretory IgA is very important biologically, but little is known of any function for serum IgA.

The IgA class of immunoglobulins contains two subclasses—IgA_1 (93%) and IgA_2 (7%). If all production of IgA on mucosal surfaces is taken into account, IgA would be the major immunoglobulin in terms of quantity.

STRUCTURAL FEATURES OF IgD. IgD is present in serum in low and variable amounts, probably because it is not secreted by plasma cells and, because, among immunoglobulins, it is uniquely susceptible to proteolytic degradation. It is not known to have any function in serum. However, together with IgM, it has been found to be a major ***surface component of many B cells***. Its presence there serves as a marker of the differentiation of B cells to a more mature form, but its exact function as a receptor for triggering or differentiation is unknown.

The IgD molecule consists of either two κ or two λ L chains and two H δ-chains. IgD is present as a monomer with a molecular weight of 180,000 daltons; it has a sedimentation coefficient of 7S, and it migrates to the fast γ-region of serum globulins. No H chain allotypes (see below) or subclasses have been reported for the IgD molecule.

STRUCTURAL FEATURES OF IgE. The IgE molecule consists of two L chains (κ or λ) and two H ϵ-chains. It has a molecular weight of approximately 200,000 daltons, its sedimentation coefficient is 8S, and it migrates electrophoretically to the fast γ-region of serum globulins. To date, no H chain allotypes or subclasses of IgE have been reported.

IgE, also called ***reaginic antibody***, is present in the lowest concentration of all immunoglobulins in serum, and it is synthesized by the lowest percentage of immunoglobulin-synthesizing plasma cells in the body. Nevertheless, its effects are out of proportion to its concentration because of the efficiency of its behavior. The H chain of IgE contains an extra domain, by which it attaches with unusually high affinity to specific receptors on ***mast cells*** and ***basophils***, where the IgE molecules may remain for weeks or months. When antigen reappears, it combines with and crosslinks the IgE molecules on the surface of mast cells. This event leads to the discharge of the contents of the mast cell granules and the ensuing symptoms of anaphylaxis (see Chapter 13).

The major physiological role of IgE is thought to involve protection against invasion by parasites, such as helminths (worms), and this protection is achieved by activation of the same acute inflammatory response seen in a more pathological form in the anaphylactic response.

Allotypes

Another form of variation in the structure of immunoglobulins is allotypy which depends on the existence of allelic forms ***(allotypes)*** of the same protein (as a result of the presence of different forms of the same gene at a given locus). As a result of allotypy, a particular constituent of any immunoglobulin can be present in some members of a species and absent in others. This situation contrasts with that of immunoglobulin classes or subclasses, which are present in *all* members of a species.

Allotypic differences at known loci usually involve changes in only one or two amino acids in the constant region of a chain. The presence of allotypic differences in two identical immunoglobulin molecules does not affect binding with antigen, but it serves as an important marker for analysis of Mendelian inheritance. There are, however, some instances in which possession of certain allotypes is linked to the ability to make certain antibody responses.

Some known allotypic markers comprise a group on the γ chain of human IgG (called ***Gm*** for IgG markers), a group on the κ-chain (formerly called ***Im,*** now called ***Km),*** and a group on the α-chain called ***Am.***

Allotypic markers have been found in the immunoglobulins of several species, usually by use of antisera generated by immunization of one member of a species with antibody from another animal of the same species. As with other allelic systems, the genes encoding the markers are expressed co-dominantly, so an individual may be homozygous or heterozygous for a given marker.

Idiotypes

As we have seen, the combining site of a specific antibody molecule is made up of a unique combination of amino acids in the variable regions of the L and H chains. Since this combination is not present in other antibody molecules, it should, theoretically, be immunogenic and capable of stimulating an immunologic response against itself in an animal of the same species. Such was actually found to be the case by Oudin and Kunkel, who showed independently that experimental immunization with a particular antibody or myeloma protein could produce an antiserum specific only for the antibody that was used to induce the response and for no other immunoglobulin of the species. These antisera contain populations of antibodies specific for several determinants, called ***idiotopes***, which are present in the variable region of the antibody used for inoculation. The collection of all the idiotopes on the inoculated antibody molecule is called the ***idiotype***. In some cases, anti-idiotypic sera prevent combination of the antibody with its antigen, in which event the idiotypic determinant is considered to be in the combining site itself. Anti-idiotypic sera, which do not block combination of antibody with antigen, are probably directed against variable determinants outside the combining site (see Fig. 4.8).

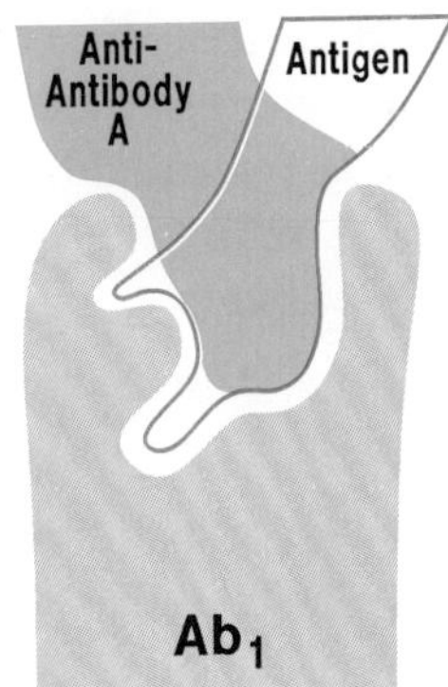

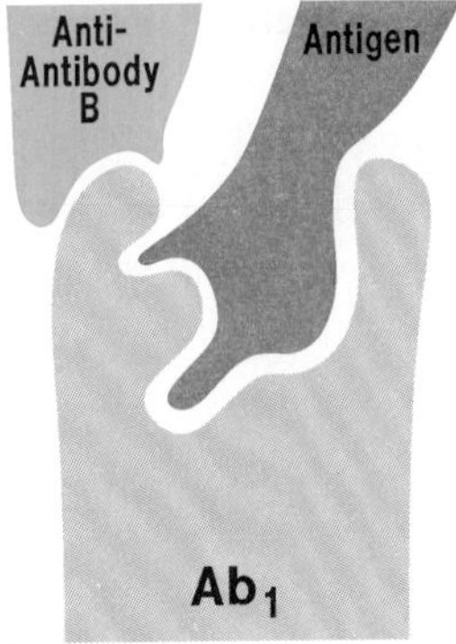

Figure 4.8.
Two anti-idiotypic antibodies to Ab_1. The anti-idiotypic antibody (**A**) on the left is directed to the combining site of Ab_1, preventing binding of Ab_1 with the antigen. The anti-idiotypic antibody (**B**) on the right binds with framework areas of Ab_1 and does not prevent its binding with antigen.

In some instances, especially with inbred species, anti-idiotypic antibodies react with several different antibodies, that have similar amino acid sequences and that share idiotypes. These idiotypes are called ***public*** or ***cross-reacting idiotypes***, and this term frequently defines families of antibody molecules. By contrast, sera that react with only one antibody molecule define a ***private idiotype***.

As we discuss in a later chapter, the presence of idiotypic determinants on immunoglobulin molecules has important consequences in the control and modulation of the immune response, as envisioned in the Jerne Network Hypothesis (see Chapter 15).

SUMMARY

1. Immunoglobulins of all classes have a fundamental four-chain structure, consisting of two identical light (L) and two identical heavy (H) chains, which are held together by disulfide bonds.

2. In the native state, the chains are coiled into domains, each of which consists of about 110 amino acids, stabilized by an intrachain disulfide bond.

3. The first domains of both H and L chains are the variable (V) regions, which, together, make up the combining site of the antibody and vary according to the specificity of the antibody.

4. The other domains are the constant (C) regions, and these domains are similar within each class of immunoglobulin molecule.

5. The classes of immunoglobulin molecules differ by virtue of the Fc regions of their H chains, which are responsible for the different biological functions carried out by each class.

6. Certain genetic markers within the C regions of the H chains, which result from differences in one or two amino acids, are called allotypes and distinguish individuals within a species. Idiotypic markers are represented by the unique combinations of amino acids that make up the combining site of an antibody molecule and that are specific for that particular antibody.

REFERENCES

Kabat EA (1976): Structural Concepts in Immunology and Immunochemistry, Ed 2. New York: Holt, Rinehart and Winston.

Nisonoff A (1984): Introduction to Molecular Immunology. Sunderland, Massachusetts: Sinauer.

REVIEW QUESTIONS

Each of the questions or incomplete statements below (questions 1–3) is followed by several suggested answers or completions. Select ONE that is BEST in each case.

1. The hinge region of an IgG heavy chain is located
   a) within the C_H1 intrachain loops.
   b) between C_H1 and C_H2.
   c) between C_H2 and C_H3.
   d) between C_H3 and C_H4.
   e) between V_H and C_H1.

2. The class-specific antigenic determinants (epitopes) of immunoglobulins are associated with
   a) L chains.
   b) J chains.
   c) disulfide bonds.
   d) H chains.
   e) variable regions.

3. The idiotype of an antibody molecule is determined by the amino acid sequence of the
   a) constant region of the L chain
   b) variable region of the L chain.
   c) constant region of the H chain.
   d) constant region of the H and L chain.
   e) variable regions of the H and L chain.

For each of the incomplete statements below (questions 4–9), ONE or MORE of the completions given is correct. Choose the appropriate answer:
A) if only *1, 2, 3* are correct
B) if only *1 and 3* are correct
C) if only *2 and 4* are correct.
D) if only *4* is correct.
E) if *all* are correct.

4. An immunoglobulin molecule contains
   1) two identical light chains.
   2) variable and constant regions on each chain present.
   3) two identical heavy chains.
   4) polypeptide chains, divided into domains.

5. Injection into rabbits of a preparation of pooled human IgG should stimulate production of
   1) anti-gamma heavy chain antibody.
   2) anti-kappa chain antibody.
   3) anti-lambda chain antibody.
   4) anti-Fc antibody.

6. Antibodies to human IgA will react with
   1) human IgM.
   2) kappa light chains.
   3) human IgG.
   4) J chains.

7. The domains of immunoglobulin H chains
   1) define separate units with different functions.
   2) probably arose from the same primordial gene.
   3) may carry allotypic markers.
   4) lack disulfide bonds.

8. The antigen binding site of an Ig molecule
   1) is in the first domain at the N-terminal end of L and H chains.
   2) is destroyed by removal of sugar residues.
   3) has a specificity determined predominantly by variations in the hypervariable regions.
   4) has a size that cannot be determined from studies on the binding of antigen fragments.

9. An individual was found to be heterologous for IgG_1 allotypes 3 and 12. The different possible IgG_1 antibodies produced by this individual may have
   1) two H chains of allotype 12.
   2) two L chains of either κ or λ.
   3) two H chains of allotype 3.
   4) two H chains, one of allotype 3 and one of allotype 12.

(*Continued on next page*)

ANSWERS TO REVIEW QUESTIONS

1. ***b*** Correct location of hinge region is between C_H1 and C_H2, where the Fc portion begins.

2. ***d*** The five classes of Ig molecules are defined by the H chains (γ, μ, α, λ, ϵ).

3. ***e*** The idiotype is the antigenic determinant of an Ig molecule, which involves its antigen-combining site, which in turn consists of contributions from the variable regions of both L and H chains.

4. ***E*** All are correct statements.

5. ***E*** All are correct statements. Since a pool of IgG is injected, it can be assumed that both κ- and λ-chains will be present, and that antibodies will be made against them, as well as against the other determinants (H chain and Fc region) present in all IgG molecules.

6. ***E*** All are correct statements. Antibody to IgA will have antibody specific for κ and λ light chains, which, of course, will react with IgG and IgM, both of which have κ- and λ-chains. Antibody will also be present against J chain if the IgA used for immunization was dimeric.

7. ***A*** 1, 2 and 3 are correct. All domains are formed around an intrachain disulfide bond; thus, statement 4 is wrong.

8. ***B*** The antigen-binding site is made up of the contribution of the hypervariable regions on the H and L chain, which are at the N-terminal ends of the chain. The size of the site can be estimated by binding studies with various fragments of antigen. Loss of sugar residues does not affect this site.

9. ***A*** In any immunoglobulin produced by a single cell, the two H chains and the two L chains are identical. Therefore, any antibody in this individual would have either allotype 3 H chains or allotype 12 H chains, not a mixture. Similarly, the antibody would have either two κ or two λ L chains.

CHAPTER

5

BIOLOGICAL PROPERTIES OF IMMUNOGLOBULINS

INTRODUCTION

Many important biological properties are attributable to antibodies. These properties include ***neutralization*** of toxins; ***immobilization*** of certain microorganisms; neutralization of viral activity; ***agglutination*** (clumping together) of microorganisms or of antigenic particles (see Chapter 7); binding with soluble antigen to form antigen–antibody ***precipitates*** (which are readily phagocytized and destroyed by phagocytic cells; see Chapter 7); binding with microorganisms to facilitate their ***lysis*** by serum complement (see Chapter 8) or their phagocytosis and destruction either by phagocytic cells or by killer lymphocytes. Still another important biological property of antibodies is their ability to ***cross the placenta*** from the mother to the fetus.

Not all antibody isotypes are equal in the performance of all of these biological roles. Indeed, prior to 1960, before the elucidation of the structure of the various isotypes, it was already recognized that antibody populations, even if directed against the same antigenic determinants, differ in their capacity to fulfill these biological functions. Consequently, those antibodies that exhibited the capacity to agglutinate particulate antigens or microorganisms were called ***agglutinating antibodies*** or ***agglutinins;*** other antibodies that activated or "fixed" complement in the presence of antigen were termed ***complement fixing*** antibodies, and so on. Today, it is well established that the differences in the various biological activities of the antibodies are attributable to their isotypic (class) structure. Although all antibody isotypes that are induced by immunization can be directed against a given antigenic determinant or epitope, the differences between the isotypes account for the different consequences of binding with antigen. Thus, a given antibody molecule has two major roles: to bind with antigen and to participate in one or more of the biological functions cited above. These two roles are performed by two different parts of the molecule, the first by the ***Fab*** and the second by the ***Fc.***

The determination of the structure of antibody, the establishment of the relationship between this structure and function, and the elucidation of the genetic organization of the Ig molecule have led to an understanding of the evolution of a sophisticated, highly specialized system in which diverse structures (immunoglobulins) all recognize the same antigen, but in which combination of immunoglobulin with antigen leads to an array of diverse biological effects. In the sections that follow, the structural characteristics of the Ig isotypes are related to their biological properties. The structural features of the immunoglobulin isotypes are described in Chapter 4, and their metabolism, distribution, and biological properties are dealt with here. ***The important features of the various immunoglobulin isotypes are presented in Tables 5.1 and 5.2.***

BIOLOGICAL PROPERTIES OF IgG

IgG is present in the serum of human adults at a concentration of approximately ***12 mg/ml,*** and it represents about 15% of the total protein in serum (other proteins include albumins, globulins, and enzymes). IgG is distributed approximately equally between the intravascular and extravascular spaces.

Except for the IgG_3 subclass, which has rapid turnover, with a ***half-life*** of 7 days, the half-life of IgG (i.e. IgG_1, IgG_2, and IgG_4) is approximately ***23 days,*** which is the longest half-life of all Ig isotypes. This longevity makes IgG the most suitable for passive immunization by transfer of antibodies. Interestingly, as the concentration of IgG in the serum increases (as occurs in cases of multiple myeloma or after the transfer of very high concentrations of IgG), the rate of catabolism of IgG increases, and its half-life decreases to 15–20 days or even less.

TABLE 5.1. The Most Important Features of Immunoglobulin Isotypes

	Isotype				
	IgG	IgM	IgA	IgE	IgD
Molecular weight	150,000	900,000	160,000 for monomer	200,000	180,000
Additional protein subunits	—	J	J and T or S	—	—
Concentration in serum					
mg/ml (adult)	12	1.0	1.8	0.0003	0.03
(newborn)	12	0.1	0.05	—	
% of total Ig	80	6	13	0.002	0.2
Distribution	~ equal—intra- and extravascular	Mostly intra-vascular	Intravascular and secretions	On basophils and mast cells; present in saliva, nasal secretions	Present on lymphocyte surface
Half-life (days)	23	5	5.5	2.0	2.8
Placental passage	++	—	—	—	—
Presence in secretion	—	—	++	—	—
Presence in milk	+	0 to trace	+	—	—
Activation of complement	+	+++	—	—	—
Binding to Fc receptors on macrophages and polymorpho-nuclear cells	++	—	—	—	—
Relative agglutinating capacity	+	+++	++	—	—
Antiviral activity	+++	—	+++	—	—
Antibacterial activity (gram-negative)	+++	+++ (with complement)	++ (with lysozyme)	—	—
Antitoxin activity	+++	—	—	—	—
"Reaginic activity"	—	—	—	++	—

TABLE 5.2. Important Differences Between Human IgG Subclasses

	IgG_1	IgG_2	IgG_3	IgG_4
Occurrence (% of total IgG)	70	20	7	3
Half-life	23	23	7	23
Complement binding	+	+	+++	—
Placental passage	++	±	++	++
Binding to monocytes	+++	+	+++	±

IgG molecules may be made to ***aggregate*** by a variety of physicochemical procedures. For example, treatment with alcohol, a method employed in the purification of IgG for passive immunization (see Chapter 20), or heating at 63°C for 10 minutes, causes aggregation. Aggregated IgG can still combine with antigen; however, many of the properties that are attributed to antigen–antibody complexes are exhibited by aggregated IgG (without antigen)—for example, attachment to phagocytic cells, as well as the activation of complement and other biologically active substances that may be harmful to the body (see Chapter 13). It is therefore imperative that no aggregated IgG be present in passively administered IgG.

Agglutination and Formation of Precipitate

IgG molecules can cause the ***agglutination*** or clumping of particulate (insoluble) antigens like microorganisms. The reaction of IgG with soluble, multivalent antigens can generate ***precipitates*** (see Chapter 7). This property of IgG is undoubtedly of considerable survival value since insoluble antigen–antibody complexes are easily phagocytized and destroyed by phagocytic cells.

Passage Through the Placenta

The IgG isotype (except for subclass IgG_2) is the only class of immunoglobulin that can pass through the placenta, enabling the mother to transfer her immunity to the fetus. Analysis of fetal immunoglobulins (see Fig. 20.2) shows that, at the third or fourth month of pregnancy, there is a rapid increase in the concentration of IgG. This IgG must be of maternal origin, since the fetus is unable to synthesize immunoglobulins at this age. Then, during the fifth month of pregnancy, the fetus begins to synthesize IgM and trace amounts of IgA. It is not until three or four months after birth, when the level of inherited maternal IgG drops as a result of catabolism (the half-life of IgG is 23 days), that the infant begins to synthesize its own IgG antibodies. Thus, the resistance of the fetus and the neonate to infection is conferred almost entirely by the mother's IgG, which passes across the placenta. It has been established that passage across the placenta is mediated by the Fc portion of the IgG molecule; $F(ab')_2$ or Fab fragments of IgG do not pass through the placenta.

While passage of IgG molecules across the placenta confers immunity to infection upon the fetus, it may also be responsible for ***hemolytic disease of the newborn (erythroblastosis fetalis)*** (see Chapter 17), which is caused by maternal antibodies to fetal red blood cells. The maternal IgG antibodies to Rh antigen pass across the placenta and attack the fetal red blood cells that carry Rh antigens (Rh^+).

Opsonization

IgG is an ***opsonizing*** antibody (from the Greek *opsonin*, which means to prepare for eating). It reacts with epitopes on microorganisms via its Fab portions; but it is the Fc portion that confers the opsonizing property, since many phagocytic cells, including macrophages and polymorphonuclear phagocytes, bear receptors for the Fc portion of the IgG molecule. These cells adhere to the antibody-coated bacteria by virtue of their receptors for Fc. The net effect is a zipper-like closure of the surface membrane of the phagocytic cell around the organism, as receptors for Fc and the Fc regions on the antibodies continue to combine, leading to the final engulfing and destruction of the microorganism (see Fig. 5.1).

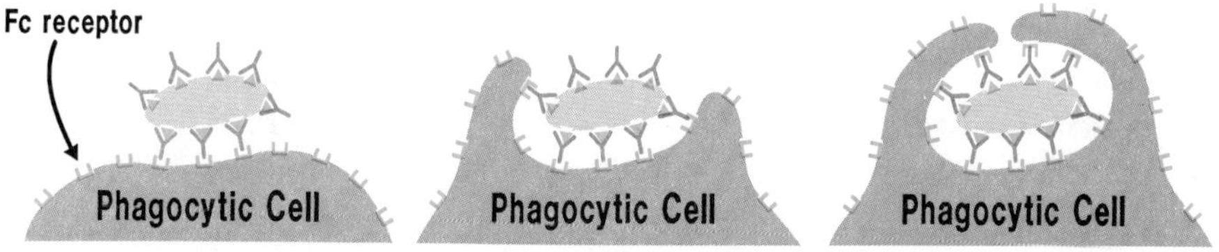

Figure 5.1.
A diagrammatic representation of phagocytosis of a particle coated with antibodies.

Antibody-Dependent, Cell-Mediated Cytotoxicity (ADCC)

The IgG molecule plays an important role in antibody-dependent, cell-mediated cytotoxicity (ADCC). In this form of cytotoxicity, the Fab portion binds with the target cell, be it a microorganism or a tumor cell, and the Fc portion binds with specific receptors for Fc that are found on certain lymphocytic cells called ***killer (or K) cells.*** By this mechanism, the IgG molecule "focuses" the killer cells on their target, and the killer cells destroy the target, not by phagocytosis but with the various substances that they release.

Activation of Complement

The IgG molecule can activate the ***complement cascade*** (see Chapter 8). Activation of complement results in the release of several important biologically active molecules and leads to lysis if the antigen is on the surface of a cell. Some of the components of complement are ***opsonins;*** they bind to the target antigen and thereby cause phagocytes, which carry receptors specific for these opsonins, to focus their phagocytic activity on the target antigen. Other components of the activation of complement are ***chemotactic;*** i.e. they attract phagocytic cells. Still other components cause the ***release of histamine*** by mast cells or basophils. All in all, the activation of complement by IgG has profound biological effects on the host and on the target antigen if it is a live cell, whether it is a microorganism or a tumor cell.

Neutralization of Toxin

The IgG molecule is an excellent antibody for the neutralization of such toxins as tetanus and botulinus, or for the inactivation of, for example, snake and scorpion venoms. Because of its ability to neutralize such poisons, and because of its long half-life, the IgG molecule is the antibody of choice for ***passive immunization*** (i.e. the transfer of antibodies) against toxins and venoms.

Immobilization of Bacteria

IgG molecules are efficient in immobilizing various motile bacteria. Reaction of antibodies specific for the ***flagella*** and ***cilia*** of certain microorganisms cause them to clump, thereby arresting their movement.

Neutralization of Viruses

The IgG antibody is an efficient virus neutralizing antibody. The antibody binds with antigenic determinants present on various portions of the viral coat, among which is the region used by the virus for attachment to the target cell. ***Inhibition of viral attachment*** effectively arrests infection.

Summary

To reiterate, the versatility in function of the IgG molecule makes it an important immunoglobulin. Its importance is accentuated in those immune deficiency disorders in which an individual is unable to synthesize IgG molecules (see Chapter 12). Such individuals are prone to infections that may result in toxemia and death.

BIOLOGICAL PROPERTIES OF IgM

IgM is present in adult human serum at a concentration of approximately ***1 mg/ml.*** It is found predominantly in the ***intravascular*** spaces. The ***half-life*** of the IgM molecule is approximately ***5 days.***

IgM antibodies do not pass across the placenta; however, since this is the only class of immunoglobulins that is synthesized by the fetus, with synthesis beginning at approximately 5 months of gestation, elevated levels of IgM in the fetus are indicative of congenital or perinatal infection.

IgM is the isotype synthesized by children and adults in appreciable amounts after immunization or exposure to thymus-independent antigens, and it is the first isotype that is synthesized after immunization with thymus-dependent antigens (see Chapter 10). Thus, elevated levels of IgM usually indicate either recent infection or recent exposure to antigen.

Agglutination

IgM molecules are efficient agglutinating antibodies. Because of their pentameric form, IgM antibodies can form macromolecular bridges between antigenic determinants (epitopes) on molecules that may be too distant from each other to be bridged by the smaller IgG antibodies. Furthermore, because of their pentameric form and multiple valency, the IgM antibodies are particularly well suited to combine with antigens that contain repeated patterns of the same antigenic determinant, as in the case of polysaccharide antigens or cellular antigens, which are multiply expressed on cell surfaces.

Isohemagglutinins

The IgM antibodies include the so-called ***natural isohemagglutinins***—the naturally occurring IgM antibodies against the red blood cell antigens of the ABO blood groups (see Chapter 17). These antibodies are presumed to arise as a result of immunization by the bacteria in the gastrointestinal and respiratory tracts, which bear determinants similar to the oligosaccharides of the ABO blood groups. Thus, without known prior immunization, people with the type O blood group have isohemagglutinins to the A and B antigens; those with the type A blood group have antibodies to the B antigens; and those with the B antigen have antibodies to the A antigen. An individual of the AB group has neither anti-A nor anti-B antibodies. Fortunately, the IgM isohemagglutinins do not pass through the placenta, so incompatibility of the ABO groups between mother and fetus poses no danger to the fetus. ***Transfusion*** reactions, which arise as a result of ***ABO incompatibility,*** and in which the recipient's isohemagglutinins react with the donor's red blood cells, may have disastrous consequences (see Chapter 17).

Activation of Complement

Because of its pentameric form, IgM is an excellent complement-fixing or complement-activating antibody. Unlike other classes of immunoglobulins, a single molecule of IgM has the ability to initiate the complement sequence. Thus, IgM is most efficient as an initiator of the complement-mediated lysis of microorganisms and other cells. This ability, taken together with the appearance of IgM as the first class of antibodies generated after immunization or infection, makes IgM antibodies very important as providers of an early line of immunological defense against bacterial infections.

In contrast to IgG, the IgM antibodies are not very versatile; they are poor toxin-neutralizing antibodies, and they are not efficient in the neutralization of viruses.

BIOLOGICAL PROPERTIES OF IgA

Serum IgA, which has no known biological function, has a ***half-life of 5.5 days.*** The concentration of serum IgA is 1.8 mg/ml. However, most IgA is present, not in the serum, but in secretions such as tears, saliva, colostrum, sweat, and mucus, where it serves an important biological function.

It has already been mentioned (see Chapter 4) that during the synthesis of IgA by plasma cells situated in various lumens of the body (e.g. in the parotid gland, along the gastrointestinal tract in the intestinal villi, in tear glands, in the lactating breast, or beneath bronchial mucosa), two monomeric IgA molecules become joined by a J chain. The J chain is attached to the IgA molecules by disulfide bonds. The IgA dimer is released into the lamina propria and transported into the lumen across the epithelial cells of the mucosa. This transport is mediated by another protein called the ***T*** (for transport) or ***S*** (for secretory) piece which is a receptor on epithelial cells that becomes attached to the dimer of IgA. The S or T piece is synthesized by epithelial cells situated near the mucous membrane, and it binds to the IgA dimer by strong, non-covalent bonds.

The IgA found in secretions (i.e. ***secretory IgA***) is always present in ***dimeric*** form (see Fig. 4.7) and has a molecular weight of 400,000 daltons. As noted before, if all secretion of IgA from various sources is taken into account, it is the major immunoglobulin synthesized in the body.

Role in Mucosal Infections

Because of its presence in secretions, such as saliva, urine, tears and gastric fluid, secretory IgA is thought to be of importance in the primary immunologic defense against local infections, such as the defense mechanisms of the respiratory or gastrointestinal tract. Thus, for protection against local infections, routes of immunization that result in local production of IgA are much more effective than routes that primarily produce antibodies in serum. For example, in the case of cholera, the pathogenic *Vibrio* organism attaches to, but never penetrates beyond, the cells that line the gastrointestinal tract, where it secretes an exotoxin responsible for all symptoms. IgA antibody, which can prevent attachment of the organism to the cells, provides protection from the pathogen.

Bactericidal Activity

The IgA molecule does not contain receptors for complement and, thus, it is not a complement-activating or complement-fixing immunoglobulin. Consequently, IgA does not induce bacterial lysis. However, IgA has been shown to possess bactericidal activity against ***gram-negative organisms,*** but only in the presence of ***lysozyme,*** which interestingly, is also present in the same secretions that contain secretory IgA.

Anti-Viral Activity

Secretory IgA is an efficient antiviral antibody, preventing viruses from entering host cells. In addition, secretory IgA is an efficient agglutinating antibody.

BIOLOGICAL PROPERTIES OF IgE

IgE or ***reaginic antibody*** has a ***half-life*** in serum of ***2 days,*** the shortest half-life of all classes of immunoglobulins. Another distinction of IgE antibodies is that they are present in serum at very low concentrations, from ***20 to 450 ng/ml serum.*** These low levels are due in part to a low rate of synthesis and, in part, to the unique ability of the Fc portion of IgE to bind with very high affinity to mast cells and basophils. Both mast cells and basophils have specific receptors for this region, and thus they effectively remove the IgE from the circulation.

Importance in Hypersensitivity Reactions

IgE is not an agglutinating or complement-activating antibody. Its role in protection against microorganisms is becoming better appreciated. Elevated levels of IgE in serum have been shown to occur during infections with certain ***parasites.*** For example, induction of IgE production has been demonstrated in cases of infestation with ***ascaris*** (a roundworm). In fact, immunization with ascaris antigen induces the formation of IgE.

The IgE class of antibodies is important in ***hypersensitivity*** or ***allergy*** (see Chapter 13). The surfaces of the highly granulated basophils or mast cells contain receptors for the Fc portion of the IgE molecule, and IgE molecules are found predominantly attached to these cells. When antigen binds with the

Fab portion of the IgE attached to these cells, the cells release the contents of their granules—histamine, heparin, leukotrienes, and other pharmacologically active compounds that trigger the hypersensitivity reaction. These reactions may be mild, as in the case of a mosquito bite, or severe, as in the case of bronchial asthma; they may even result in systemic anaphylaxis, which can cause death within minutes.

BIOLOGICAL PROPERTIES OF IgD

IgD is present in the serum in very small amounts, with a concentration between ***0*** and ***0.04 mg/ml.*** Serum IgD has a ***half-life of 2.8 days,*** possibly as a result of its susceptibility to enzymatic degradation, which is greater than that of any of the other classes of immunoglobulins. Its rate of turnover is unknown.

Although there are isolated reports of serum IgD with specificity against certain antigens, generally, the antibodies in serum that belong to this class of immunoglobulins have not been demonstrated to bind with antigen or to serve a protective function. Nevertheless, IgD serving as an antigen-specific receptor on the surface of ***B lymphocytes*** has been shown to be involved in the differentiation of these cells (see Chapter 9).

SUMMARY

1. There are many biological functions that antibodies carry out in addition to binding with antigen.

2. These properties are conferred upon the antibody by the heavy chain, and the biological functions (excluding binding with antigen) are mediated by the Fc portion of the antibody and by the hinge region.

3. IgG is the most versatile class of antibody, capable of carrying out numerous biological functions that range from neutralization of toxin to activation of complement and opsonization. IgG is the only class of immunoglobulin that passes through the placenta and confers maternal immunity on the fetus.

4. IgM antibody is present in pentameric form; of all classes of immunoglobulins it is the best agglutinating and complement-activating antibody.

5. IgA antibody is present in monomeric as well as in dimeric form. The dimeric IgA found in secretions and referred to as secretory IgA is an important anti-viral immunoglobulin.

6. IgE, also called reaginic antibody, is of paramount importance in hypersensitivity reactions. It also appears to be of importance in protection against parasitic infections. The Fc portion of IgE binds with high affinity to receptors on mast cells and, on contact with antigen, it triggers the degranulation of mast cells.

7. IgD antibodies are present on the surface of B lymphocytes at certain developmental stages of these cells and appear to be involved in their differentiation.

REFERENCES

Davies DR, Metzger H (1983): Structural basis of antibody function. Annu Rev Immunol 1:87.
Ishizaka K, Dayton DH (eds) (1973): The Biological Role of the Immunoglobulin E System. Bethesda, Maryland: National Institute of Child Health and Human Development.
Koshland ME (1975): Structure and function of J-chain. Adv Immunol 20:41.
Nisonoff A, Hopper JR, Spring SB (1975): The Antibody Molecule. New York: Academic Press.
Walker WA, Isselbacher KJ (1977): Intestinal antibodies. N Engl J Med 297:767.

REVIEW QUESTIONS

Each question or incomplete statement below (questions 1–3) is followed by several suggested answers or completions. Select ONE that is BEST in each case.

1. Agglutinins are useful in detection of infection caused by *Mycoplasma pneumoniae*. They are mainly IgM molecules. Assuming that successful treatment of infection caused abrupt cessation of synthesis of agglutinins, how long would it take for a four-fold drop in the concentration of IgM molecules in serum to take place?
   a) approximately 2 days
   b) approximately 10 days
   c) approximately 2 months
   d) approximately 2 years
   e) approximately 2 hours

2. The antibody isotype that acts in concert with lysozyme against gram negative organisms is

a) IgA.
b) IgG.
c) IgD.
d) IgM.
e) IgE.

3. The first immunoglobulin synthesized by the fetus is
   a) IgA.
   b) IgE.
   c) IgG.
   d) IgM.
   e) The fetus does not synthesize immunoglobulins.

For the following incomplete statement, ONE or MORE of the completions given is correct. Choose the appropriate answer:
A) if only *1, 2, 3* are correct
B) if only *1 and 3* are correct
C) if only *2 and 4* are correct
D) if only *4* is correct
E) if *all* are correct

4. The properties of human IgG are such that
   1) it can pass the placenta.
   2) it can be cleaved by pepsin and yet remains divalent.
   3) its half-life is approximately 23 days.
   4) it induces the formation of leukocytes.

ANSWERS TO REVIEW QUESTIONS

1. ***b*** The half-life of serum IgM is approximately 5 days. Therefore a four-fold drop will occur after two half-lives—i.e. after approximately 10 days.

2. ***a*** Secretory IgA works in concert with lysozyme, which is found in many secretions.

3. ***d*** The first (and only) immunoglobulin synthesized by the fetus is IgM. The IgG present in the fetus is maternal IgG which has passed through the placenta. No other immunoglobulins are found in the fetus.

4. ***A*** (1, 2 and 3 are correct). Human IgG is the only Ig that passes across the placenta. It has a half-life of 23 days. It can be cleaved by pepsin to yield a divalent antibody portion $(Fab')_2$. It does not induce the formation of leukocytes.

CHAPTER

6

THE GENETIC BASIS OF ANTIBODY STRUCTURE

INTRODUCTION

Estimates of the repertoire, in a given individual, of antibody molecules with different specificities range from 10^6 to 10^8. An understanding of the genetic mechanism by which this remarkable diversity is achieved has only recently been acquired, largely as a result of the enormous advances in molecular biology. One discovery with major implications is the ability of genes to move and to rearrange themselves within the genome. Thus, a gene can be located in one position in the DNA of the germ line, and then be moved to another position prior to transcription into RNA and translation into protein. The variable and constant regions of an immunoglobulin chain are encoded by separate genes. During the differentiation of B cells, an appropriate set of genes for the variable and constant regions of an immunoglobulin chain is strung together to make a "complete" gene, which is translated into a complete H or L chain of an antibody molecule.

Each of the chains (κ, λ, and H) involved in the formation of antibody is encoded by a cluster of genes on a separate chromosome, the identity of which varies with the species (2, 22, and 14 for human; and 6, 16, and 12 for mouse).

In addition, the recently discovered chains that are part of receptors on T cells, and that contain regions with significant homologies to the antibody chains, are on still other chromosomes. Thus, while all these chains may have originated from a common precursor and may possess many structural and functional characteristics in common, in the process of evolution they have moved to various chromosomal locations. A complex and coordinated series of events is therefore required for synthesis of a complete immunoglobulin molecule. In the paragraphs that follow, this process is examined in greater detail.

GENES INVOLVED IN THE SYNTHESIS OF IMMUNOGLOBULIN CHAINS

κ-Chain

By analysis of recombinant DNA and techniques of DNA hybridization, Tonegawa and Leder and their colleagues demonstrated that, despite the large number of different antibody molecules, there is only a ***small number of genes*** involved in the synthesis of κ-chains. This limitation is offset by the fact that some or all of those genes are ***used repeatedly*** in different combinations. For any particular κ light chain, for example, there are ***separate genes for the V and C regions***, and those genes are found to be much closer together in the DNA from a mature B cell than in the DNA of an embryo or a non-lymphoid cell. This greater proximity indicates that, in the process of differentiation of a B cell, ***somatic rearrangement*** must occur, whereby the genes that encode the V and C regions are brought closer together.

These initial discoveries were rapidly extended to give the current picture of the events that occur during synthesis of κ-chains, which involve ***somatic rearrangement of DNA, splicing of RNA,*** and ***limited proteolysis*** of polypeptides to generate the final peptide chain.

The genes for the V region of the κ-chain have been found to exist in a linear array of 50–200 separate genes. The DNA sequences that are translated into peptides are called ***exons,*** and the intervening sequences between them, which are excised and remain untranslated, are called ***introns.*** Polypeptide chains must penetrate membranes in order to leave the endoplasmic reticulum, where they are synthesized. For this purpose, they contain a ***leader sequence*** that is cleaved from the chain as it leaves the membrane. As shown in Figure 6.1, the V genes of the κ-chain are aligned linearly on embryonic DNA, and

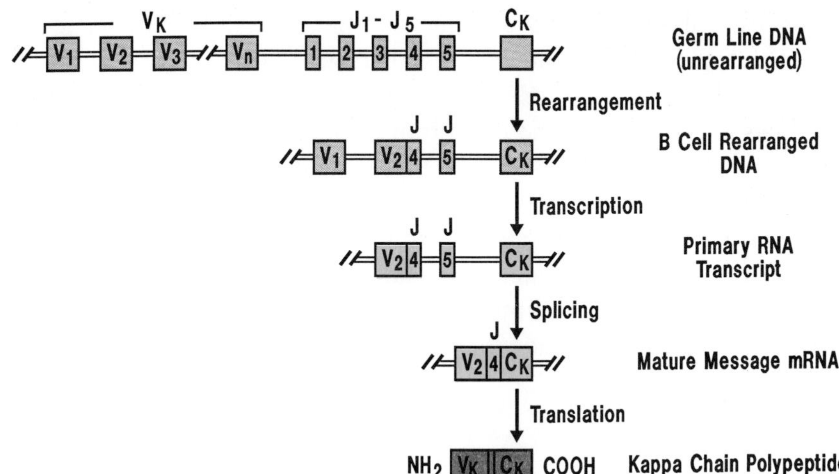

Figure 6.1.
The genetic events leading to the synthesis of κ light chain.

each has its own leader sequence. The different V genes are separated by untranslated (intron) stretches of DNA, and each of the V gene exons codes for only the first ***95 amino acids*** of the V region. Adjacent to the V gene region, after a long intron, is a cluster of about ***5 small exons***, each of which codes for a short segment of amino acids called the ***J (joining) region*** (not to be confused with the J chain in IgM and IgA molecules), which completes the V segment of the κ-chains. Another long intron separates the J regions from a single C region that is characteristic of all κ-chains.

In the differentiation of a pre-B cell to an antibody-forming plasma cell, the first step in the synthesis of κ-chains is the ***rearrangement*** of one of the genes that codes for a V region to a position adjacent to one of the J genes. This rearrangement occurs by a complex process of ***transposition,*** in which the two exons are aligned by their flanking sequences, the intervening intron loop is excised, and one end of the V gene is joined to one end of the J gene. The existence of several genes for J regions provides another degree of variability, since it permits each V gene to combine with any J gene. Thus, if there are 200 separate V genes that can combine with any of 5 different J genes, then there is a total of 1,000 (200 $\times$ 5) possible V regions. Transposition, therefore, permits the economical use of DNA in the generation of the enormous diversity of antibiodies that is required.

After transposition, the entire sequence—one V gene, with its leader sequence spliced to one J sequence, together with the ***single C gene***—is transcribed into a large, ***primary RNA transcript***. These events all occur in the nucleus, as does the ***splicing*** of the RNA transcript, from which all the introns and the unused J chains are excised, and the remaining coding sequences are then joined into a continuous strand of messenger RNA. This mRNA is ***transported to the cytoplasm***, where it is ***translated*** on ribosomes into κ-chain polypeptide. After passage through the endoplasmic reticulum, the leader sequence is ***clipped off***, and the completed κ-chain is available for combination with the H chain and export outside the plasma cell.

λ-Chain

The synthesis of λ-chains is similar in principle to the synthesis of κ-chains, in that it involves rearrangements of Vλ, Jλ, and Cλ genes. However, whereas in a κ-chain there is a cluster of J regions available for V–J recombination with the single C region gene, in the λ-chain there are ***several genes encoded for a constant*** λ ***region, each with its own J region***. Thus, in the mouse, the λ region is amplified to give four J regions, each associated with its own C region. Fewer genes for Vλ regions seem to be available for recombination, in keeping with the very limited level of synthesis of λ-chains in the mouse (95% κ, 5% λ). The organization of the human λ-chain genes has not been fully elucidated, but it probably involves degrees of complexity commensurate with the greater production of λ-chains found in humans (60% κ, 40% λ).

Heavy Chains

Although mechanisms for genetic rearrangement similar to those just discussed are involved in the synthesis of H chains, greater complexity is involved because of the presence of additional exons that encode a ***diversity (D) segment,*** in addition to the presence of ***multiple C region genes.*** The organization in the germline of the gene for H chains is illustrated in Figure 6.2. Between approximately ***100 and 200 V genes*** have been identified for H chains, each with its own leader sequence and intron spacing. The V genes are adjacent to approximately ***4 functional genes for J segments.*** However, in contrast to the organization of κ-chains, ***an additional cluster of 12 gene***

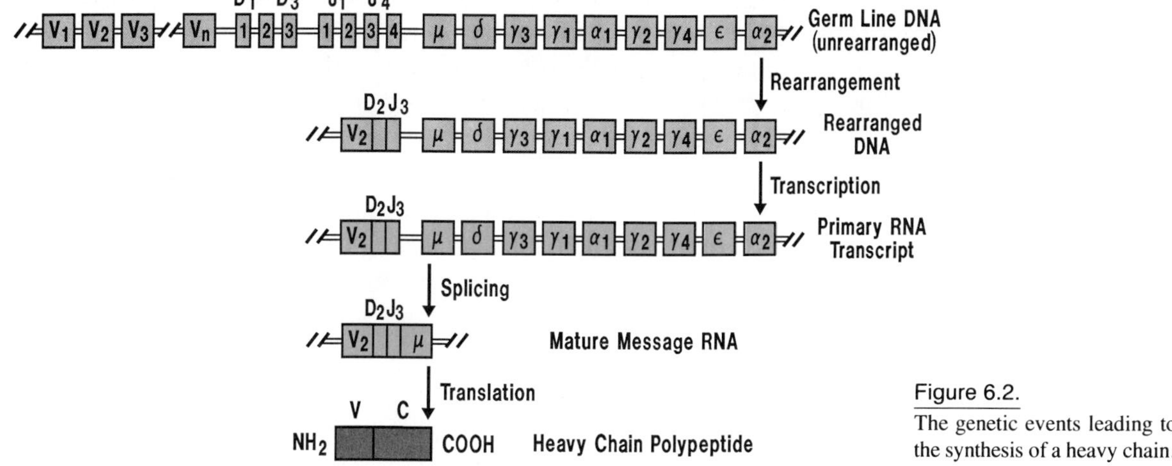

Figure 6.2.
The genetic events leading to the synthesis of a heavy chain.

segments that encode a short stretch of amino acids between the V and J regions of H chains is present. These small genes are the D (for diversity) genes and, as their name implies, they provide an additional degree of variability in the possible permutations of genetic sequences, while at the same time economizing on the amount of DNA used to generate antibody diversity. As an example, if we assume that there are 150 V genes, 12 D genes, and 4 J genes in the H chain gene complex, and if random association of any of these genes is possible, we can calculate that 7,200 ($150 \times 12 \times 4$) different H chains are possible. If these H chains could, in addition, associate randomly with any of the 1,000 possible κ-chains mentioned above, the total number of different antibody molecules that could be synthesized from this gene pool would be 7.2×10^6 (7,200 H $\times$ 1,000 κ). This large number is the result of a calculation that is based on the assumption of random recombination among only 371 genes (150 V_H + 12 D_H + 4 J_H and 200 $V\kappa$ + 5 $J\kappa$), and it demonstrates effectively how a limited amount of DNA can generate a large number of different polypeptides and antibodies.

The final group of genes that contribute to the H chain in embryonic DNA consists of the genes that encode the C regions, which are required by all known classes of immunoglobulins. In humans, the C genes occur in the following order μ, δ, γ_3, γ_1, α_1, γ_2, γ_4, ϵ, and α_2, each gene being flanked by introns.

The assembly of the H chain follows the general principles already described. First, a rearrangement of the germline DNA occurs, and a particular set of genes (e.g V_2, D_2, and J_3) are spliced together, and all the intervening sequences are excised. An RNA transcript is made from this spliced set of genes. The RNA transcript itself is then spliced to bring the entire V region (made up of V, D, and J segments) adjacent to a particular C region gene, again with the excision of all the intervening sequences. The spliced RNA then serves as the mRNA from which the complete H chain is synthesized.

ANTIBODY DIVERSITY

We have already seen how rearrangement of germline genes allows the synthesis of the enormous array of different antibodies required for an animal to deal with the variety of antigenic challenges that it confronts. Still more mechanisms for generating diversity exist, each of which is discussed briefly below.

Multiple V Genes in the Germline

The number of different genes for the V region in the germline constitutes the baseline from which antibody diversity is derived and represents the minimum numbers of different antibodies present.

Recombination With J and D Regions

As we have already seen, recombination of V genes with any of several J genes in κ- or λ-chains, and with D genes, as well as J genes, in the synthesis of H chains, is possible. Since the third hypervariable region has large contributions from the D and J segments, this recombination introduces significant diversity in antibody specificity.

Imprecise Recombinations

The precise positions at which the genes for the V and J, or the V, D and J, segments are spliced together are not constant, and imprecise recombination can lead to changes in the amino acids at these junction sites. The absence of precision in splicing leads, via the RNA transcript, to insertions, deletions, or changes of amino acids that affect the antigen-binding site, since they occur in parts of the hypervariable region, where complementarity to antigen is determined.

Random Assortment of H and L Chains

Since the genes for the H and L chains are separately encoded in DNA and synthesized independently, virtually any L chain may pair with any H chain to give a further, enormous amplification of diversity.

Somatic Cell Mutation

Mutations that occur in the genes of the germline during the lifetime of an individual B cell can increase the variety of antibodies produced by the B cell. It is only recently that evidence has accumulated to suggest that such mutations may provide the major means for fine tuning an immune response. It has been shown by sequencing of DNA and polypeptides that the antibody formed in a ***primary response*** follows very closely the sequence of the protein that would be encoded by ***germline DNA.*** As the response matures, after ***secondary stimulation*** by the antigen, an increase in affinity of the antibody for the antigen occurs, and a divergence is found from the amino acid sequence that is encoded in germline DNA. This divergence occurs as a result of ***point mutations,*** which affect individual amino acids in the hypervariable regions. Thus, it is believed that an immune response commences with the formation of low-affinity, prototypic antibodies, built according to information provided by germline genes. As the immune response continues, somatic mutations occur that are positively selected for, since they lead to the production of antibody with greater affinity for antigen. Mature antibody of high affinity therefore shares many features of the prototypic antibody, but it differs in ways that can be explained by point mutations, which alter single base pairs in DNA encoding for different amino acids in the complementarity-determining regions of H or L chains.

ALLELIC EXCLUSION

Diploid organisms possess two copies of each gene, one derived from each parent. Usually, both copies are expressed co-dominantly. A major exception to this rule is found in the production of antibodies. A given stem cell differentiates into an immunoglobulin-producing B cell, which makes antibody of only a single specificity by a process called ***allelic exclusion,*** the mechanism of which is still not completely understood. It seems that, in the differentiating cell, one cluster of H chain genes on one chromosome begins to rearrange. If a successful (i.e. productive) splicing of V, D, and J gene DNA occurs in one of the parental germline genes, then the other parental DNA remains in its embryonic form as a result of some kind of suppressive mechanism. If the first attempt to splice the V, D, and J genes is unsuccessful (i.e. if it fails to produce a peptide chain), then the second parental copy undergoes rearrangement. Thus, even though there are two chromosomal copies of the H chain in each cell, ***only one is functionally expressed.*** The same process then occurs first with the κ and then with the λ chain genes. Successful rearrangement by V to J splicing of any one of these genes causes the others to remain in embryonic form. In this way, the cell progresses through some or all of its chromosomal copies until it has successfully completed the productive rearrangement of genes for one H and one L chain. These chains then become the basis of the antibody specificity of that particular cell, modified by subsequent somatic mutations. This mechanism of ***gene exclusion*** prevents formation of antibody with two different L or two different H chains, and it therefore ***ensures the functional divalence*** of the synthesized antibody, which gives the antibody enhanced ability to agglutinate or increased ***avidity*** (which is the summation of individual affinities). A cell that fails to make the requisite rearrangements makes no immunoglobulin receptors; it is incapable of responding to further stimulation and it dies. These events occur in the absence of antigenic stimulation and are the basis for the formation of a library of B lymphocytes that contains all the specificities from which clonal selection operates (see Chapter 9).

CLASS OR ISOTYPE SWITCHING

It is known that, while ***a single B cell makes antibody of a single specificity*** that is determined by the nature of the rearrangements of the VJ gene of the L chain and the VDJ gene of the H chain, as just described, the particular class of antibody that this cell makes can change from IgM to IgG, IgA, or IgE. The mechanism of this ***class switch*** also involves ***rearrangement*** at the DNA level. In the earliest stage of differentiation, after completion of a successful rearrangement of the VDJ gene of its H chain, the B cell rearranges this segment to the gene for the μ constant region and then makes a primary RNA transcript from this rearranged DNA. This is followed by further RNA splicing to give an mRNA containing the VDJ and μ genes. This mRNA is then translated into the complete H chain protein. Class switching, which occurs under the influence of antigen and factors from helper T cells involves ***transposition*** of this same VDJ segment to another of the C region genes at the DNA level (e.g. γ_1) eliminating all the loci (μ, δ, γ_3) in between (Fig. 6.3).

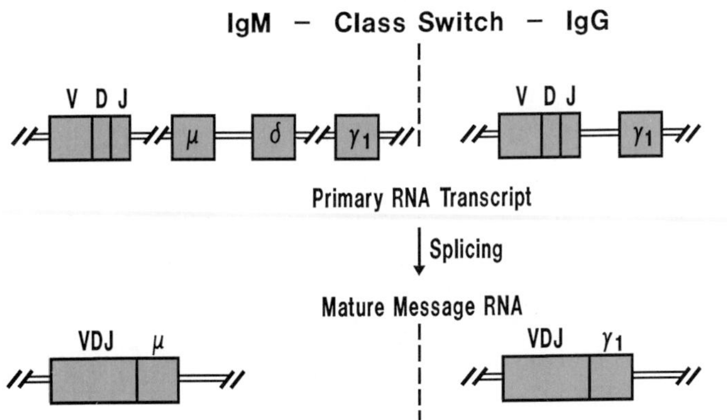

Figure 6.3.
The genetic events involved in immunoglobulin class switching.

This VDC gene is then transcribed and processed to give an mRNA for an H chain of IgG_1. Transposition is thought to be ***sequential,*** so that, in the same B cell clone, a particular VDJ segment of DNA might move downstream from μ to γ_1 to α (Fig. 6.3), as the immunological response matures. Once a switch is made at the DNA level, however, a cell ***cannot return to synthesis of an earlier (upstream) class,*** since the intervening DNA has been spliced out and lost. The mechanism of class switching provides flexibility to the immune response, since antibodies of identical specificity but with different biological properties may be made to defend against a particular pathogen.

SUMMARY

1. The DNA for the synthesis of the L and H chains of immunoglobulin molecules consists of a series of separate genes (exons), each of which codes for a different V region, and all of which are separated from one another by stretches of untranslated DNA (introns), as well as from other genes that code for joining (J) regions and the constant (C) region.

2. In the process of B cell differentiation, a cell first rearranges its germline DNA in such a way that one V region gene is spliced to a J region gene to encode an L chain.

3. The same type of rearrangement occurs for production of a gene for an H chain, and involves splicing of V, D, and J regions.

4. When splicing of DNA has occurred, the specificity of that particular cell is fixed. RNA transcripts are made from the rearranged DNA, and further splicing of the RNA brings the VJ of the L chain and the VDJ of the H chain adjacent to a particular C region gene. Messenger RNA, made from this spliced RNA, is then translated into the L and H chains of the antibody molecule, and the proteins are assembled for export.

5. Diversity in antibody specificity is achieved by 1) multiple genes for the V regions of both L and H chains; 2) recombination with multiple J and D regions; 3) absence of precision in the splicing of these regions; 4) random assortment of all the possible different L and H chains; and 5) somatic mutation, which occurs after stimulation by antigen, leading to selection for mutations that endow the antibody with higher affinity for the antigen.

6. This mechanism of splicing separate genes to generate the gene for a complete protein molecule also accounts well for the phenomena of allelic exclusion and class switching during an immune response.

REFERENCES

Baltimore D, Davies DR (1986): Immunoglobulins. Progress in Immunol 6:121.

Honjo T (1983): Immunoglobulin genes. Annu Rev Immunol 1:499.

Leder P (1982): The genetics of antibody diversity. Sci Am 246:102.

Tonegawa S (1983): Somatic generation of antibody diversity. Nature 302:575.

REVIEW QUESTIONS

For each of the incomplete statements below, ONE or MORE of the completions given is correct. Choose the appropriate answer:
A) if only *1, 2, 3* are correct
B) if only *1 and 3* are correct
C) if only *2 and 4* are correct
D) if only *4* is correct
E) if *all* are correct

1. The structural genes that encode a complete immunoglobulin heavy chain and light chain
   1) exist as several discrete segments in the germline DNA.
   2) require several somatic translocation events before transcription into mRNA.
   3) use a combinatorial association scheme to achieve greater diversity.
   4) are all on the same chromosome.

2. Differences in the specificities of combining sites of antibodies have been ascribed to
   1) multiple V genes in the germline.
   2) random assortment of L and H chains.
   3) imprecise recombination of V and J or V, D, and J segments.
   4) ability of antibody to fold around any antigenic determinant.

3. Which of the following statement(s) concerning the organization of immunoglobulin genes is/are correct?
   1) Once V to J joining of light chains and V, D, and J joining of heavy chain DNA segments has occurred in a B cell, the antigenic specificity of that B cell is fixed.
   2) V and J regions of embryonic DNA have already undergone a rearrangement.
   3) The VDJ segments of an immunoglobulin V region may be expressed in association with different heavy chain constant regions.
   4) The light chain of the immunoglobulin molecule can be switched after surface IgM is expressed.

4. If you could analyze, at the molecular level, a plasma cell that is making IgA antibody, you would find the following:
   1) a DNA sequence for V, D, and J genes translocated near the αDNA exon.
   2) mRNA specific for either κ or λ light chains.
   3) mRNA specific for J chains.
   4) mRNA specific for both κ and λ light chains.

(Continued on next page)

5. If you had 200 V and 5 J regions in a light chain and 300 V, 10 D, and 5 J regions in a heavy chain, you could have
   1) exactly 1,000 antibody specificities.
   2) exactly 15,000 antibody specificities.
   3) exactly 15,000,000 specificities.
   4) more than 15,000,000 specificities.

6. Antibody specificity of a particular B cell
   1) is encoded in the genome of the B cell.
   2) may switch from one idiotype to another during differentiation.
   3) may switch from one isotype to another during differentiation.
   4) is induced by interactions with antigen.

7. The switch mechanism for changing IgM to various classes of IgG involves
   1) use of genes that code for the same V, D, and J regions.
   2) recombination at the DNA level at certain points in the intervening sequences.
   3) loss of DNA segments for genes between the V region of the H chain and the gene to which the switch occurs.
   4) selection of a new L chain.

ANSWERS TO REVIEW QUESTIONS

1. ***A*** Only 4 is incorrect since genes for L and H chain are on different chromosomes.

2. ***A*** 1, 2, and 3 are all involved in development of multiple specificities. 4 was a concept in the "Instructional Theory" of antibody specificity, which is no longer tenable.

3. ***B*** 1 and 3 are the processes that fix specificity for a particular B cell and allow class switching to occur. 2 and 4 are incorrect since embryonic DNA is unrearranged and allelic exclusion prevents synthesis of a different light chain.

4. ***A*** 1 would be the rearranged H chain DNA present, 2 and 3 would represent the other chains being synthesized for IgA, while allelic exclusion would prevent expression of both κ and λ genes.

5. ***D*** While 15,000,000 would be the product of all possible combinations of genes, there would still be many other possibilities due to imprecise recombinations of VJ or VDJ segments as well as somatic mutation.

6. ***B*** Once splicing to give V to J and V, D, and J joining occurs, the specificity and idiotype of that particular B cell are fixed. These events occur in the absence of antigen, but when the cell is exposed to antigen, differentiation may result in class (isotype) switching, with retention of specificity and idiotype.

7. ***A*** The only thing not occurring in the switch mechanism is the selection of a new L chain.

CHAPTER

7

ANTIGEN–ANTIBODY INTERACTIONS

INTRODUCTION

Antibodies constitute the humoral arm of acquired immunity which provides protection against infectious organisms and their toxic products. Therefore, the interaction between antigen and antibody is of paramount importance. Because of the exquisite specificity of the immune response, the interaction between antigen and antibody in vitro is widely used for diagnostic purposes, for the detection and identification of either antigen or antibody. The exploitation of the in vitro reaction between antigen and serum antibodies is termed ***serology***. An example of the use of serology for the identification and classification of antigens is the ***serotyping*** of various microorganisms by the use of specific antisera.

The interaction of antigen with antibodies can result in a variety of consequences, including ***precipitation*** (if the antigen is soluble in saline), ***agglutination*** (if the antigen is particulate), ***neutralization of toxin,*** and ***activation of complement.*** Most, if not all, of these outcomes are caused by the interactions between multivalent antigens and antibodies that have at least two combining sites per molecule.

The consequences of antigen–antibody interaction listed above do not represent the primary interaction between antibodies and a given epitope but, rather, depend on secondary phenomena, which result from the interactions between multivalent antigens and antibodies. Such phenomena as the formation of precipitate, agglutination, and complement fixation would not occur if the antibody with two or more combining sites reacted with a hapten (i.e. a unideterminant, univalent antigen), nor would these secondary phenomena occur as a result of the interaction between a univalent fragment of antibody, such as Fab, and an antigen, even if the antigen were multivalent. The reasons for these differences are depicted in Figure 7.1 (A–E). ***Cross-linking*** of various antigen molecules by antibody is required for precipitation, agglutination, or complement fixation, and it is possible only if the antigen is multivalent and the antibody is divalent [either intact, or $F(ab')_2$] (see Fig. 7.1B, D, and E). In contrast, no cross-linking is possible if either the antigen or the antibody is

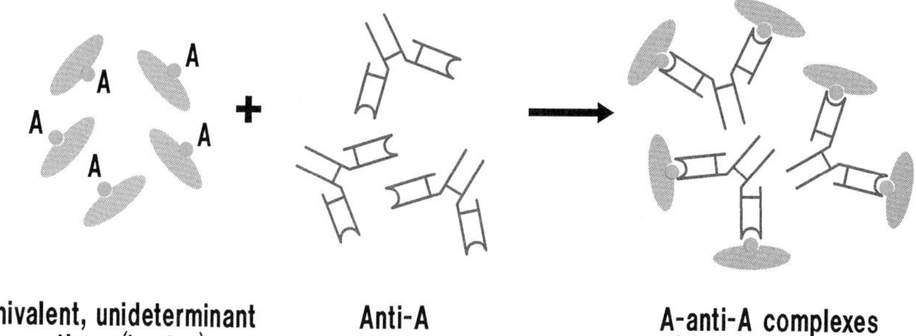

Figure 7.1A.
The reaction between antibody and a hapten.

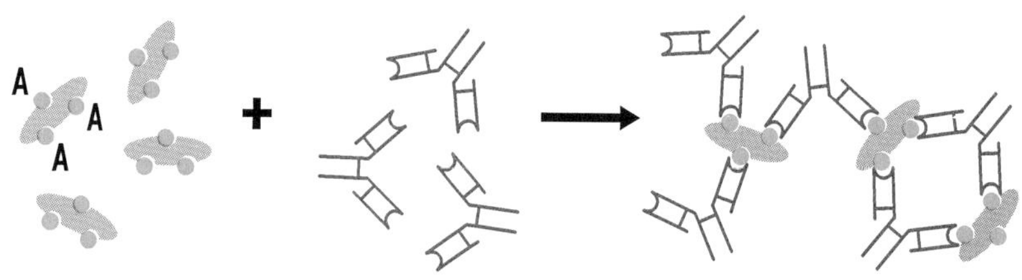

Figure 7.1B.
The reaction between antibody and a unideterminant, multivalent antigen.

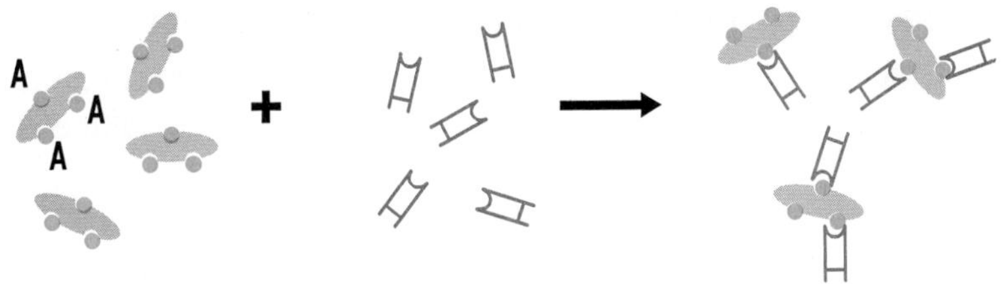

Figure 7.1C.
The reaction between Fab and a unideterminant, multivalent antigen.

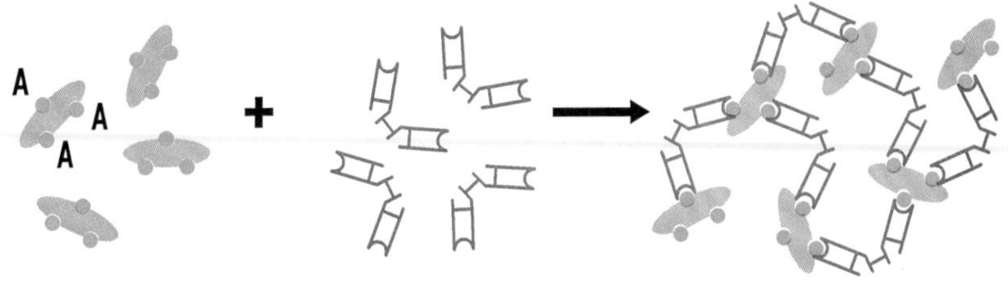

Figure 7.1D.
The reaction between $F(ab^{1})_2$ and a unideterminant, multivalent antigen.

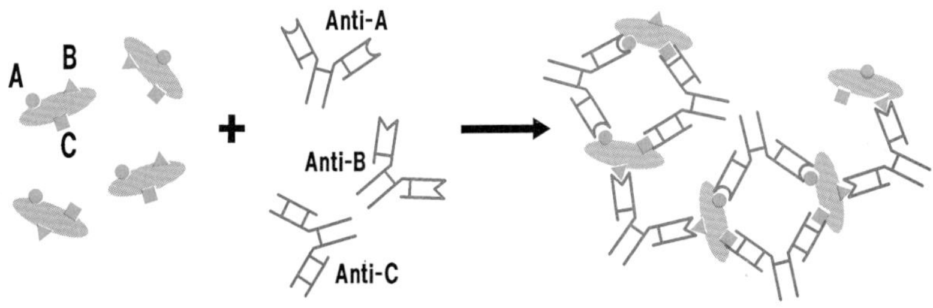

Figure 7.1E.
The reaction between antibodies to determinants A, B, C, and a multivalent, multideterminant antigen with determinants A, B, and C.

univalent (see Fig. 7.1A, and C). Agglutination, precipitation, and activation of complement require cross-linked antigen–antibody complexes, and the formation of such complexes is possible only with multivalent antigens and antibodies.

There are many serological reactions that demonstrate the binding between antigen and antibodies. This chapter describes selected reactions that are widely used in diagnosis; many others, not included here, are mostly variations of the reactions described here.

PRIMARY INTERACTIONS BETWEEN ANTIBODY AND ANTIGEN

The reaction between an antibody and an epitope of an antigen is exemplified by the reaction between antibody and a univalent hapten. Because an antibody molecule is symmetrical, with two identical Fab antigen-combining sites, one antibody molecule binds with two identical hapten molecules, each Fab binding in an independent fashion with one hapten molecule. The binding of a hapten (H) with each site can be represented by the equation

$$\mathrm{Ab} + \mathrm{H} \rightleftharpoons \mathrm{AbH}$$

and the association constant between the reactants is expressed as

$$\mathrm{K} = \frac{[\mathrm{AbH}]}{[\mathrm{Ab}][\mathrm{H}]}$$

When all the antibody molecules binding to a given hapten or epitope are identical (as in the case of monoclonal antibodies), then K represents the ***intrinsic association constant***. However, because serum antibodies—even those binding to a given epitope—are heterogeneous an ***average association constant*** of all the antibodies to the epitope is referred to as K_o.

No covalent bonds are involved in the interaction between an antibody and an epitope, so the binding forces between an antibody molecule and its specific epitope are relatively weak. They consist mainly of ***Van der Waal forces***, ***electrostatic forces***, and ***hydrophobic forces***, all of which require a very close proximity between the interacting moieties. Thus, the interaction requires a very close fit between an epitope and the antibody, a fit that is often compared to that between a lock and key.

Because of the low levels of energy involved in the interaction, antigen–antibody complexes can be readily ***dissociated*** by ***low or high pH,*** by ***high salt concentrations,*** or by ***chaotropic ions,*** such as cyanates, which efficiently interfere with the hydrogen bonding of water molecules.

The interaction between antibodies and each epitope of a multivalent antigen follows the same kinetics and energetics as those involved in the interaction between antibodies and haptens, because each epitope of the antigen reacts with its corresponding antibody in the same manner as that described above.

Affinity and Avidity

The intrinsic association constant that characterizes the binding of an antibody with an epitope or a hapten is termed ***affinity***. When the antigen consists of many repeating identical epitopes or when antigens are multivalent, the association between the entire antigen molecule and antibodies depends not only on the affinity between each epitope and its corresponding antibody but also on the sum of the affinities of all the epitopes involved. For example, the affinity of binding of anti-A with multivalent A (Fig. 7.1B) may be 4 or 5 orders of magnitude higher than between the same antibody (i.e. anti-A) and univalent A (Fig. 7.1A). This is because the pairing of anti-A with A (where A is multivalent) is influenced by the increased number of sites on A with which anti-A can react.

While the term ***affinity*** denotes the intrinsic association constant between antibody and a univalent ligand such as a hapten, the term ***avidity*** is used to denote the overall binding energy between antibodies and the multivalent antigen. Thus, in general, IgM antibodies are of higher avidity than IgG antibodies, although the binding of each Fab in the IgM antibody with ligand may be of lower affinity than that of the Fab from IgG.

SECONDARY INTERACTIONS BETWEEN ANTIBODY AND ANTIGEN

Agglutination Reactions

The reactions of antibody with a multivalent antigen that is ***particulate*** (i.e. an insoluble particle) results in the cross-linking of the various antigen particles by the antibodies. This cross-linking eventually results in the clumping, or ***agglutination,*** of the antigen particles by the antibodies (see Fig. 7.2). The example given in Figure 7.2A depicts a particulate antigen that is multivalent but unideterminant, since it has, on its surface, many identical epitopes, each of the A specificity. This antigen is agglutinated by anti-A antibodies. Similarly, if the particle carried different antigenic determinants on its surface, such as A, B, C, it would be agglutinated by a mixture of anti-A, anti-B, and anti-C antibodies (Fig. 7.2B).

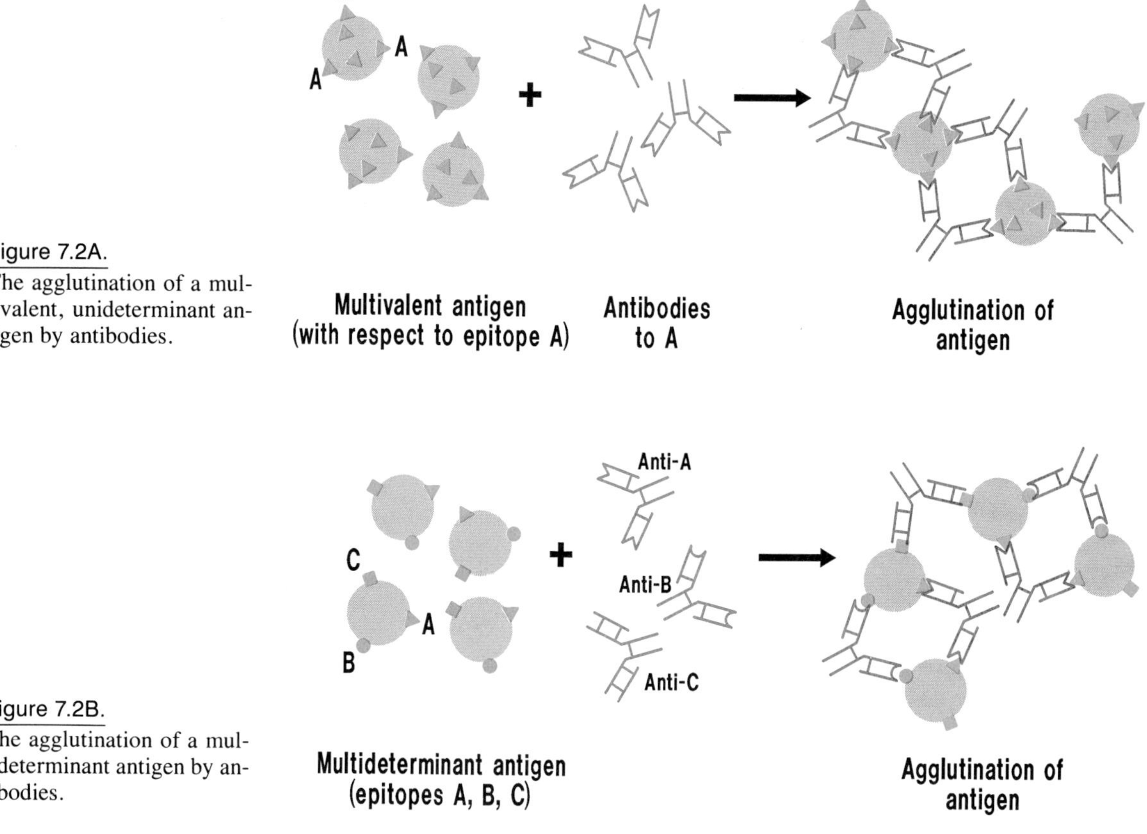

Figure 7.2A.
The agglutination of a multivalent, unideterminant antigen by antibodies.

Figure 7.2B.
The agglutination of a multideterminant antigen by antibodies.

TITER. The agglutination of an antigen as a result of cross-linking by antibodies is dependent on the correct proportion of antigen to antibody. Figure 7.3 depicts ten tubes, each of which contains precisely the same volume and the same amount of a particulate antigen, for example, a suspension of the bacterium *Brucella abortus*. Antiserum containing antibodies to *B. abortus* is added to each tube successively. A certain volume of antiserum is first added to the tube at the far left, with the same volume of a twofold serial dilution of the serum added to each successive tube to the right, until an identical volume of antiserum at a dilution of 1:2048 is added to the last tube. The plus and minus signs denote the presence and absence of agglutination. The results of the test (shown below each tube), indicate that agglutination occurs at dilutions of serum of 1:16 to 1:1024. There is no agglutination at higher dilutions because at such dilutions there are not enough antibodies to cause appreciable, visible agglutination. The highest dilution of serum that still causes agglutination, but beyond which no agglutination occurs, is termed the ***titer.*** In the example depicted in Figure 7.3, the titer is 1:1024.

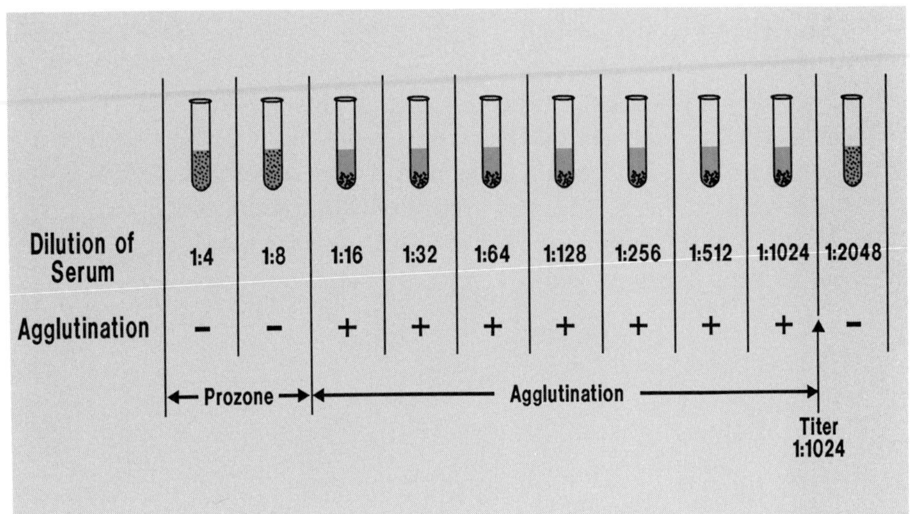

Figure 7.3.
A representation of the agglutination test.

The agglutinating titer of a certain serum is only a ***semiquantitative*** expression of the antibodies present in the serum; it is not a quantitative measure of the concentration of antibody (weight/volume). Rather, the titer represents the ability of a certain dilution (i.e. volume) of the antibodies in the serum to cause agglutination. As such, the agglutinating titer of a given antiserum may be used for comparison with the agglutinating titer to another antiserum to the same antigen. For example, after one immunization of an animal with *B. abortus* the serum titer of anti-*B. abortus* antibodies may be 1:64, while, after an additional booster injection, the titer may rise to 1:1024 or higher. Thus, agglutination titers are useful for comparisons of the relative concentrations of agglutinating antibodies in various sera. Since the titer in any agglutination assay depends on a variety of factors, such as size, charge, and density of epitopes on an antigen, it is of little use to compare titers of antisera to different antigens.

PROZONE. The left-hand side of Figure 7.3 shows tubes containing a suspension of antigen into which concentrated serum (diluted only 1:4 or 1:8) has been added. It is a common observation that agglutination does not occur at high concentrations of antibody, even though it does take place at higher dilutions of serum. The tubes with high concentrations of serum, where agglutination does not occur, represent a ***prozone.*** At the prozone antibodies are present in excess, so that the ratio of antigen to antibody is out of balance. Agglutination cannot occur at high concentrations of antibody, because the individual antibodies may bind with every epitope on one particle and thus interfere with the crosslinking between different particles (see Fig. 7.4).

Because of the prozone phenomenon, in testing for the presence of agglutinating antibodies to a certain antigen, it is imperative that the antiserum be tested at several dilutions. Testing serum at only one concentration may give misleading results if no agglutination occurs, because the absence of agglutination might reflect a prozone, and not a lack of antibody.

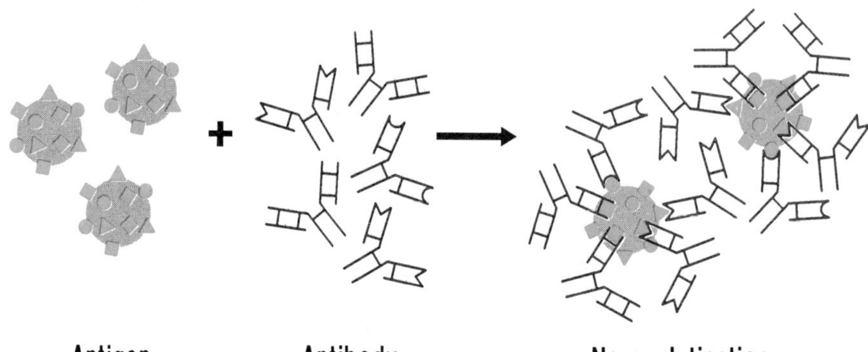

Figure 7.4.
A representation of a prozone (when antibody is present in excess) in the agglutination reaction.

ZETA POTENTIAL. The surfaces of certain particulate antigens may possess an electrical charge, as for example the net negative charge on the surface of red blood cells caused by the presence of sialic acid. When such charged particles are suspended in saline solution, an electrical potential termed the ***zeta potential*** is created between particles, preventing them from getting very close to each other. This electrical potential introduces a difficulty when attempts are made to agglutinate charged particles by antibodies, in particular when attempts are made to agglutinate red blood cells by IgG antibodies. The distance between the Fab portions of the IgG molecule, even in its most extended form, is too short to allow effective bridging between two red blood cells across the separation caused by the zeta potential. Thus, although IgG antibodies may be directed against antigens on the charged erythrocytes, no agglutination occurs because of the zeta potential. On the other hand, ***IgM*** pentamers contain Fab areas that are far enough apart so that it is possible to bridge between red blood cells separated by the zeta potential. This property of IgM antibodies, together with their pentavalence, is a major reason for their ***effectiveness as agglutinating antibodies.***

Through the years attempts were made to improve agglutination reactions by decreasing the zeta potential in various ways, none of which was universally applicable or effective. However, an ingenious method was devised in the 1950s by Coombs to overcome the problems imposed by the zeta potential. This method, described below, facilitates the agglutination of erythrocytes by IgG antibodies specific for erythrocyte antigens. It is also useful for the detection of antibodies that are present on the surface of erythrocytes but that are unable to agglutinate them.

THE COOMBS' TEST. The Coombs' test employs antibodies to immunoglobulins (hence, it is also called the ***anti-immunoglobulin test).*** It is based on two important facts: 1) that immunoglobulins of one species (e.g. human) are immunogenic when injected into another species (e.g. rabbit) and lead to the production of antibodies against the immunoglobulins; and 2) that many of the anti-immunoglobulins (e.g. rabbit anti-human Ig) bind with antigenic determinants present on the Fc portion of the antibody, and leave the Fab portions free to react with antigen. Thus, for example, if human IgG antibodies are attached to their respective epitopes on the erythrocyte, then the addition of rabbit antibodies to human IgG will result in their binding with the Fc portions of the human antibodies, which are bound to the erythrocyte by their Fab portion (see Fig. 7.5). These rabbit antibodies not only bind with the human

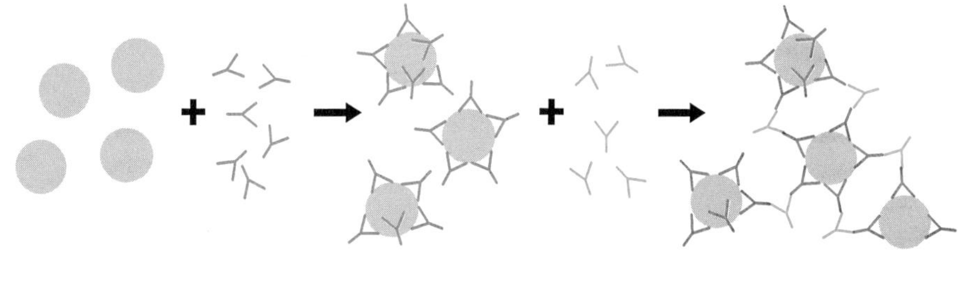

Figure 7.5.
A representation of the anti-immunoglobulin (Coombs') test.

antibodies bound to the erythrocyte but also, by doing so, they cross-link (form bridges) between human IgG on relatively distant erythrocytes, across the separation induced by the zeta potential, and cause agglutination.

The addition of anti-immunoglobulin brings about agglutination, even if the antibodies directed against the erythrocytes are present at an excessive concentration that causes the prozone phenomenon.

There are two versions of the Coombs' test: the ***direct Coombs' test*** and the ***indirect Coombs' test.*** The two versions differ somewhat in the mechanics of the test but both are based on the same principle: using heterologous anti-immunoglobulins to detect a reaction between immunoglobulins and antigen.

In the ***direct Coombs' test,*** anti-immunoglobulins are added to the particles (e.g. red blood cells) that are suspected of having antibodies bound to antigens on their surfaces. For example, a newborn baby is suspected of having hemolytic disease of the newborn caused by maternal anti-Rh IgG antibodies that are bound to the baby's erythrocytes. If that suspicion proved to be correct, the direct Coombs' test would have the following results: the addition of anti-immunoglobulin to a suspension of the baby's erythrocytes would result in the binding of the anti-immunoglobulin to the maternal IgG on the surface of the erythrocytes, and would cause agglutination (Fig. 7.6A).

In contrast to the direct Coombs' test, where anti-immunoglobulins are added to particles suspected of having immunoglobulins bound to their surfaces, the ***indirect Coombs' test*** is used to detect the presence ***in the serum*** of antibodies specific to antigens on the particle itself. The serum antibodies, when added to the particles, fail to cause agglutination because of the zeta potential. The subsequent addition of anti-Ig will cause agglutination. A common application of the indirect Coombs' test is in the detection of anti-Rh IgG

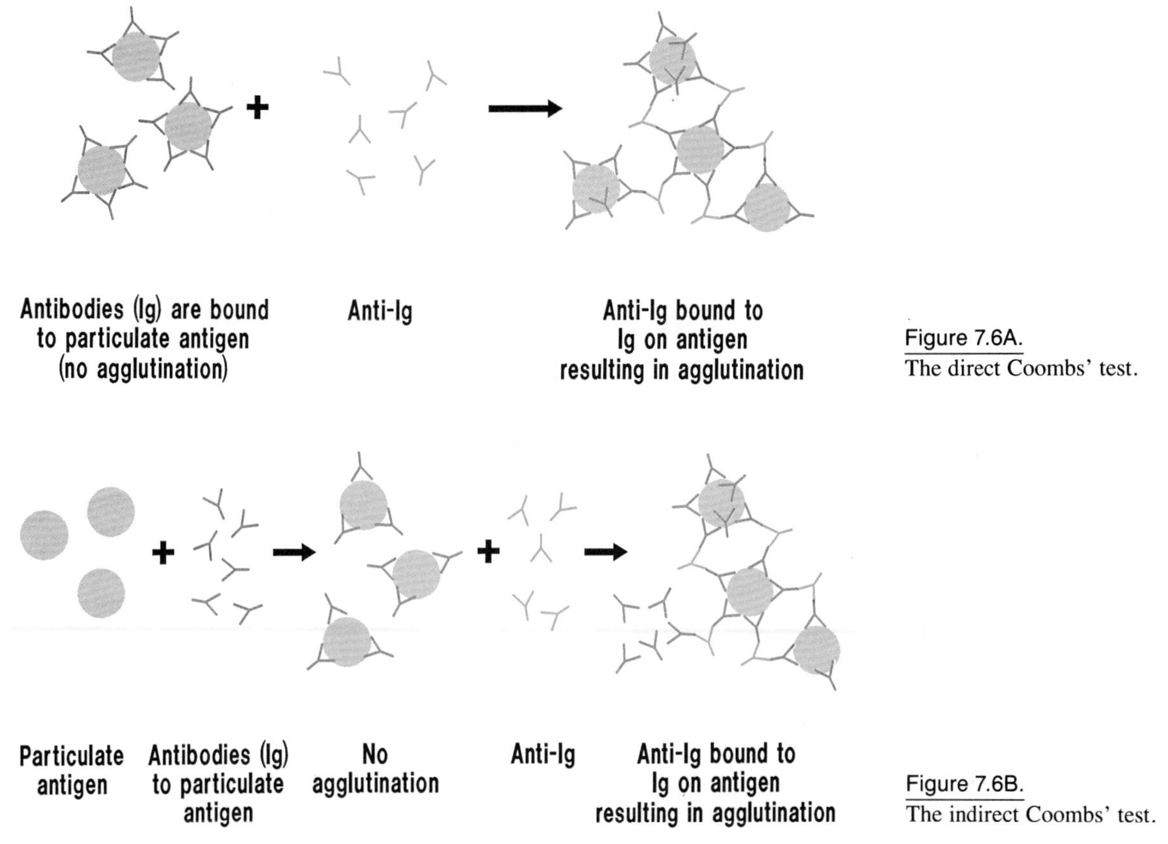

Figure 7.6A.
The direct Coombs' test.

Figure 7.6B.
The indirect Coombs' test.

antibodies in the blood of an Rh-negative woman. The indirect Coombs' test consists, first, of reaction of the antibodies with the particulate antigen (in the present example, the reaction of the woman's serum with Rh^+ erythrocytes), and then the addition of the anti-immunoglobulins (as in the direct Coombs' test) (Fig. 7.6B).

Originally, the Coombs' test was used for the detection of human antibodies on the surface of erythrocytes. Today the term "Coombs' test" (direct or indirect) is applied to the detection by the use of anti-immunoglobulin, of any Ig that is bound to antigen.

PASSIVE AGGLUTINATION. The agglutination reaction can be used not only with particulate antigens (e.g. erythrocytes or bacteria) but also with soluble antigens, provided that the soluble antigen can be firmly attached to insoluble particles. For example, the soluble antigen thyroglobulin can be attached to latex particles, so that the addition of antibodies to the thyroglobulin antigen will cause agglutination of the particles coated with thyroglobulin.

In contrast to cases of ***direct agglutination,*** where the antigen is a natural constituent of the particle, agglutination that uses particles to which soluble antigens have been attached is referred to as ***passive agglutination.*** Latex particles and sheep red blood cells are widely used as insoluble supports for soluble antigens in tests that involve passive agglutination. When red blood cells are used, the test is referred to as ***passive hemagglutination.***

Precipitation Reactions

THE PRECIPITIN REACTION. In contrast to the agglutination reaction, which takes place between antibodies and particulate antigen, the ***precipitation reaction*** takes place when antibodies and ***soluble antigen*** are mixed in the correct proportions. As in the case of agglutination, precipitation of antigen–antibody complexes occurs because the divalent antibody molecules cross-link multivalent antigen molecules to form a ***lattice***. When it reaches a certain size, this antigen–antibody complex loses its solubility and precipitates out of solution. The phenomenon of precipitation is termed the ***precipitin reaction***.

Figure 7.7 depicts a quantitative precipitin reaction. When increasing concentrations of antigen are added to a series of tubes that contain a constant concentration of antibodies, variable amounts of precipitate form. The weight of the precipitate in each tube may be determined by a variety of methods. If the weight of the precipitate is plotted against the amount of antigen added, a precipitin curve like the one shown in Figure 7.7 is obtained.

There are three important areas under the curve shown in Figure 7.7: the ***zone of antibody excess,*** the ***equivalence zone,*** and the ***zone of antigen excess.*** In the equivalence zone, the proportion of antigen to antibody is optimal for maximal precipitation; in the zones of antibody excess or antigen excess, the proportions of the reactants are not optimal for efficient cross-linking and formation of precipitate.

It should be emphasized that the zones of the precipitin curve are based on the amounts of antigen–antibody complex precipitated. However, each zone may also contain soluble antigen–antibody complexes, particularly the zone of antigen excess where, although a minimal amount of precipitate is formed, large amounts of ***soluble antigen–antibody complexes*** are present. In fact, insoluble antigen–antibody precipitates can be dissolved by the addition of

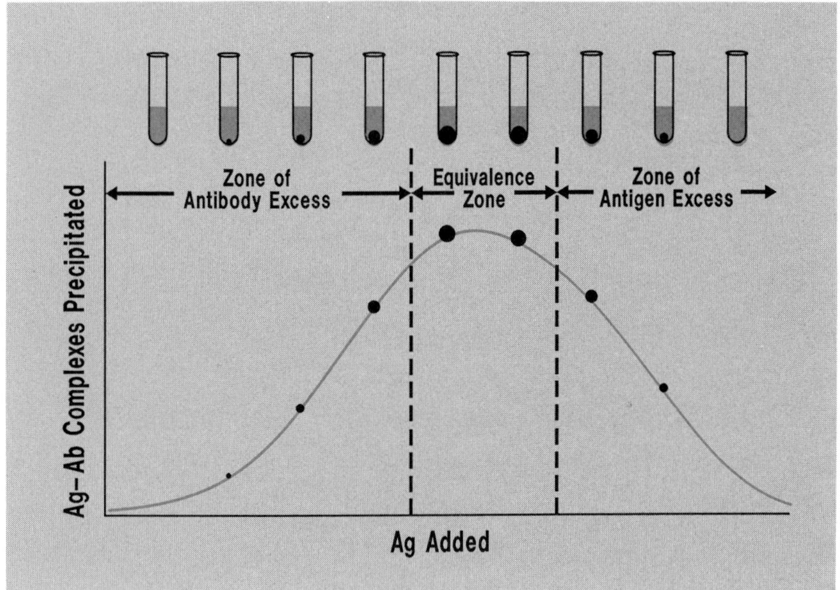

Figure 7.7.
A representation of the precipitin reaction.

more antigen. Conversely, if antibodies are added to the soluble antigen–antibody complexes, in the supernatant of the tube where excess antigen is present, then additional precipitation will occur. Thus, the precipitin reaction is dependent upon the proportions of the reactant antigens and antibodies: the correct proportions of the reactants result in maximal formation of precipitate; excess of antigen (or antibody) results in soluble complexes.

PRECIPITATION REACTIONS IN GELS. Precipitation reactions between soluble antigens and antibodies can take place not only in solution but also in semi-solid media such as agar gels. When soluble antigen and antibodies are placed in wells cut in a gel (Fig. 7.8A), the reactants diffuse in the gel and form gradients of concentration, with the highest concentrations closest to the wells. Somewhere between the two wells, the reacting antigen and antibodies will be present at proportions that are optimal for formation of a precipitate.

If the antibody well contains antibodies 1, 2, and 3 specific for antigens 1, 2, and 3, respectively, and if antigens 1, 2, and 3, placed in the antigen well, diffuse at different rates (with diffusion rates of $1>2>3$), then three distinct precipitin lines will form. These three precipitin lines form because anti-1, anti-2, and anti-3, which diffuse at the same rate, react independently with

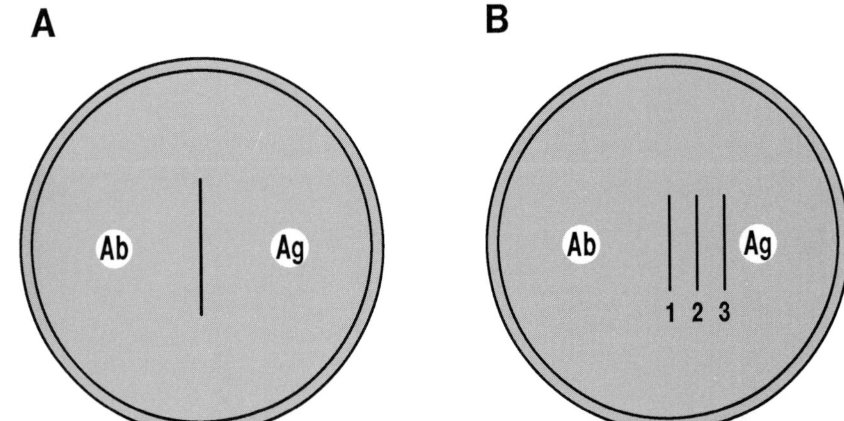

Figure 7.8.
Gel diffusion by *A* antibodies and a single antigen and *B* antibodies to antigens 1, 2, 3 and the respective antigens.

antigens 1, 2, and 3, respectively, to form three equivalence zones and thus three separate lines of precipitate (Fig. 7.8B). Different rates of diffusion of the antigen result from differences in concentration, molecular size, or shape.

This ***double-diffusion*** method, developed by Ouchterlony, where antigen and antibody diffuse toward each other, is very useful for establishing the antigenic relationship between various substances, as shown in Figure 7.9.

Three patterns of reactions are seen in gel diffusion, each of which is illustrated in Figure 7.9: patterns of identity, patterns of non-identity, and patterns of partial identity.

Patterns of Identity. In the example given on the left of Figure 7.9, the central well contains antibodies and the peripheral wells contain identical antigens. The antibodies diffuse from the central well toward the antigens which, since they are identical, diffuse at an equal rate from the peripheral

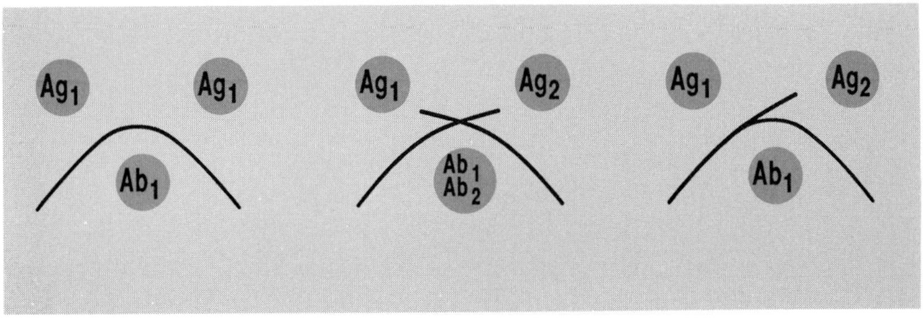

Figure 7.9.
Double gel diffusion patterns showing pattern of identity (left), pattern of non-identity (center), and pattern of partial identity (right).

wells. As a result, one ***continuous, coalescing*** precipitin line is formed. This pattern, formed when the two antigens are identical is termed a ***pattern of identity.***

Patterns of Non-Identity. In the example in the center of Figure 7.9, the central well contains antibodies to antigen-1 and antigen-2, two non-related antigens, and the peripheral wells contain the two non-related antigens, antigen-1 and antigen-2. The two antibody (immunoglobulin) populations diffuse at the same rate toward the peripheral wells. Antigen-1 and antigen-2 diffuse from the two peripheral wells toward the antibodies. Each antigen forms a precipitin line with its corresponding antibody, independent of the other antigen-antibody reaction, and the precipitin lines cross each other. A pattern where the precipitin lines ***cross each other*** denotes ***non-identity*** of the two antigens.

Patterns of Partial Identity. This pattern is shown in the right-hand part of Figure 7.9, where the center well contains antibodies to various epitopes of antigen-1. The reaction of these antibodies with antigen-1 results in a precipitin line. Antigen-2, however, contains some (but not all) of the epitopes present on antigen-1. Thus, some of the antibodies to antigen-1 will also combine with antigen-2. This ***partial identity*** between the two antigens is responsible for the coalescence of the two lines to give a line of identity. However, antibodies that do not bind with antigen-2 will pass through this line of precipitate, combine with antigen-1 and form a ***spur.*** This pattern, with the formation of a spur, denotes partial identity, signifying that antigen-1 and antigen-2 share epitopes, with antigen-1 having more epitopes (and being able to react with more antibodies) than antigen-2.

RADIAL IMMUNODIFFUSION. The radial immunodiffusion test, depicted in Figure 7.10, represents a variation of the diffusion test. The wells contain antigen at different concentrations, while the antibodies are distributed uniformly in the agar gel. Thus, the precipitin line is replaced by a precipitin ring around the well. The distance of the periphery of the precipitin ring from the center of the antigen well is directly proportional to the concentration of antigen in the well. The relationship between concentration of antigen in a well and the diameter of the precipitin ring can be plotted as shown in Figure 7.10. If wells, such as F and G, contain unknown amounts of the same antigen, the concentration of that antigen in these wells can be determined by comparing the diameter of the precipitin ring with the ***diameter*** of the ring formed by a known concentration of the antigen.

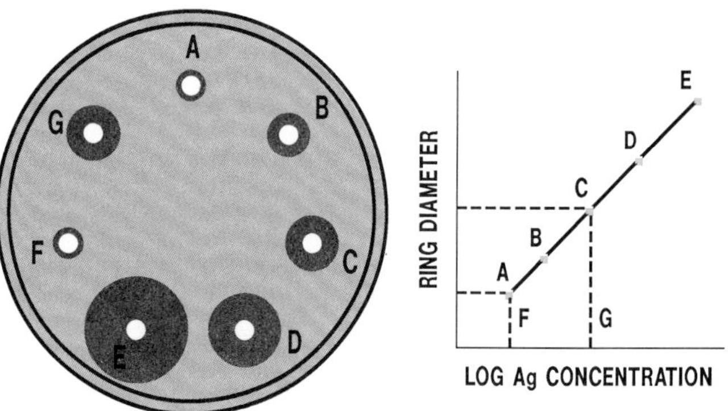

Figure 7.10.
Radial diffusion. A, B, C, D, E represent known concentrations of antigen; F and G represent unknown concentrations that can be determined from the graph.

IMMUNOELECTROPHORESIS. ***Immunoelectrophoresis*** consists of moving proteins in an electrical field (electrophoresis) followed by gel diffusion. It is very useful for the analysis of a mixture of antigens by an antiserum that contains antibodies to the antigens in the mixture. A good example of the usefulness of immunoelectrophoresis is its clinical use for the characterization of human serum proteins. A small drop of human serum is placed in a well cut in the center of a slide that is coated with agar gel. The serum is then subjected to electrophoresis, which separates the various components according to their mobilities in the electrical field. After electrophoresis, a trough is cut along the side of the slide, and antibodies to human serum proteins are placed into the trough. The antibodies diffuse in the agar, as do the separated serum proteins. At an optimal antigen–antibody ratio for each antigen and its corresponding antibodies, each serum protein forms a precipitin line with its antibodies. The result is a pattern similar to that depicted in Figure 7.11. Comparison of the pattern and intensity of lines of normal human serum with the patterns and intensity of lines obtained with sera of patients may reveal an absence, overabundance, or other abnormality of one or more serum proteins.

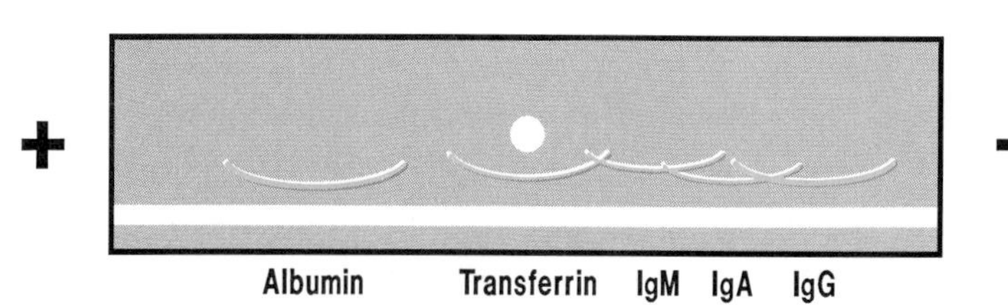

Figure 7.11.
Patterns of immunoelectrophoresis.

IMMUNOASSAYS

Radioimmunoassay (RIA) employs isotopically labeled molecules and permits measurements of extremely small amounts of antigen, antibody, or antigen–antibody complexes. The concentration of such labeled molecules is determined by measuring their radioactivity, rather than by chemical analysis. The sensitivity of detection is thus increased by several orders of magnitude.

The principle of radioimmunoassy is illustrated in Figure 7.12. A known amount of radioactively labeled antigen is reacted with a limited amount of antibody. The solution now contains antibody-bound labeled antigen, as well as some unbound labeled antigen. The antibody-bound antigen is separated from the free antigen, and the radioactivity bound to antibody is determined (Fig. 7.12A). The test continues with performance of a similar procedure; however, this time the same amount of labeled antigen is pre-mixed with unlabeled antigen (Fig. 7.12B). The mixture is reacted with the same amount of antibody as before, and the antibody-bound antigen is separated from the unbound antigen. The unlabeled antigen ***competes*** with the labeled antigen for the antibody and, as a result, less label is bound to antibody (or more unbound labeled antigen remains free in the reaction mixture) than in the absence of unlabeled antigen. The more unlabeled antigen present in the reaction mixture, the smaller the ratio of antibody-bound, radiolabeled antigen to free, radiolabeled antigen. This ratio can be plotted as a function of the concentration of the unlabeled antigen used for competition. A typical plot is shown in Figure 7.13.

To determine an unknown concentration of antigen in a solution, a sample of the solution that contains the unknown concentration of antigen is mixed with predetermined amounts of labeled antigen and antibody. The ratio of ***bound/free radioactivity*** is compared with that obtained in the absence of unlabeled antigen (the latter value is set at 100%).

An important step in performing a radioimmunoassay, as described above, is the separation of free antigen from that bound to antibody. Depending upon the antigen, this separation is usually performed in one of two ways: by the Farr technique or by the anti-immunoglobulin procedure.

The Farr Technique

The ***Farr technique*** is based on the fact that immunoglobulins precipitate out of solution in ***33% saturated ammonium sulfate,*** and that the binding of antibodies with antigen is unaffected by this concentration of ammonium

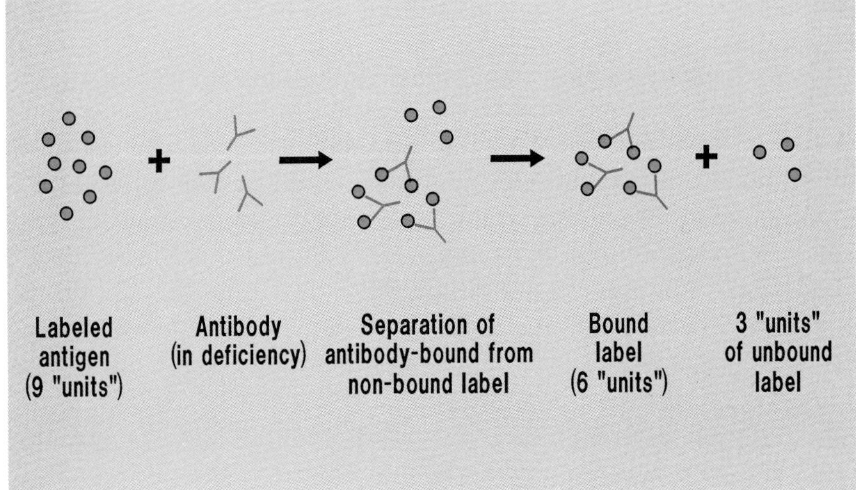

Figure 7.12A.
Amount of label bound to antibody after incubation of constant amounts of antibody and labeled antigen.

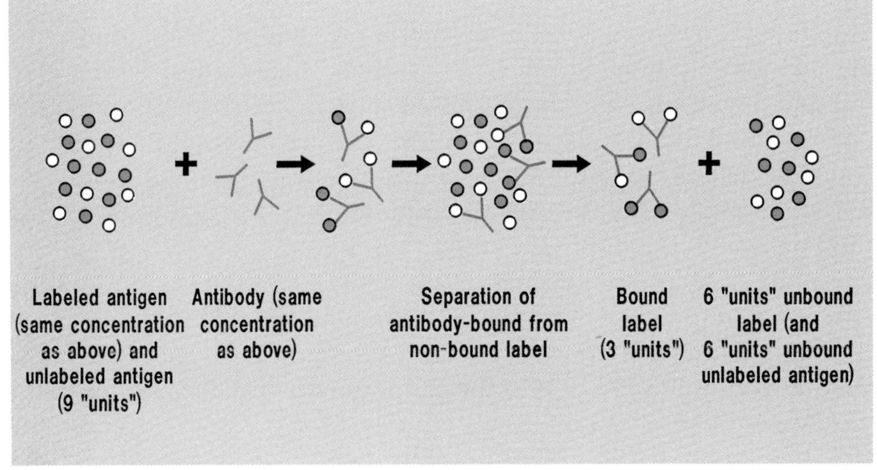

Figure 7.12B.
Radioimmunoassay, based on the competition of nonlabeled and labeled antigens for antibody.

sulfate. Thus, if a given (free) antigen does not precipitate in 33% saturated ammonium sulfate, the antigen that is bound to antibody will be precipitated, and thus separated, from free antigen. The precipitate is removed by centrifugation, and the radioactivity present in the separated precipitate (which consists of radioactive antigen bound to antibody) or the radioactivity of the supernatant (which contains free antigen) is measured.

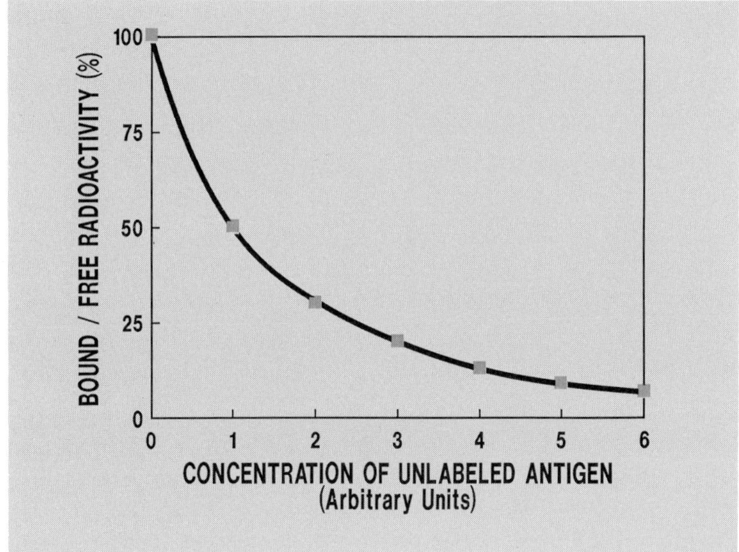

Figure 7.13.
A standard curve showing the inhibition of binding of labeled antigen to antibodies by non-labeled antigen.

The Farr technique is used extensively in the radioimmunoassay of antigens of relatively ***low molecular weight,*** such as ***drugs*** and ***hormones,*** which normally do not precipitate in 33% saturated ammonium sulfate.

The Anti-Immunoglobulin Procedure

The antiglobulin procedure is based on the fact that immunoglobulins, even if bound to antigen, react with antibodies to the immunoglobulins that have been made in another species, and form a precipitate. Antigen (labeled or unlabeled) bound to these immunoglobulins will also be precipitated, so that only unbound antigen remains in the supernatant. Radioimmunoassays commonly employ rabbit antibodies to the desired antigens. The rabbit antibody–antigen complexes may be precipitated by the addition of goat antibodies raised against rabbit immunoglobulins.

It is important to recognize that the amounts of antigen and antibody required for radioimmunoassy are extremely small. The antigen–antibody complexes, either precipitated out at 33% saturated ammonium sulfate, or reacted with anti-immunoglobulin, would form only tiny precipitates. It is difficult, if not impossible, to recover these precipitates quantitatively by conventional means, in order to determine their radioactivity. To overcome this problem, it is customary to add non-specific immunoglobulins to the reaction mixture, thereby increasing the amount of total immunoglobulins to an amount that can easily be precipitated by ammonium sulfate, or by anti-immunoglobulins, and recovered quantitatively. Such precipitates consist mainly of non-specific immunoglobulins to which radioactive antigen does not bind. However, they also contain the extremely small amount of antigen-specific immunoglobulin and any radioactive antigen bound to it.

Solid Phase Immunoassays

Solid phase immunoassays employ the property of various plastics (e.g. polyvinyl or polystyrene) to adsorb monomolecular layers of proteins onto their surfaces. Although the adsorbed molecules may lose some of their antigenic determinants, enough molecules remain unaltered and can still react with their corresponding antibodies. The presence of these antibodies, bound to antigen adsorbed onto the plastic, may be detected by the use of anti-immunoglobulins (Fig. 7.14) labeled with a radioactive tracer. A solid phase assay, which uses radioactive anti-immunoglobulins, is termed ***solid phase radioimmunoassay (SPRIA)***. If the test uses anti-immunoglobulins that are labeled with an enzyme, the test is called an ***enzyme-linked immunosorbent assay (ELISA);*** the test is described below.

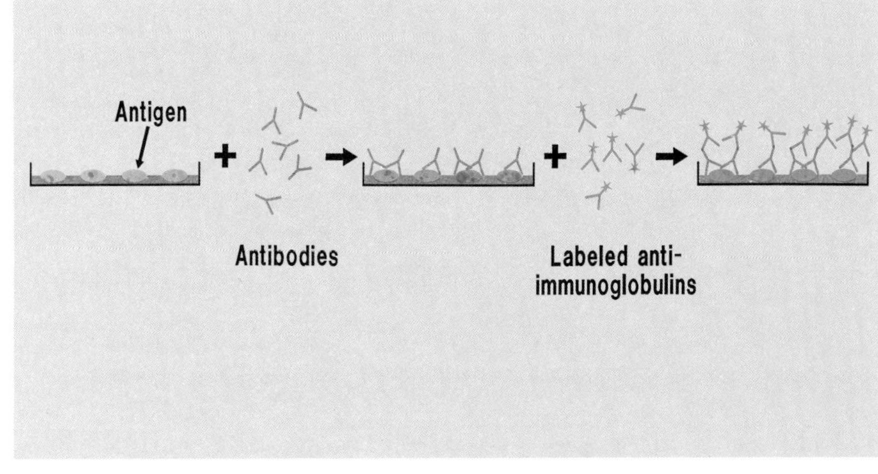

Figure 7.14.
A schematic representation of a solid phase immunoassay.

It should be emphasized that, after the coating of the plastic surface with antigen, it is imperative to ***"block"*** any uncoated plastic surface to prevent it from adsorbing the antibodies. Such "blocking" ensures that the antibodies bind only to the antigen and not to free plastic surfaces, and is achieved by coating the plastic surface with a high concentration of an unrelated protein, such as gelatin.

Solid phase immunoassay may be used to detect the presence of antibodies to the antigen that coats the plastic. Since the plastic wells are usually coated with relatively large amounts of antigen, the higher the concentration of antibodies bound with the antigen, the higher the amount of labeled anti-immunoglobulin that can bind to the antibodies. Thus, it is important always to use an excess of labeled anti-immunoglobulin.

Solid phase immunoassay is a semi-quantitative test. It is useful for comparisons of the concentrations of antibody present in various sera, but it does not provide an absolute determination of the concentration of antibody (wt/volume) in the serum.

Solid phase immunoassay may be used for the qualitative and quantitative determination of antigen. Such determinations are performed by mixing the antiserum with varying known concentrations of antigen, before adding the antiserum to the antigen-coated plastic wells. This preliminary procedure results in the binding of the antibodies with the soluble antigen, decreasing the availability of antibodies for binding with the antigen that is coating the plastic. The higher the concentration of antigen that reacts with antibodies prior to addition of the antibody to the wells, the lower the number of antibodies that can bind with the antigen on the plate, and the lower the number of labeled anti-immunoglobulin that can bind to these antibodies. The decrease in the amount of bound label as a function of the concentration of antigen used to cause this decrease can be plotted, and the amount of antigen in an unknown solution can then be determined from the graph by a comparison of the decrease in bound label caused by the unknown solution to the decrease caused by known concentrations of pure antigen.

ELISA—Enzyme-Linked Immunosorbent Assay

The anti-immunoglobulin used in this solid phase immunoassay is conjugated to an enzyme, usually one that reacts with an added substrate to yield a colored product. Detection of enzyme-linked anti-immunoglobulins is therefore achieved by addition of substrate to the reaction. Appearance of the characteristic color that results from the activity of the enzyme on its substrate signifies the presence of anti-immunoglobulin. This solid phase immunoassay, which employs an enzyme-linked anti-immunoglobulin, is termed the ***enzyme-linked immunosorbent assay (ELISA).*** The ELISA is rapidly replacing many assays in which radioactive label is used, because it is less expensive. Also, it does not require special precautions for the handling of radioactivity, and it is, in general, just as sensitive.

Radioallergosorbent (RAST) Test

The ***RAST*** test, illustrated in Figure 7.15, is basically a solid phase radioimmunoassay especially designed for the detection of IgE (reaginic) antibodies in the serum of a patient suspected of having an IgE-mediated hypersen-

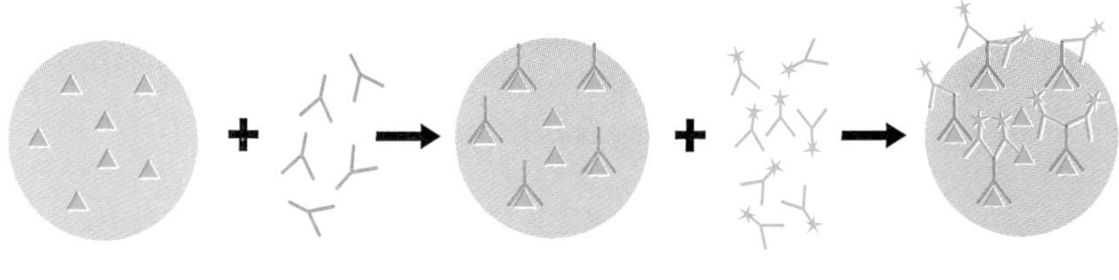

Figure 7.15.
The radioallergosorbent (RAST) test.

sitivity or allergy to a certain antigen or allergen (see Chapter 13). The test employs a paper disc to which the suspected allergen has been covalently linked (the allergen may be pollen extract, bee venom, etc.). The patient's serum is then applied to the paper. After washing the paper disc with saline, radioactively labeled anti-serum specific for human IgE is applied to the disc. After several additional washings, the radioactivity bound to the disc is determined. Radioactivity present on the paper disc indicates that the patient's IgE antibodies have bound to the antigen and have, in turn, bound labeled antibodies to human IgE.

Immunofluorescence

A fluorescent compound has the property of emitting light of a certain wavelength when it is excited by exposure to light of a shorter wavelength.

Immunofluorescence is a method for localizing an antigen by the use of fluorescent labeled antibodies. The procedure, originally described by Coons, employs antibodies to which fluorescent groups have been covalently linked without any appreciable change in antibody activity.

One fluorescent compound that is widely used in immunology is ***fluorescein isothiocyanate (FITC),*** which fluoresces with a visible greenish color when excited by ultraviolet light, and is easily coupled to free amino groups. Another widely used fluorescent compound is ***tetramethyl rhodamine isothiocyanate (TRITC),*** which fluoresces red-orange and is also easily coupled to free amino groups. There are specially constructed microscopes that permit visualization of fluorescent antibody on a microscopic specimen, and fluorescent antibodies are widely used to localize antigens on various tissues and microorganisms.

There are two important and related procedures that employ fluorescent antibodies (see Fig. 7.16A).

DIRECT IMMUNOFLUORESCENCE. In direct immunofluorescence the target tissue (or microorganism) is reacted with fluorescently labeled specific antibodies as shown in Figure 7.16A.

INDIRECT IMMUNOFLUORESCENCE. Another procedure, indirect immunofluorescence, first involves reacting the target with specific antibodies. That reaction is followed by an additional reaction with fluorescently labeled anti-immunoglobulin (see Fig. 7.16B).

The indirect immunofluorescence method is more widely used than the direct method, because a single fluorescent anti-immunoglobulin antibody can be used to the localize many different antibodies. Moreover, since the anti-immunoglobulins contain antibodies to many epitopes on the specific immunoglobulin, the use of fluorescent anti-immunoglobulins amplifies many-fold the fluorescent response.

Immunoabsorption and Immunoadsorption

Because of the specific binding between antigen and antibody, it is possible to "trap," or selectively absorb, an antigen against which an antibody is directed, from a mixture of antigens in solution. By the same token, it is

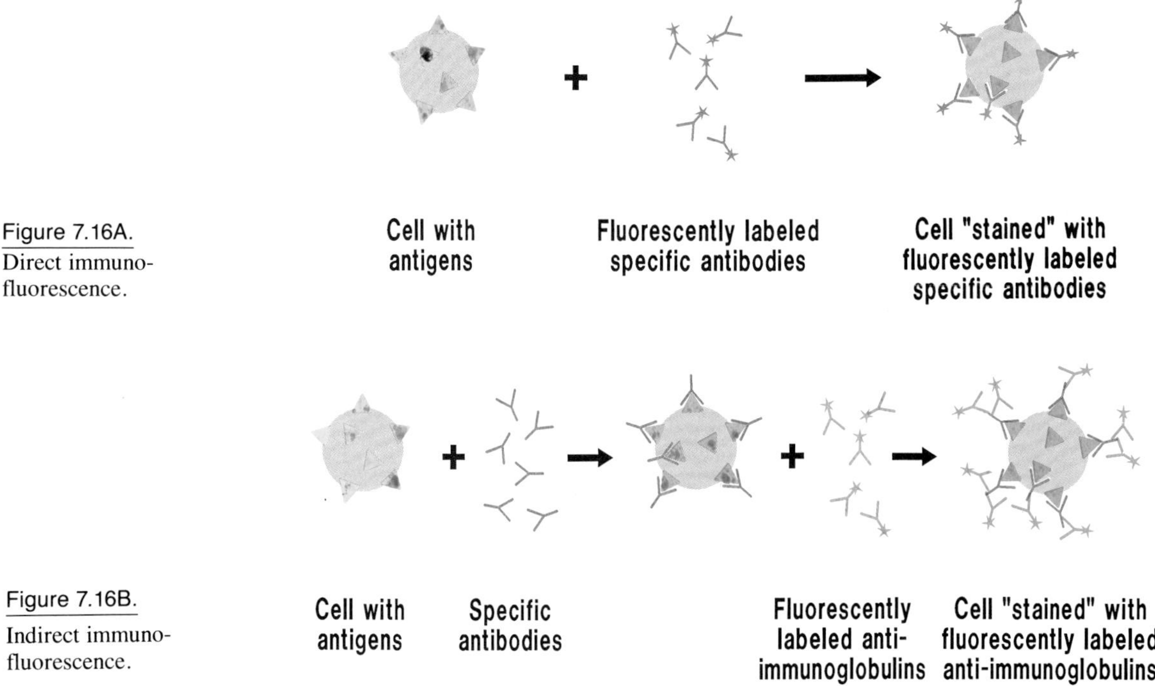

Figure 7.16A. Direct immunofluorescence.

Figure 7.16B. Indirect immunofluorescence.

possible to trap or absorb selectively the antigen-specific antibodies from a mixture of antibodies, using the specific antigen.

There are two methods by which this absorption can be achieved. The methods are related but, in one method, the absorption is done with both reagents in solution ***(immunoabsorption)*** and, in the second method, it is performed with one reagent attached to an insoluble support ***(immunoadsorption).***

After immunoabsorption or immunoadsorption, the adsorbed material can be recovered from the complex by careful treatments that dissociate antigen–antibody complexes, such as lowering the pH (HCl-glycine or acetic acid, pH 2–3) or adding chaotropic ions.

MONOCLONAL ANTIBODIES

The specificity of the immune response has served as the basis for serological reactions in which antibody specificity is used for the qualitative and quantitative determination of antigen. The discriminating power of serum antibody is not without limitations, however, because the immunizing antigen, which usually has many antigenic determinants, leads to production of antisera that contain a mixture of antibodies with varying specificity for all the determinants. Indeed, even antibodies to a simple determinant are usually mixtures of immunoglobulins with different ***fine specificities,*** and therefore different affinities for the determinant.

A quantum leap in the resolution and discriminating power of experimentally produced antibodies was provided in the 1970s with the development of methods for the synthesis of monoclonal antibodies by Milstein and Kohler, who shared the Nobel prize for this development. ***Monoclonal antibodies*** are homogeneous populations of antibody molecules in which all antibodies are identical and of the same precise specificity for a given epitope.

In general, immunization with an antigen expands various populations of antibody-forming lymphocytes (see Chapter 10). These cells can be maintained in culture only for a short time (on the order of days), so that it is impractical, if not impossible, to grow normal cells and obtain clones that produce antibodies of a single specificity. In contrast, malignant plasma cells, which are poor producers of antibody are "immortal" and can be maintained in culture for years. It is possible to select a population of malignant plasma cells that is deficient in the enzyme hypoxanthine phosphoribosyl transferase (HPRT), and that will die unless HPRT is reintroduced. The biotechnology for the production of ***hybridomas***, developed by Kohler and Milstein (and illustrated in Figure 7.17) makes use of these properties of the selected cell populations by ***fusing*** antibody-producing cells, which have HPRT, with the malignant cells which do not. The fusion may be accomplished by the use of ***polyethylene glycol (PEG)*** or by inactivated ***Sendai virus.*** The nuclei of the hybrids also fuse, and the hybridoma cells then possess both the capacity to manufacture immunoglobulins and the ability to survive in culture in select media such as that which contains hypoxanthine, aminopterin, and thymidine (HAT). The enzyme deficiency of the selected malignant cell results in its death in this medium unless that deficiency is corrected by the acquisition of the enzyme-producing genes derived from the antibody-producing cell. Thus, the hybrids can be separated from the contaminating malignant cells, which do not survive, because they have not acquired the enzyme.

Those hybrid cells synthesizing specific antibody are selected by some test of antigen reactivity and then ***cloned*** from single cells and propagated in tissue culture, each clone synthesizing antibodies of a ***single specificity.*** These highly specific, monoclonal antibodies are used as reagents for numerous procedures, ranging from specific diagnostic tests to "magic bullets" in immunotherapy of cancer. In immunotherapy, various drugs or toxins are conjugated to monoclonal antibodies, which, in turn, "deliver" these substances to the tumor cells against which the antibodies are specifically directed (see Chapter 19).

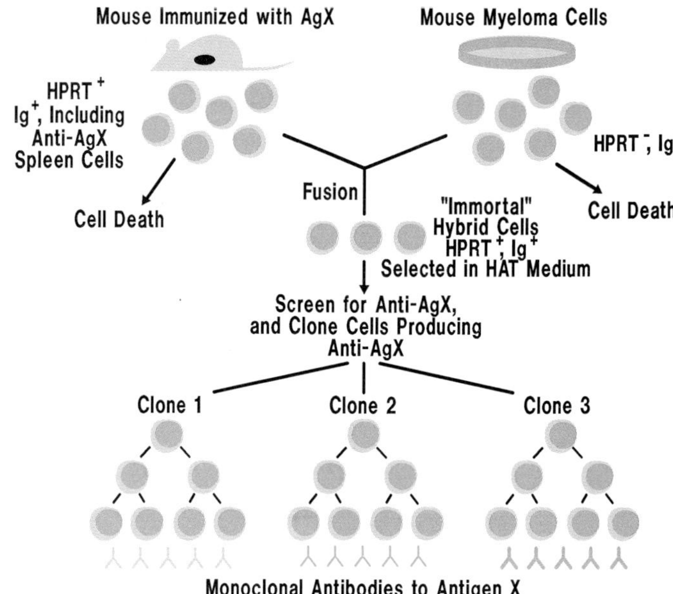

Figure 7.17.
A schematic representation of the production of monoclonal antibodies.

The production of hybridomas as described above is based on the fusion of cells of the B cell lineage (B cells or plasma cells). In the late 1970s, methods for producing hybridomas were also developed for T cells, using lines of malignant T cells and non-malignant, antigen-specific T lymphocytes whose populations have been expanded by immunization with antigen. ***T-cell hybridomas*** and ***T-cell clones*** are extremely useful for the production of large quantities of the soluble products of T cells ***(lymphokines).*** Furthermore, because of their uniformity, T cell clones have been very valuable in the characterization of various T cell structures, in particular the antigen receptor (see Chapter 11).

SUMMARY

1. The reaction between an antibody and an epitope does not involve covalent forces; it involves weak forces of interaction such as electrostatic, hydrophobic, and Van der Waal forces. Consequently, for a significant interaction, the combining sites on the antibody and the epitope require a close steric fit, like a lock and key.

2. Only the reaction between a multivalent antigen and at least a divalent antibody can bring about the secondary antigen–antibody reactions that depend upon cross-linking of antigen molecules by antibodies. These secondary reactions do not take place with haptens or monovalent Fab.

3. The interaction between a soluble antibody and an insoluble, particulate antigen results in agglutination. The extent of agglutination depends upon the proportions of the interacting antibody and antigen. When there is a great excess of antibody, agglutination may not occur. This phenomenon is referred to as a prozone. The term titer refers to the highest dilution of serum at which agglutination still takes place and beyond which no agglutination occurs.

4. Because of the zeta potential, which prevents some antigenic particles from approaching beyond a certain distance, IgG antibodies are incapable of causing agglutination. IgM antibodies, however, have properties that enable them to overcome the zeta potential and to agglutinate charged antigenic particles.

5. The use of heterologous anti-immunoglobulin antibodies may bridge between antigenic particles which are bound to non-agglutinating antibodies, leading to agglutination. This sequence of events is the basis for the Coombs' test.

6. Precipitation reactions occur upon the mixing, in appropriate proportions, of soluble multivalent antigen and (at least) divalent antibodies. The reaction may take place in aqueous media or in gels.

7. The reaction between soluble antigen and antibodies in gels may be used for the qualitative and quantitative analysis of antigen or antibody. Examples are gel diffusion tests, radial diffusion tests, and immunoelectrophoresis.

8. Radioimmunoassay. This test is based on competitive inhibition of nonlabeled and labeled antigen for antibody (at limiting concentrations of antibody). It necessitates the separation of antibody-bound from non-bound,

labeled antigen. Separation is usually achieved by the Farr technique (precipitation in 33% saturated ammonium sulfate) or by the anti-immunoglobulin procedure.

9. Solid phase immunoassay. This test employs the property of many proteins to adhere to plastic and form a monomolecular layer. Antigen is applied to plastic wells, antibodies are added, the well is washed, and any antibodies bound to antigen are measured by the use of radiolabeled or enzyme-linked anti-immunoglobulins.

10. ELISA. This enzyme-linked immunosorbent assay is essentially a solid phase immunoassay in which an enzyme is linked to the anti-immunoglobulin. Quantitation of enzyme-linked anti-immunoglobulins is achieved by colorimetric evaluation, after the addition of a substrate, which changes color upon the action of the enzyme.

11. Radioallergosorbent (RAST) test. This test is a solid phase immunoassay in which antigen (allergen) is covalently linked to a solid support (e.g. paper), and serum containing IgE to the allergen is applied to the antigen. The amount of IgE (reaginic antibodies) specific to the allergen is determined after the addition of radioactively labeled anti-human IgE, by quantitation of label bound to the insoluble support.

12. Immunofluorescence. In immunofluorescence, the antigen is detected by the use of fluorescent labeled immunoglobulins. In direct immunofluorescence, the antibody to the antigen in question carries a fluorescent label. In indirect immunofluorescence, the antigen-specific antibody is not labeled; it is detected by the addition of fluorescently labeled anti-immunoglobulin.

13. Monoclonal antibodies are highly specific reagents consisting of homogeneous populations of antibodies, all of precisely the same specificity toward an epitope.

REFERENCES

Huzzell JGR (ed) (1982): Monoclonal Hybridoma Antibodies: Techniques and Application. New York: CRC Press.

Mishell BB, Shiigi SM (eds) (1980): Selected Methods in Cellular Immunology. San Francisco: W.H. Freeman and Co.

Rose NR, Friedman H, Fahey J (1986): Manual of Clinical Immunology, Ed 3. Washington, D.C.: American Society for Microbiology.

Stites DP (1984): Clinical Laboratory Methods for Detection of Antigens and Antibodies. In Stites DP, Stobo JD, Fudenberg HH, Wells JV (eds): Basic and Clinical Immunology, Ed 5. Los Altos, California: Lange Medical Publications.

Weir DM (ed) (1985): Handbook of Experimental Immunology, Vol. 12, Ed 4. Oxford: Blackwell Scientific Publications.

REVIEW QUESTIONS

Each of the questions or incomplete statements (questions 1–2) below is followed by several suggested answers or completions. Select ONE that is BEST in each case.

1. A pregnancy test for luteinizing hormone releasing hormone (LHRH) was performed by radioimmunoassy on a sample of urine, using standardized rabbit antiserum and radioactive LHRH with specific radioactivity of 100,000 cpm/μg. The antiserum (0.1 ml), representing a slight antibody deficiency, and 1 μg of LHRH were allowed to react together first. Analysis of antibody-bound LHRH revealed 50,000 cpm bound. The urine (1.0 ml) was mixed with 1 μg of radioactive LHRH and the mixture was reacted with 0.1 ml of the antiserum. Analysis of antibody-bound radioactivity revealed 25,000 cpm bound to antibody. The concentration (μg/ml) of LHRH in the urine is
   a) 20 μg/ml.
   b) 10 μg/ml.
   c) 2 μg/ml.
   d) 1 μg/ml.
   e) 0 μg/ml.

2. The RAST test is
   a) a skin test for IgE.
   b) a bioassay for IgE.
   c) a radioimmunoassay for antigen-specific IgE.
   d) a test based on degranulation of mast cells.
   e) a test for allergen.

For each of the incomplete statements below, questions 3–8, ONE or MORE of the completions given is correct. Choose the appropriate answer:
A) if only *1, 2, 3* are correct
B) if only *1 and 3* are correct
C) if only *2 and 4* are correct
D) if only *4* is correct
E) if *all* are correct

3. Which of the following reaction(s) require(s) multivalent antigens and divalent antibodies:
   1) precipitin.
   2) radioimmunoassay using 33% saturated ammonium sulfate.
   3) radioimmunoassay using anti-antibody.
   4) the reaction between Fab and hapten.

4. In the indirect immunofluorescent antibody test for syphilis, the reactants involved are

(*Continued on next page*)

1) patient's serum, fluorescein-labeled killed *Treponema pallidum*.
2) patient's penile exudate, fluorescein-labeled rabbit anti-human antibody.
3) fluorescein-labeled patient's serum, rabbit anti-human antibody, killed *Treponema pallidum*.
4) patient's serum, killed *Treponema pallidum*, fluorescein-labeled rabbit anti-human antibodies.

5. The specificity of the reaction of antigen with antibody is usually highly dependent upon
   1) molecular weight of the antigen.
   2) charge of the antibody.
   3) immunoglobulin isotype.
   4) conformation of the reactants.

6. Convalescence from bubonic plague is followed by performing agglutination reactions on sera. The following results were obtained:

serum dilution

1:2	1:4	1:8	1:16	1:32	1:64	1:128	1:256
−	−	+	+	+	+	+	+

Which of the following conclusions can be drawn?
1) The test antigen is too concentrated.
2) The patient's convalescence is satisfactory.
3) The patient should be actively immunized against plague.
4) The titer cannot be determined.

7. The forces involved in antigen-antibody interaction
   1) depend upon the presence of complement.
   2) involve covalent interactions.
   3) operate between antigen in solution and antibody within the cytoplasm of plasma cells.
   4) may involve electrostatic interactions.

8. A quantitative precipitin reaction between an antigen and serum was performed. No precipitate was formed between the reactants. The absence of precipitate may be due to the fact that
   1) the serum does not contain antibodies to the antigen.
   2) the antigen is monovalent.
   3) the proportions of the reactants are such that there is a great excess of antigen.
   4) the pH of the reaction is too low.

ANSWERS TO REVIEW QUESTIONS

1. ***d*** When antibody is present in limited quantity, the radioactive antigen and non-radioactive antigen compete for antibody. As stated, when a given amount of antibody (0.1 ml) is allowed to react with 1 μg of radioactive LHRH (100,000 cpm) 50,000 cpm are bound to antibody (i.e. 0.5 μg). Pre-mixing the non-labeled sample with 1 μg of radioactive LHRH reduces the amount of radioactivity bound by the same amount of antibody (0.1 ml) to 25,000 cpm, because the mixture contains 2 μg of LHRH (of which 1 μg is non-radioactive and 1 μg is radioactive; i.e. 2 μg with radioactivity of 100,000 cpm or 50,000 cpm/μg). The antibody is still capable of binding only 0.5 μg of antigen. However, this time the 0.5 μg of antigen is of specific radioactivity 50,000 cpm/μg. Thus the "unknown" sample contains a concentration of non-radioactive antigen identical to that of the radioactive antigen (1 μg/ml) with which the antibodies are allowed to react.

2. ***c*** The RAST (radioallergosorbent) test employs a filter disc onto which antigen (or allergen) is covalently linked. Patient's serum is placed on the disc and the disc is washed. If the serum contains antibodies to the antigen, these antibodies will bind to the disc and will not be removed by washing the disc. Radioactive antibodies to human IgE are then applied to the disc and bind with any human IgE bound to the disc. Thus, the RAST test is a solid phase radioimmunoassay for antigen-specific IgE.

3. ***B*** A precipitin reaction requires multivalent antigen and at least divalent antibodies. A radioimmunoassay, in which antibodies bound to radioactive antigen are precipitated by anti-antibodies, also requires that the two sets of antibodies be more than univalent, so that they can generate a lattice of cross-linked complexes that is large enough to form a precipitate. In contrast, 33% saturated ammonium sulfate causes precipitation of immunoglobulins. Under these conditions, the antibodies will precipitate in the salt solution, even if they are reacted with univalent antigens, which, when mixed with antibodies, do not precipitate because of their inability to cross-link antibody molecules. Similarly, Fab or haptens are univalent, cannot cross-link and do not form precipitates.

4. ***D*** In the indirect method, the antibody to the antigen is not fluorescent. However, the anti-antibody (in this case, rabbit anti-human antibody) is fluorescent.

(Continued on next page)

5. ***D*** The specificity of the reaction between antigen and antibody is highly dependent upon a close fit between the epitope and the combining site on the antibody. This close fit is greatly dependent upon the conformation of the reactants.

6. ***D*** A titer is defined as that dilution of serum beyond which no agglutination occurs. Since there is agglutination with a serum dilution of 1:256, and since it is impossible to tell whether the next dilution would result in agglutination, the titer of the serum cannot be determined from the data given.

7. ***D*** From all the possibilities given, only the 4th, namely that the Ag–Ab reaction may involve electrostatic interactions, is correct. Ag–Ab interactions *do not* involve covalent bonds. The other possibilities are irrelevant for the interaction.

8. ***E*** No precipitation will occur if there are no antibodies with which antigen can react, or if the antigen is monovalent and incapable of cross-linking antibody molecules. Precipitation occurs maximally at the equivalence zone. Excess antigen will reduce precipitation, resulting in soluble complexes. Antigen-antibody complexes, whether soluble or not, dissociate at low pH.

CHAPTER

8

COMPLEMENT

INTRODUCTION

In 1894 Pfeiffer discovered that cholera bacilli (*Vibrio cholerae*) were dissolved or lysed in vitro by the addition of guinea pig anti-cholera serum. Heating of the serum at 56°C for 30 minutes abolished this activity, but heating did not abolish the activity of antibodies against the bacilli, since the heated serum could still transfer immunity passively from one guinea pig to another. Pfeiffer discovered that the addition of normal, fresh serum to the heat-treated antiserum restored its lytic activity. From these experiments, he concluded that antibodies to the bacilli, plus a heat-labile component present in immune as well as in normal serum, were necessary for the lysis of *V. cholera* in vitro.

A few years later, Bordet confirmed that bacteriolysis by immune serum required a heat-labile component that he termed "Alexine." The term ***complement,*** applied some years later by Ehrlich, displaced "Alexine" and is used to denote the heat-labile components in normal serum which, together with antigen-bound antibodies, exhibit a variety of biological properties, one of which is the ability to lyse cells or microorganisms. Complement consists of a group of serum proteins, that act in concert, and in an orderly sequence, to exert their effect. These proteins are not immunoglobulins, and their concentrations in serum do not increase after immunization. Like antibodies, they appear to have arisen late in evolution and are found only in vertebrates.

Bordet discovered that the action of complement, in the presence of the appropriate antiserum, results in the lysis of red blood cells. Based on this observation, he developed the ***complement fixation test,*** which constitutes a powerful serological test that is used today in a variety of diagnostic procedures.

This chapter describes the complement fixation test, as well as the properties of the complement components and their biological relevance.

THE COMPLEMENT FIXATION TEST

The complement fixation test is based on the competition, for complement, between various antigen–antibody complexes and red blood cell-specific antibodies, which attach to the red blood cells (RBC) and which, together with complement, bring about the lysis of RBC.

The complement fixation test is shown in Table 8.1. The test consists of an ***indicator system*** composed of predetermined amounts of sheep red blood cells (SRBC), antibodies to SRBC (also termed ***hemolysin***), and complement (C′), which is generally supplied as guinea pig serum. The amounts of each reagent are predetermined in such a way that the introduction of a given amount of complement to SRBC–anti-SRBC complexes ("sensitized" SRBC) results in almost complete (e.g. 95%) lysis. The degree of lysis can be determined spectrophotometrically by measuring the intensity of the red color of hemoglobin released into the solution.

TABLE 8.1. The Complement Fixation Test

		Indicator system					Result
Test system		C′ (complement)	+	Sheep RBC (SRBC)	+	Anti-sheep RBC (hemolysin)	Hemolysis (release of hemoglobin)
Antigen X	+	C′	+	SRBC	+	Anti-SRBC	Hemolysis
Antibody to X	+	C′	+	SRBC	+	Anti-SRBC	Hemolysis
X-Anti X complex	+	C′	+	SRBC	+	Anti-SRBC	No hemolysis

Since the concentration of complement is limiting, any loss of complement would be reflected by a decrease in the extent of lysis. Such a loss could occur during preincubation of the fixed amount of complement with an antigen–

antibody system (not related to SRBC and anti-SRBC) that would result in the attachment of complement to the antibody in this antigen–antibody system. This attachment or ***fixation*** of complement results in the activation of the ***complement cascade.*** The complement system is activated and consumed by the antigen–antibody complexes, so that subsequent introduction of sensitized SRBC into the mixture does not result in lysis of the SRBC, because complement has been fixed by the first antigen–antibody system. The greater the concentration of the antigen–antibody complexes, the more complement would be fixed by this system, and the more limited would be the lysis of the SRBC.

Complement cannot be fixed or activated by antibodies alone. Fixation or activation requires that the antibody be complexed to antigen in such a way as to expose, or bring together, the receptors for complement that are close to the hinge regions of several antibody molecules (see Chapter 4). Complexed with antigen, ***IgG*** and ***IgM*** antibodies, which have receptors for complement, fix complement most efficiently and are the classes of immunoglobulins that are normally measured in the complement fixation test.

The fixation of complement by an antigen–antibody system can be plotted as a function of the concentration of antigen, if the amount of antibody is constant; or as a function of the concentration of antibody, if the amount of antigen is constant. It should be noted that, as in the case of the precipitation and agglutination reactions, there is a reduction in the amount of complement fixed when antigen is present in excess. This reduction occurs because, when there is a considerable excess of antigen, fewer antibodies are cross-linked by the antigen molecules, and the necessary aggregation or conformational changes do not occur to allow binding of complement to its receptors on the antibodies. Furthermore, since no cross-linking occurs with small haptens or monovalent antigens, complement is not fixed or activated by antibodies to which haptens are bound. Complement is not fixed by monovalent Fab or by divalent fragments of antibodies that lack the receptor for complement on the Fc portion.

It is important to note that appropriate ***controls*** have to be set up in every complement fixation assay, because some antigens (usually of very high molecular weight or highly aggregated) are capable of binding complement by themselves, in the absence of antibodies. Also, there are some sera that contain substances capable of binding complement and are, thus, ***anti-complementary***. Finally, since the serum to be tested also contains complement, it is essential that the serum be inactivated by heating at 56°C for 30 minutes, in order to destroy its own complement activity and to ensure that this serum complement does not interfere in the complement fixation test.

THE COMPLEMENT SYSTEM

There are two pathways for the activation of complement, the so-called ***classical pathway*** and the ***alternative pathway.*** Although both pathways have many common components, they differ in the ways in which they are initiated. The classical pathway requires antigen–antibody complexes for initiation, while the alternative pathway does not. In the sections that follow, both pathways, their activation, and their products are described.

The Classical Complement Pathway

The ***classical complement system*** consists of nine major protein components designated C1 through C9. During complement activation these proteins become activated in an orderly fashion. For several steps in the activation, the product is an enzyme that catalyzes the subsequent step. This cascade provides amplification and activation of large amounts of complement by a relatively small initial signal. The series of reactions also provides several sites for regulation. In addition, products with activities other than just the ability to lyse cells are formed at various stages of complement activation.

The sequence of the classical complement pathway is given in Figure 8.1 and is discussed below.

ACTIVATION OF C1. The first component to become activated is the C1 complex. C1 is a trimolecular complex consisting of three proteins, C1q, C1r, and C1s, with molecular weights of approximately 400,000, 95,000 and 85,000 daltons, respectively. The complex is held together by calcium ions.

C1q itself consists of 6 identical subunits. The activation of C1q requires the binding of C1q subunits to at least two adjacent Fc portions of IgG_1, IgG_2 or IgG_3. However, C1q can become activated by binding to two or more Fc regions of a single pentameric IgM molecule, so that IgM is an efficient complement-activating antibody. IgG_4, IgA, and IgE cannot activate C1q. Activated C1q activates C1r which, in turn, activates C1s. Activated C1s has esterolytic and proteolytic properties. It activates the next component of complement, namely C4.

ACTIVATION OF C4. C4 is the second component of complement to be activated. It is called C4 because of the order in which the components of complement were discovered. C4 is a glycoprotein of molecular weight 180,000

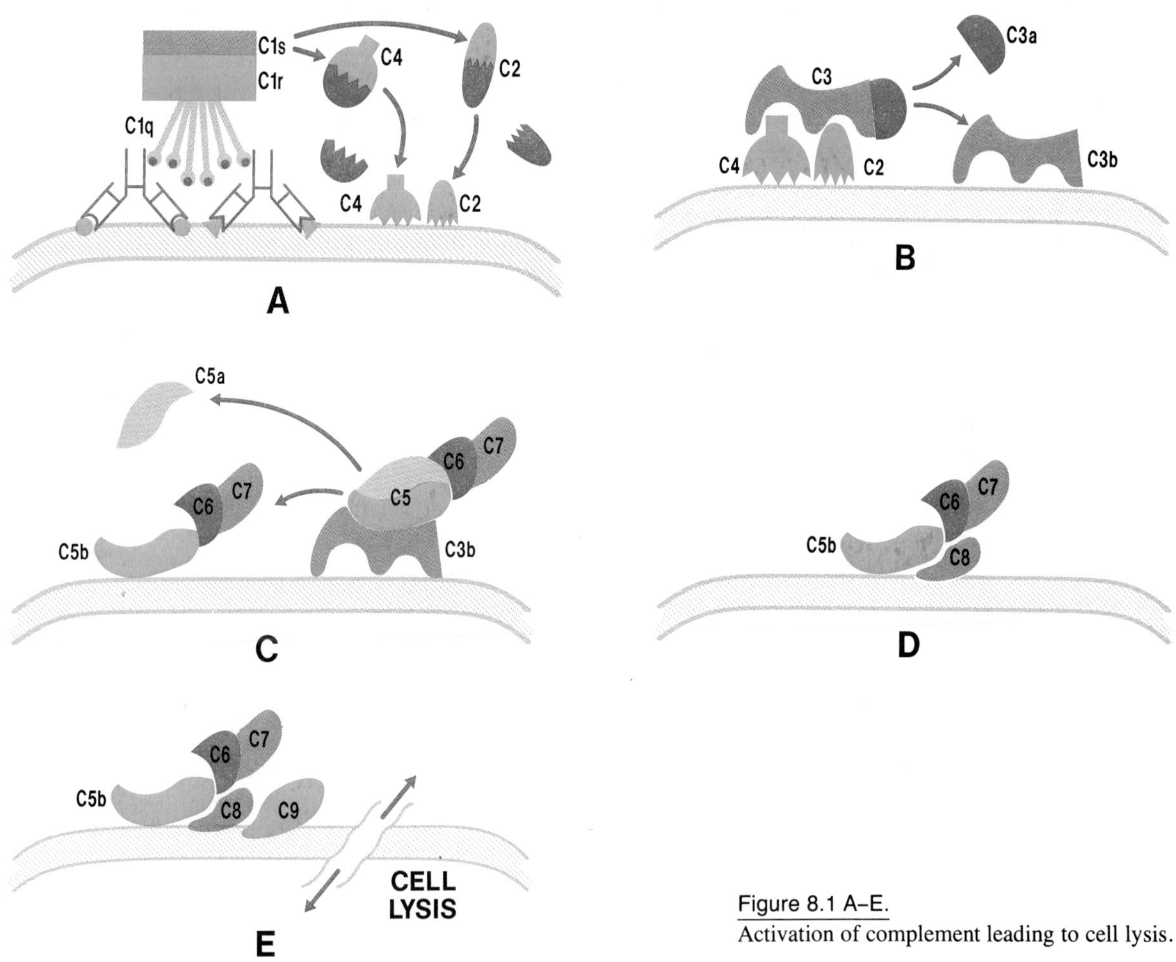

Figure 8.1 A–E.
Activation of complement leading to cell lysis.

daltons. It is synthesized by macrophages. The action of C1s on C4 cleaves a fragment from C4 and thereby activates C4. The activated C4 has several functions, one of which is to bind to the cell membrane adjacent to the antibody (which is bound to the epitope of the antigen and to C1q). Another function of activated C4 is to interact with C1s. Somehow, this interaction induces a more efficient cleavage of C2, which is the next component of complement to become activated.

ACTIVATION OF C2. C2 is a glycoprotein with a molecular weight of approximately 115,000 daltons. It is cleaved by the action of C1s and C4, but activated C2 remains associated with activated C4. This complex is a new enzyme designated $C\overline{42}$ (a bar above the numbers designates an active complex of the components under the bar), also called ***C3 convertase.*** It acts upon and activates C3.

ACTIVATION OF C3. C3 is a β-globulin with a molecular weight of 180,000 daltons. It is secreted (as pro-C3) by macrophages. C3 becomes activated by C3 convertase ($C\overline{42}$) which splits C3 into a small fragment, C3a, and a larger fragment, C3b. It has been determined that a single, biomolecular complex of $C\overline{42}$ (i.e. C3 convertase) is able to activate hundreds of C3 molecules to yield hundreds of C3a and C3b fragments. Thus, the action of C3 convertase upon C3 constitutes a very important ***amplification*** step in the complement cascade, as it generates C3a and C3b fragments.

Both C3a and C3b have several important biological properties and functions, some of which will be described later. However, one of the functions of C3b is its attachment to the cell membrane in the immediate vicinity of its site of activation. Thus, through the action of C3 convertase, many C3b molecules are split from C3 and become attached to the target cell membrane. These C3b fragments can also become attached to membranes of many different types of cells, such as red blood cells, bacteria, polymorphonuclear cells, macrophages and platelets, all of which have receptors for C3b. C3b also combines with $C\overline{42}$ to form $C\overline{423}$, an enzyme that is also called C5 convertase because it activates C5. The C3a fragment remains in the fluid phase and, as we shall see later, it has its own important biological properties.

ACTIVATION OF C5, C6, AND C7. C5, C6, and C7 are globular proteins of molecular weight 180,000, 130,000, and 120,000 daltons, respectively. By the action of C5 convertase ($C\overline{423}$), C5 is split into two fragments: a small fragment, C5a (molecular weight 11,000 daltons), which has several important biological properties (described later), and C5b, which binds stoichiometrically with C6 and C7 to form a $C\overline{567}$ complex on the cell membrane. This complex, especially the part consisting of C6 and C7, focuses the activities of the next components, C8 and C9, onto the target cell membrane.

ACTIVATION OF C8 AND C9. C8 and C9 consist of proteins with molecular weights of approximately 160,000 and 80,000 daltons respectively. The actions of these molecules, which have detergent properties, are directed against the membrane by $C\overline{567}$ and produce "holes," which result in cell lysis.

The exact mechanism that leads to lysis is still not completely understood. It appears, however, that lysis is caused by perturbations of the cell's lipid bilayer, which produce holes of diameter 80–100 μm, that can be observed on the surface of the cell. These holes are tubular, transmembrane channels through which ions can pass. This passage of ions disturbs the osmotic equilibrium, and there is a rapid influx of water into the cell. As the cell swells, the membrane becomes permeable to macromolecules, which can then escape from the cell.

The Alternative Complement Pathway

The classical pathway of complement activation involves the activation of components C1 through C9 via the mediation of antibody. One important aspect of this classical pathway is that the antibody focuses the activities of the components of complement on the membrane of the target cell. Another important aspect is that the activation of C3 by C3 convertase ($C\overline{142}$) results in the release of various physiologically active substances at the site of the reaction. Thus, the activation of C3 is an important event in the classical pathway of complement activation.

C3 can also be activated by another route, termed the ***alternative pathway*** of complement activation. It arose in evolution earlier than the classical pathway, and it does not require antigen–antibody interaction for initiation. The alternative pathway of complement activation (shown in Fig. 8.2) may be triggered by ***lipopolysaccharide*** (LPS) or endotoxin from the cell walls of gram-negative bacteria, by the ***cell walls of some bacteria, by cell walls of yeasts (zymosan)***, by ***aggregated IgA***, and by a factor present in ***cobra venom***.

C3b exists in trace amounts in normal serum. It combines with a serum factor called ***factor B,*** forming a complex, C3bB. The complex is further activated by serum ***factor D,*** which cleaves factor B while it is attached to C3b to generate the enzyme complex, C3bBb, which acts as a C3 convertase and releases C3a and C3b from C3. The C3b fragment complexes with factor B and becomes activated by factor D to yield more C3 convertase, thereby amplifying the amount of C3 convertase and the amount of C3 that becomes activated. This amplification is delicately balanced by the fact that the C3bBb complex dissociates rapidly. However, this dissociation is regulated by a serum protein called ***properdin,*** which acts to stabilize the C3bBb complex.

As mentioned above, C3b is present in trace amounts in normal serum. It probably originates from a low level of activity of factors B and D on C3, which causes the release of C3b. The released C3b is largely inactivated by

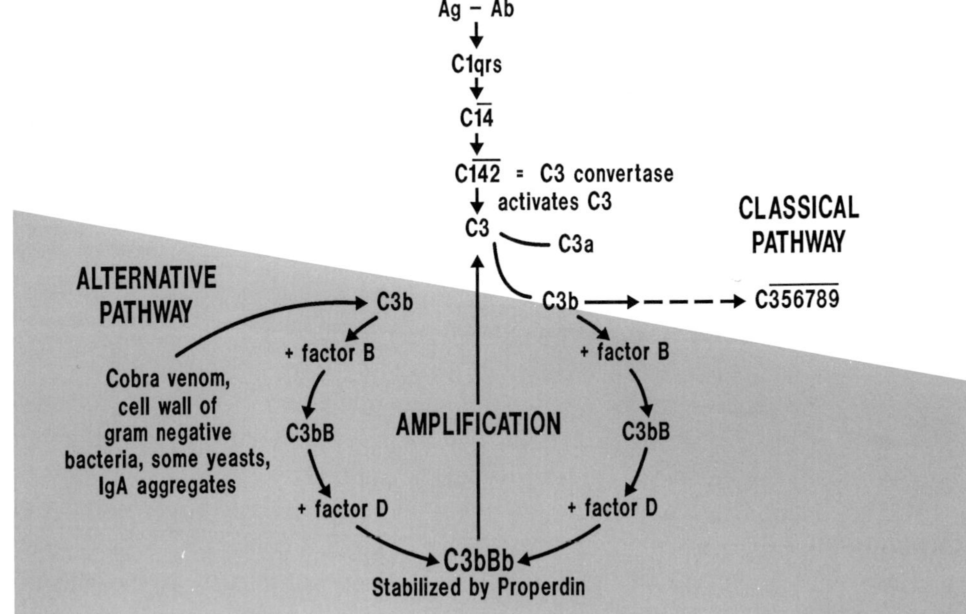

Figure 8.2.
The relationship between the classical and the alternative pathways of complement activation.

yet two other factors, namely factor H and factor I (the C3b inactivator). It is believed that lipopolysaccharides of gram-negative bacteria and other substances that initiate the alternative pathway of complement activation somehow protect the small amounts of C3b from inactivation, so that the presence of these substances triggers the alternative pathway.

C3b promotes ***immune adherence***, especially between bacteria and macrophages, an activity that enhances phagocytosis. C3b also activates C3, an event that is followed by the activation of the remaining components of the complement cascade.

The two pathways of complement are interconnected; in fact, the amplification process involved in the alternative pathway of activation is also operative in the classical pathway. Thus, the alternative pathway amplifies both antibody-dependent and antibody-independent cleavage of C3.

BIOLOGICAL ACTIVITY OF THE COMPONENTS OF COMPLEMENT

In addition to cell lysis, the activation of complement yields fragments of complement components that possess various biological activities. These activities are summarized below.

Anaphylatoxins

An ***anaphylatoxin*** is a substance (usually of low molecular weight) that induces the degranulation of mast cells and/or basophils, causing, among other things, release of histamine. Histamine has several important physiological functions (e.g. it increases capillary permeability and causes contraction of smooth muscle) that are associated with ***anaphylaxis*** and other allergic reactions (see Chapter 13).

The anaphylatoxins that are elaborated during the activation of complement are C3a and C5a. Recently C4a has also been shown to possess weak activity as an anaphylatoxin. The increase in capillary permeability caused by histamine results in ***local edema*** (accumulation of fluid) in the tissue. The influx of edema fluid, which contains more antibodies and more components of complement, causes additional release of anaphylatoxins, thus amplifying the reaction.

Chemotaxins

Chemotaxins are substances that attract phagocytic cells and cause their migration from an area of lesser concentration to an area of higher concentration (chemotaxis). The chemotaxins produced during complement activation are C3a and C5a.

Immune Adherence

Immune adherence is a phenomenon in which a particulate antigen, coated with antibodies and in the presence of complement, adheres to various surfaces. In vivo, these surfaces include the walls of blood vessels. Its adherence to the walls of blood vessels makes the particulate antigen easy prey for circulating phagocytic cells. The complement component C3b is responsible for immune adherence.

Opsonization

Opsonization refers to the coating of particulate antigen by antibody, and/or by complement components that render the particle more attractive to phagocytic cells and allows them to be phagocytized more readily. The attachment is facilitated by the presence, on the surface of the phagocytic cells, of receptors for the Fc portion of the antibody and for the C3b component of complement. Thus, not only are antibodies, notably IgG, referred to as ***opsonins*** but also the C3b component of complement is called an opsonin.

REGULATION OF COMPLEMENT ACTIVATION

The serum proteins that are components of the classical or the alternative activation routes of complement are synthesized in the liver, by macrophages and blood monocytes, and by intestinal epithelial cells. They are released into the serum in their inactive forms and become activated during the events of the complement cascade.

On the one hand, complement activation necessitates the formation of stable molecular complexes for short periods. On the other hand, this activation generates physiologically powerful molecules. Consequently, the activation of complement requires careful control and regulation by a variety of mechanisms, in order to prevent adverse reactions. Indeed, there are many inactivators of the various components of complement, such as C1 esterase inhibitor, C3b inhibitor, anaphylatoxin inactivator, and C4b inhibitor, among others.

There are rare genetic disorders that result in deficiencies in the proteins that regulate the complement pathways. One such disorder is associated with a deficiency of C1 esterase inhibitor ***(C1INH)***. This deficiency leaves the action of activated C1 on C4 and C2 uncontrolled, and allows production of more and more fragments that are, in turn activated by ***plasmin*** to yield a vasoactive peptide. Thus, a small stimulus that activates C1 may trigger a large response that cannot be interrupted.

C1INH deficiency is transmitted in an autosomal dominant manner. Individuals with this disorder have ***hereditary angioneurotic edema.*** They suffer from local edema in various organs, such as skin, gastrointestinal tract, and the upper respiratory tract. The edema may become life-threatening when it occurs in the larynx and obstructs the air passage (see Chapter 13).

COMPLEMENT DEFICIENCY

Genetic deficiencies in complement components have been reported for almost all of the major components of the system. Heterozygous individuals, with a defective allele for any complement component, have about half the normal level of that component in their serum. Individuals with a homozygous defect in a given complement component are rare, but they do exist. As would be expected, many of the latter individuals suffer from recurrent infections, most notably gonococcal and meningococcal infections.

The consequences of a deficiency in a particular component of complement vary, depending on the deficient component. Thus, for example, deficiency in C2 does not appear to be particularly harmful to some individuals, probably because the mechanism for activation of the alternative complement pathway is not affected. In contrast, individuals deficient in C3 usually suffer from recurrent infections with pyogenic and gram–negative bacteria, probably because of the absence of chemotactic, opsonizing, and bactericidal activities from their serum complement. Disorders that result from complement deficiency are discussed in more detail in Chapter 12.

SUMMARY

1. Complement consists of a group of serum proteins that activate each other in an orderly fashion to generate biologically active molecules, such as enzymes, opsonins, anaphylatoxins, and chemotaxins.

2. Complement can be activated through two pathways: a) the classical pathway that is initiated by antigen–antibody complexes and b) the alternative pathway, in which complement components become activated by the cell walls of some bacteria and yeasts, in combination with several serum factors.

3. The activation through the classical pathway requires C1q for initiation; the alternative pathway requires C3b, serum factors B and D, and properdin.

4. The activity of complement and its components is tightly regulated by various inhibitors.

5. The level of complement does not increase after immunization.

6. The complement fixation test is based on the competition for complement between immune complexes consisting of anti-sheep red blood cell antibody and sheep red blood cells, in which the sheep erythrocytes lyse, and a second antigen–antibody system. The greater the amount of the second system present, the more it will fix complement and inhibit the lysis of the sheep erythrocytes.

REFERENCES

Boackle RJ (1986): The complement system. In Virella G, Goust JM, Fudenberg HH, Patrick CC (eds): Introduction to Medical Immunology. New York: Marcel Dekker, Inc.

Fearon DT, Austen KF (1980): The alternative pathway of complement—A system for host resistance to microbial infection. N Engl J Med 303:259.

Mayer MM (1973): The complement system. Sci Am 229:54.

Muller-Eberhard HJ (1975): Complement. Annu Rev Biochem 44:697.

Muller-Eberhard HJ (1983): Chemistry and function of the complement system. In Dixon FW, Fisher DW (eds): The Biology of Immunologic Disease. Sunderland, Massachusetts: Sinauer.

Muller-Eberhard HJ, Colten HR (1986): The complement system. Progress in Immunol 6:267.

Muller-Eberhard HJ, Schreiber R (1980): Molecular biology and chemistry of the alternative pathway of complement. Adv Immunol 29:1.

REVIEW QUESTIONS

For each of the incomplete statements below, ONE or MORE of the completions given is correct. Choose the appropriate answer:
A) if only *1, 2, 3* are correct
B) if only *1 and 3* are correct
C) if only *2 and 4* are correct
D) if only *4* is correct
E) if *all* are correct

1. Complement is required for
   1) lysis of erythrocytes by lecithinase.
   2) lysis of erythrocytes by specific antibodies.
   3) phagocytosis.
   4) bacteriolysis by specific antibodies.

2. Complement activation by an immune complex may result in
   1) precipitation.

2) release of anaphylatoxins.
3) release of macrophage-inhibiting factor.
4) opsonization.

3. Active fragments of C5 can lead to
1) contraction of smooth muscle.
2) vasodilation.
3) attraction of leukocytes.
4) attachment of lymphocytes to macrophages.

4. The alternative pathway of complement activation is characterized by
1) activation of complement components beyond C3 in the cascade.
2) participation of properdin.
3) generation of anaphylatoxin.
4) utilization of C4.

5. In the complement fixation test, the hemolysin–sheep erythrocyte complex
1) is the test system.
2) is the indicator system.
3) fixes complement in a positive test.
4) is used to detect any non-complexed complement.

6. Immunoglobulins that activate the first component of complement (C1q) via their Fc portions include
1) IgG.
2) IgA.
3) IgM.
4) IgE.

7. The following activate(s) the alternative pathway of complement
1) endotoxin.
2) monomeric IgG.
3) yeast cell wall.
4) C1.

8. Which component(s) of complement could be missing and still leave the remainder of the complement system capable of activation by the alternative pathway
1) C1, 2 and 3.
2) C3 only.
3) C2, 3, and 4.
4) C1, 2, and 4.

ANSWERS TO REVIEW QUESTIONS

---

1. ***C*** 2 and 4 are correct. Complement is required for the lysis of erythrocytes by anti-erythrocyte antibody (IgG or IgM) and for lysis of bacteria by specific antibacterial IgM or IgG. Complement is not required for phagocytosis or lysis of erythrocytes by lecithinase, which can take place without complement. (How-

(Continued on next page)

ever, the C3b opsonins, which are generated during complement activation, enhance phagocytosis of the opsonized particle.)

2. ***C*** 2 and 4 are correct. C3a and C5a are activated during complement activation. Both are anaphylatoxins, and their presence leads to the degranulation of mast cells. C3b, which is generated during complement activation, is an opsonin; it coats particles and enhances phagocytosis by phagocytic cells that have receptors for C3b.

3. ***A*** 1, 2, and 3 are correct. C5a is an anaphylatoxin, causing degranulation of mast cells, with the release of histamine, which causes vasodilation and contraction of smooth muscles. C5a is also a chemotaxin, attracting leukocytes to the area of its release (where the antigen is reacting with antibodies and activates the complement system).

4. ***A*** 1, 2, and 3 are correct. The alternative pathway of complement activation connects with the classical pathway at the activation of C3. Thus, it does not require C1, C4, and C2. Properdin is essential for the activation through the alternative pathway, since it stabilizes the complex (C3bBb), formed between C3b and activated serum factor B, which acts as a C3 convertase and activates C3. During the activation of the alternative pathway both C3a and C5a are generated; both are anaphylatoxins and cause degranulation of mast cells.

5. ***C*** 2 and 4 are correct. The hemolysin–sheep erythrocyte complex, in the presence of complement, will result in lysis of the erythrocytes. A non-related, antigen–antibody system would compete for complement with the hemolysin–sheep erythrocyte system. Thus, the hemolysin–sheep erythrocyte system serves as an indicator system. Fixation of complement by another antigen–antibody system would result in less lysis in the indicator system. Thus, the indicator system is used to detect complement that is free or uncomplexed (not fixed) by another antigen–antibody system.

6. ***B*** Only IgG and IgM have receptors for C1q.

7. ***B*** Endotoxin (lipopolysaccharide) from cell walls of gram-negative bacteria and cell walls of yeasts can activate the alternative pathway of complement.

8. ***D*** C3 is required for the alternative pathway of complement activation, while C1, C2, or C4 is not required.

CHAPTER

9

THE CELLULAR BASIS OF THE IMMUNE RESPONSE

INTRODUCTION

In previous chapters we have described the structural and genetic mechanisms by which the immune response is able to achieve its diversity (i.e. its ability to respond to many different antigenic determinants, or epitopes). We will now consider briefly the cellular basis for several other, major characteristics of the immune response, as follows:

Specificity: The ability to discriminate among different antigenic epitopes, and to respond only to those that necessitate a response rather than to make a random, undifferentiated response.

Memory: The ability to recall previous contact with a particular antigen, such that subsequent exposure leads to a more rapid and larger production of antibody.

Affinity maturation and changes in classes of immunoglobulins: As the immune response proceeds, the affinity of antibody for antigen tends to increase, and additional classes of immunoglobulin (IgG, IgE, etc.) tend to be produced.

Adaptiveness: The ability to respond to previously unseen antigens, which may never have existed before on earth.

Discrimination between "self" and "non-self": The ability to respond to those antigens that are not "self" but to avoid making responses to those antigens which are part of "self."

The most widely accepted theory that best explains these features of the immune system is the ***Clonal Selection Theory*** proposed and developed by Jerne and Burnet (both Nobel Prize winners) and by Talmage. The essential postulates of this theory may be summarized as follows:

1. Antibodies of all specificities are produced *prior* to contact with antigen.
2. B lymphocytes, participating in the immune response, have receptors on their surface membranes that are immunoglobulin molecules of the same specificity as that of the antibodies that will be produced by their activated and differentiated progeny.
3. Each lymphocyte carries immunoglobulin molecules of only a single specificity on its surface.
4. Circulating self-antigens that reach the developing lymphoid system prior to its maturation are recognized as "self," and no subsequent immune response will be induced against them.
5. Immunocompetent lymphocytes, which are not shut off or deleted in this process, can be stimulated under appropriate conditions by antigen to proliferate and differentiate into clones of antibody-producing plasma cells and memory cells.

In this and succeeding chapters, we will explore the evidence that establishes the Clonal Selection Theory as a general paradigm for immunology. Although this theory was developed for antibody-producing cells, it applies equally to T cells, except that T cells do not make antibodies but have receptors that are immunoglobulin-like in their structure and synthesis by genetic rearrangements.

CELLS INVOLVED IN THE IMMUNE RESPONSE

In mammalian species, circulating blood cells have their common origin in a small cluster of cells that move from the primitive yolk sac to the fetal liver, and finally to the bone marrow, where they take up permanent residence. These cells are the ***hematopoietic stem cells***, so called because they are the undifferentiated cells from which all the other specialized cells in the blood develop (see Fig. 9.1). One pathway of differentiation (***myeloid differentiation***) starts from a bone marrow stem cell that gives rise to differentiated precursors and culminates with erythrocytes, thrombocytes (platelets), and the various granule-containing cells of the granulocyte–monocyte series. The other pathway of differentiation (***lymphocytic differentiation***) leads to two distinct cell types called B and T lymphocytes.

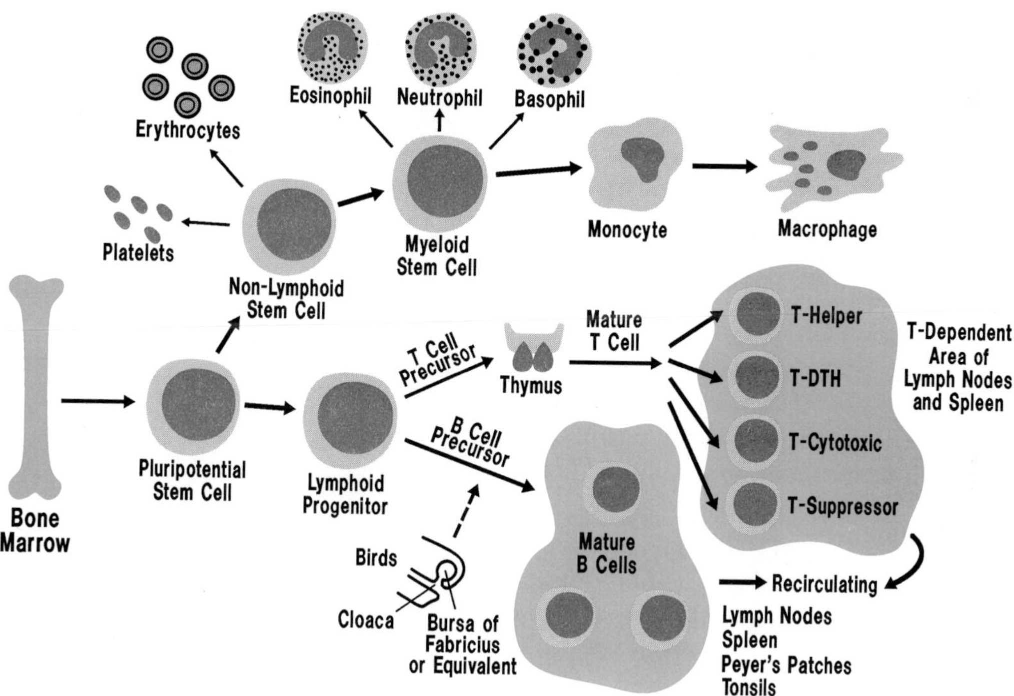

Figure 9.1.
The developmental pathway of various cell types from a pluripotential bone marrow stem cell.

The undifferentiated stem cells are characterized by an ability to proliferate throughout life as a self-renewing reservoir that replenishes the pool of more mature cells as they are used up during normal activity. These early stem cells are considered to be ***pluripotent***; that is, they are capable of developing into any of the more differentiated lines of cells, under the influence of a variety of soluble factors that control both the extent and the direction of maturation. Once differentiation in any direction has occurred, the cells become committed to make only a single type of cell; i.e. they become ***unipotent***. This chapter focuses primarily on the cells of the two lymphoid lines: the B cells and the T cells.

ONTOGENY OF THE B LYMPHOCYTE

B cells are the cells concerned with the synthesis of antibody, and they owe their name to their historical origins. In early experiments with birds, it was found that the two lymphocytic lines of cells underwent maturation and differentiation in two separate primary lymphoid organs. Antibody-forming cells developed in an organ called the ***bursa of Fabricius***, an outpouching of the cloacal epithelium. Stem cells migrating to this organ and proliferating into mature, antibody-forming cells were called bursal or B cells. No single analog of the bursa has yet been found in evolutionarily more advanced species such as mammals. Instead, the maturation into B cells of precursor stem cells derived from bone marrow takes place either in the bone marrow itself or in an undiscovered location. Maturation culminates with migration of the B cells to lymphoid organs such as spleen, lymph nodes, and tonsils.

The ***differentiation*** of a stem cell into a mature, antibody-producing ***plasma cell*** can be divided into several stages (see Fig. 9.2). The stem cell itself has no known distinguishing features, and the first sign of its progression along the pathway toward maturation into a B cell is seen in the ***rearrangement*** of its V, D, J genes to generate the gene for an H chain of an immunoglobulin molecule (see Chapter 6). Once successful rearrangement has occurred; the heavy chain of IgM (μ) is synthesized in the cytoplasm. The presence of this ***cytoplasmic μ-chain*** serves to allow characterization of the cell by immunological techniques as a ***pre-B cell***. In the next stage, genes for L chains rearrange, a complete L chain is synthesized, and a monomeric form of IgM is made and inserted into the cell's membrane. This monomeric surface receptor, ***sIgM***, for the first time, permits the cell to recognize and respond to antigen, because of its specific ability to bind antigen. However, contact between this ***immature B cell*** and antigen leads, not so much to further expansion and differentiation, as to the shutdown and deletion of this clone.

Our understanding of the next stage of development is still a little vague, but it is generally agreed that immunoglobulin D (IgD) is made by construction of a large nuclear RNA transcript that contains both μ and δ genes and is then processed into either μ mRNA or δ mRNA and then into IgM or IgD for

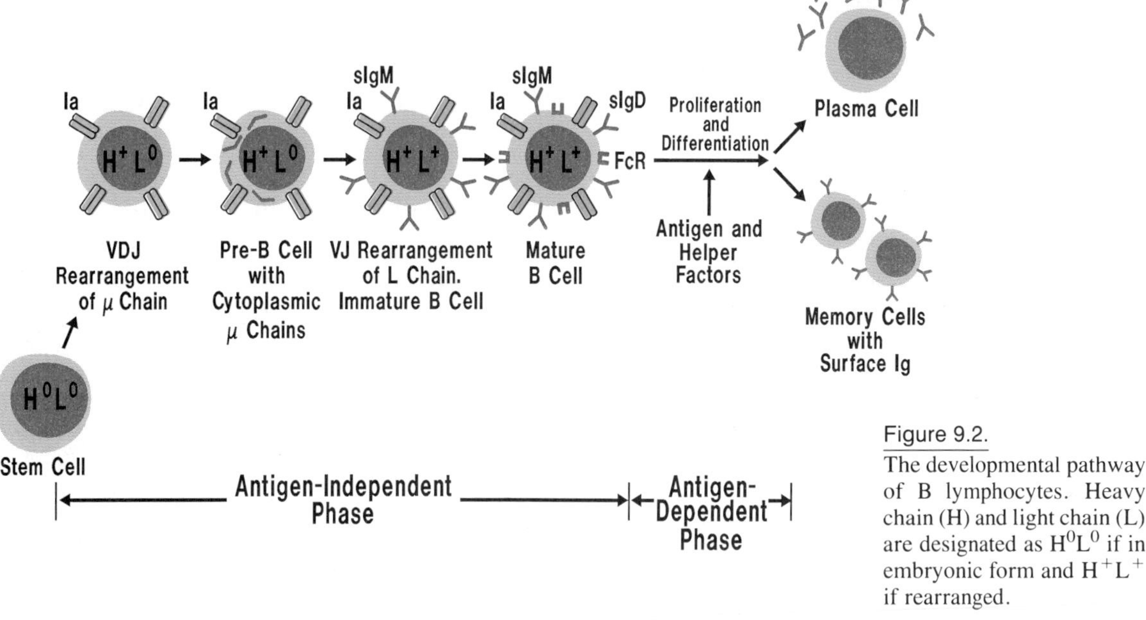

Figure 9.2.
The developmental pathway of B lymphocytes. Heavy chain (H) and light chain (L) are designated as H^0L^0 if in embryonic form and H^+L^+ if rearranged.

insertion into the membrane. The cell, which has IgM and IgD receptors of identical specificities on its surface, is now considered mature and fully capable of responding to stimulation by the specific antigen. It is important to note that all the maturation up to this point has taken place in the absence of specific antigen and proceeds constantly in cells derived from the pool of stem cell progenitors. Thus, the organism builds up a constantly replenished library of diverse specificities (a ***repertoire***) directed against a similarly diverse array of antigens. Subsequent response now depends on selection by contact with specific antigen and help from T cells, and each mature B cell is now capable of responding to antigens of only a single specificity.

During ***antigen-dependent development*** (the stage in differentiation triggered by specific antigen) a complex series of events may occur. Those cells selected specifically by reaction with antigen and appropriate help from T cells (see later) are triggered to differentiate further in one of two ways. These B cells may proliferate and differentiate into ***plasma cells***, which are the specialized, fully differentiated cells capable of synthesizing and secreting antibody of the same specificity as that of the receptors on their precursor surface membranes. At the same time, a proportion of daughter cells, produced in this proliferative response, transform back into resting, mature B cells that are capable of being activated for a subsequent and even more rapid response. These resting cells are called ***memory B cells***.

Concurrently with these antigen-induced processes, the phenomenon of ***class switching*** occurs. Progeny of the B cell that was involved in the initial response begin to synthesize IgG, IgA, or IgE molecules. A multiplicity of cells is generated, producing a variety of immunoglobulin classes, but with all progeny of a particular clone having the same specificity. Some question remains about the exact nature of the immunoglobulin isotype that serves as a receptor on the memory cells produced. Some evidence suggests that it changes to IgG; other evidence indicates it becomes the isotype that the cell is destined to make (e.g. IgA). In the absence of the ability to follow a single B-cell clone through the proliferative and class switching process, it may be difficult to answer this question. In any event, succeeding contact with antigen triggers an expanded population of memory cells to differentiate into plasma cells, and to synthesize IgG or IgA or IgE that is all of one specificity. Thus, genetic rearrangement provides a clone of a unique specificity, but class switching provides offspring of diverse biological function.

B-Cell Markers

All lymphocytes are relatively indistinguishable by light microscopy, but various markers have been found that serve to identify their ***phenotypes***. Most useful among these markers are those on the surface of the cell, and although their function is in many cases unknown, their presence can be exploited for purification, as well as characterization, of these cells.

SURFACE IMMUNOGLOBULIN (sIg). All B cells are characterized by the presence of immunoglobulin molecules on their cell surfaces. Antisera directed against any portion of the immunoglobulin molecule (L chain, Fab, etc.) serve as reagents for identification of B cells, for separating them from other lymphocytes, and as triggers to activate them in the absence of antigen. B cells can be divided into subsets by use of such antisera (e.g. cells that carry only IgM or only IgG, etc.).

Fc RECEPTORS (FcR). Virtually all B cells carry receptors for the Fc portion of IgG, and these receptors serve to distinguish B cells from a variety of other cells. These receptors are best observed if sheep red blood cells (SRBC) coated with an IgG antibody are mixed with B cells. The protruding

Fc portion of the antibody on the surface of the SRBC is bound by an Fc receptor on a B cell. As a result, a halo ***(rosette)*** of SRBC is formed around each B cell.

C3 RECEPTORS. B cells also have receptors that bind some of the activated components of complement, most notably C3b (see Chapter 8). Therefore, B cells can be studied by rosette formation, in a similar manner to that described above, using C3-coated SRBC.

EBV RECEPTORS. Epstein-Barr virus (EBV) appears to have the capacity, unique among viruses, to bind to B cells by attachment to a specific receptor (the C3d receptor). Infection with this virus frequently produces "***immortalization***," with the development of a stable continually replicating line of B cells.

Ia AND DR ANTIGENS. In common with several other specialized types of cells, such as macrophages and dendritic cells, B cells possess, on their surface, antigens of the class II major histocompatibility complex (Ia in the mouse and DR in humans) (see Chapter 11). As we shall describe later, these antigens are essential for the triggering of T cells and the generation of help for the activation of B cells.

ONTOGENY OF THE T LYMPHOCYTE

The second pathway of differentiation of bone marrow stem cells that differentiate into lymphocytes passes through the ***thymus***. This anterior, mediastinal organ derives embryonically from the 3rd and 4th pharyngeal pouches (see Chapter 2). Precursor cells from the bone marrow, arriving in the thymus late in fetal development or soon after birth—and to a lesser extent throughout life—pass through the mesh of cortical epithelial cells in this organ and are induced, by direct contact or humoral factors, to undergo a burst of proliferation and differentiation (see Fig. 9.3). During this process, the cells acquire distinct surface markers and functions, and they move to the medullary region of the thymus. In a process that is analogous to events in B cells, the genes coding for the two chains (α and β) that comprise the antigen-specific part of the T cell receptor undergo ***rearrangement*** at this stage. While the details of the individual steps are not yet completely understood, it is known that genes for V, D, J regions, very similar to but wholly separate from those coding for

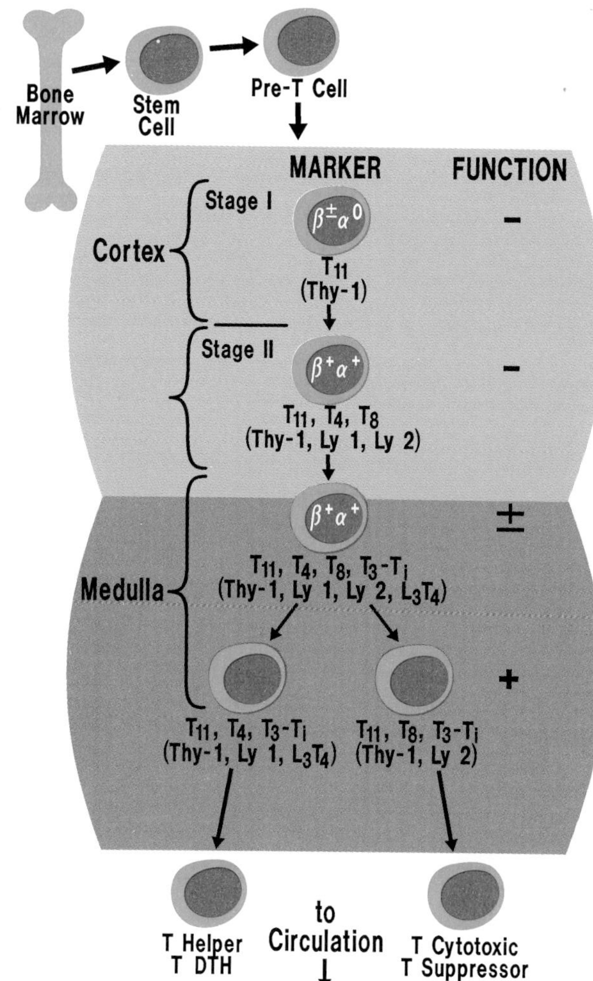

Figure 9.3.
The developmental pathway in the thymus of T lymphocytes and their markers in humans and in mice. (Mouse markers are given in parentheses.) α and β chains are designated as α° and β° if not rearranged, and as α^{+} and β^{+} if rearranged.

the immunoglobulin molecules, rearrange and are spliced to encode the polypeptide chains that make up the particular combining site that fixes the specificity of that particular T cell and its progeny. Little is known, as yet, about genes for the constant regions of T cell receptors, and whether there is a maturation of the T cell response by somatic cell mutation or by some other process. This antigen-specific part of the receptor is known as ***Ti***, since it contains an idiotype similar to the one on an Ig molecule.

After completing the maturation process in the thymus, the T cells leave the medulla by passing between the endothelial cells of small venules. They then enter the general circulation, where they become the major component of the recirculating pool of lymphocytes. By retaining the capacity to pass through postcapillary venules, T cells are able to cycle continuously from blood through the lymph nodes, spleen, etc., exiting into the lymphatics, whence they return to the general circulation via the thoracic duct.

Loss of certain specific molecules (designated ***MEL-14***) from the surface of T cells results in loss of ability to recirculate by this functionally essential route. T cells without MEL-14 become trapped and sequestered in the reticuloendothelial organs, such as liver and lung, where they cannot carry out their immunologic functions. It is probably as a result of this entrapment that long-term cultures or clones of T cells lose many of their functions in vivo, while they retain the ability to function perfectly in vitro.

One of the curious but poorly understood features of the thymus is that, in early life, it is one of the most active sites of cell proliferation in the whole body. However, many more cells are produced by multiplication in the thymus than actually leave it or can be accounted for in the circulation. In fact, it is estimated that as many as 90% of the thymocytes produced are somehow destroyed. The reasons for this apparent wastage are unknown but may represent a selection process for the elimination of cells that have failed to acquire functional receptors because of faulty rearrangement of genes. Alternatively, the wasted cells may carry receptors specific for self-antigens and are consequently deleted upon initial contact with those antigens, before maturation is complete.

T-Cell Markers

HUMANS. As in the case of B cells, the process of maturation of T cells is accompanied by the acquisition of new properties and ***differentiation markers*** that include enzymes, glycoproteins, and specific receptors. Tracing the gain or loss of these markers by use of specific monoclonal antibodies has allowed the processes involved in the differentiation of T cells to be reconstructed, as follows:

T-11. In the development of human T cells (see Fig. 9.3), one of the earliest markers that has been found is a receptor capable of binding to sheep red blood cells and forming rosettes. It is clear that this ability to bind SRBC could not have been the function for which this receptor was developed, yet it remains a useful marker for following differentiation of T cells, since it is the first marker to appear in ontogeny, and it persists through maturity in all T cells. The receptor has been characterized by a specific monoclonal antibody and is designated ***T-11***. It may represent an early form of the receptor whose engagement, under some circumstances, can trigger either the proliferation or the self-destruction of T cells, depending on the stage of maturation.

T4 and T8. In the next stage of differentiation, the genes coding for the α- and β- chains of the receptors on the surface of the T cell rearrange in preparation for synthesis of the antigen-specific receptor (Ti) of the T cell. At this stage, two additional markers, T4 and T8, appear. These markers are glycoproteins of molecular weights 62,000 and 76,000 daltons, respectively, whose functions are not completely understood, but whose presence on the surface of the T cell bears a striking correlation with the ability of the cell to recognize and respond to certain restricting elements, in association with antigen. This response is discussed later, but for the present, it is sufficient to understand that ***T4*** is associated with recognition of class II MHC (major histocompatibility complex) molecules and that ***T8*** is associated with recognition of class I molecules.

Ti. At the next stage of differentiation, the complex of proteins representing the complete T cell receptor appears. This receptor, called Ti, consists of an antigen-specific, variable part that comprises the previously mentioned α- and β-chains (of molecular weights 43,000 and 49,000 daltons, respectively). The α- and β-chains, like the immunoglobulin molecules, have V regions, formed by rearrangement of V, D, J genes that differ among clones of T cells of different specificities. Antisera specific for these receptors recognize idiotopes analogous to those of the combining sites on immunoglobulins and are called ***anti-idiotypic antisera*** or ***clonotypic antisera***. They serve to characterize an individual T cell or its progeny.

T3. Production of the antigen-specific receptor requires the concurrent synthesis of an invariant cell-surface complex that contains at least three different polypeptide chains. This complex, detected by a monoclonal antibody, is called ***T3*** and is present on *all* mature T cells (regardless of their function), in very close association with their antigen-specific receptors (Ti). The T3 complex appears to be an essential portion of the receptor required for triggering T cells.

TdT. Terminal deoxyribonucleotidyl transferase, ***TdT***, is an enzyme whose presence is useful for detection of very early stem cells or pre-T cells. It is found in cortical, but not in medullary thymic lymphocytes.

In the final stages of differentiation in the thymic medulla, prior to their leaving it, T cells acquire functional abilities for the first time. This acquisition occurs concurrently with loss of either T4 or T8 markers. Thus, less mature cells that were both $T4^+$ and $T8^+$ but had little functional ability now become $T4^+T8^-$ (the cells primarily responsible for helper functions and delayed hypersensitivity) or $T4^-T8^+$ (the cells primarily responsible for cytotoxic or suppressor function). This classification of $T4^+$ and $T8^+$ cells into functional categories was a useful first approximation, but it is now known to be invalid. The characteristic of $T4^+$ or $T8^+$ is now known to be associated primarily with the class of MHC molecule that serves as a recognition element (see Chapter 11), and not with function; in fact, the molecules T4 and T8 are thought to be the structures that allow this recognition to occur.

MICE. In mice, the earliest indicator of T cell lineage is acquisition of a surface glycoprotein called ***Thy-1.*** This antigen, although it decreases in level somewhat in more mature T cells, is characteristic of the whole class of T cells and is useful for purification of T cells. Other useful markers, detected by appropriate antisera, are ***Lyt-1*** and ***Lyt-2***. (There is also a Lyt-3 antigen but it is probably only a separate determinant on the Lyt-2 molecule.) By use of antisera to these markers, murine T cells have been placed on an ontogenetic pathway that is similar to, but less firmly established than, the one in humans. There are three major phenotypes. Lyt-1^+2^+ cells appear to be less differentiated precursor cells that differentiate into Lyt-1^+2^- cells (the major class of helper cells) and Lyt-1^-2^+ cells (most of the cytotoxic and suppressor cells). Once again, the association of Lyt-1^+ or Lyt-2^+ is only a first approximation and it is now known to coincide more strictly with the recognition element associated with the antigen (Lyt-1^+ with class II and Lyt-2^+ with class I). This recognition is discussed more fully in Chapter 11. A recently discovered marker, ***L3T4***, appears to be the murine analog of the human T4 marker and is believed to represent an invariant component of receptors on T cells that have class II MHC molecules as restriction elements.

Functional Markers

MITOGENS AND LECTINS. There are several naturally occurring materials that have the capacity to bind to, and to trigger proliferation and differentiation of, many clones of lymphocytes. These substances, called ***mitogens,*** are often referred to as ***polyclonal activators*** because they stimulate whole classes of lymphocytes and not just clones of particular specificity. Two plant glycoproteins (***lectins***), ***concanavalin A (con A)*** and ***phytohemagglutinin (PHA),*** are potent mitogens for T cells and are useful in the identification and study of the function of this class of cells. ***Lipopolysaccharide (LPS)***, isolated from gram-negative bacterial cell walls, has a similar mitogenic effect on B cells. ***Pokeweed mitogen*** is considered to be mitogenic for both T cells and B cells.

CELLS THAT PROCESS AND PRESENT ANTIGEN

The third major component of the immune response is a class of mononuclear cells of the ***monocyte–macrophage series***. These cells arise from a ***myeloid/erythroid precursor*** stem cell that is probably distinct from the ***lymphoid precursor*** that gives rise to the B and T cells discussed earlier in this chapter (see Fig. 9.1). After entering the blood as monocytes, these cells migrate to various tissues where they undergo further differentiation into a variety of histologic forms that are included in the so-called ***reticuloendothelial system (RES)***, which is widely distributed throughout the body (see Chapter 2).

The monocyte itself is a small, spherical cell with few projections, abundant cytoplasm, little endoplasmic reticulum, and many granules. Once settled in a particular tissue, the monocyte takes on many of the characteristics of a specialized set of macrophages and assumes many forms, as follows:

Kupffer cells: large cells with many cytoplasmic projections, in the liver
Alveolar macrophages, in the lung
Splenic macrophages, in the white pulp
Peritoneal macrophages, free–floating in peritoneal fluid
Dendritic cells, in spleen and lymph nodes
Langerhans cells, dendritic cells in the skin
Microglial cells, in the central nervous tissue

While associated with so many diverse names and locations, many of these cells share common features, such as the ability to ***bind and engulf particulate materials and antigens***. Their locations along capillaries makes them the cells most likely to make first contact with invading pathogens and antigens, and the performance of these cells, as we shall see later, plays a large part in the success of the immune response.

In general, cells of the macrophage series have two major functions. One of their functions, as their name ("large eater") implies, is to ***engulf*** and, with the aid of all the degradative enzymes in their lysosomal granules, ***break down*** trapped materials into simple amino acids, sugars, etc., for excretion or re-utilization.

The second major function of the macrophages is to take up antigens, ***process*** them by denaturation or by partial digestion, and ***present*** them, on their surfaces, to specific T cells. This function is described in some detail in Chapter 11.

Just as there is great diversity in the histologic appearance and location of these cells, so too is there diversity in their function. Some of them perform best in one or the other of the roles just described, and some perform efficiently in both. Common characteristics that are used as markers for these cells include the ability to adhere to glass or plastic surfaces, and their possession of receptors for Fc and C3, which enable them to engulf antibody or complement-coated material.

SUMMARY

1. The Clonal Selection Theory best explains the general features of an immune response. Its cardinal feature is that antibody exists as a receptor on B lymphocytes prior to exposure of the individual to antigen.

2. In the differentiation of B cells, the first stage is rearrangement of the V, D, and J genes of the H chain in the embryonic DNA and formation of a cytoplasmic H chain. This event is followed by rearrangement of the genes for L chains and formation of an IgM molecule, which appears on the surface of the cell and characterizes the cell as a B cell of a particular specificity.

3. Further development depends on exposure to specific antigen, which leads to proliferation and differentiation of the B cell into plasma cells, which are mature cells that serve as factories for the synthesis and export of antibody.

4. T cells follow a different path in ontogeny and pass through the thymus gland, where they acquire specific markers and differentiate into cells with a variety of functions.

5. T cells also undergo rearrangement of the genes that encode the two chains that form an antigen-specific receptor analogous to the immunoglobulins on the surface of B cells.

6. The third type of cell involved in the immune response is the monocyte–macrophage series, which is derived from myeloid precursors, and which processes and presents antigens to T cells.

7. The coordinated action of these three types of cell is generally necessary for a successful immune response.

REFERENCES

Cantor H (1984): T-lymphocytes. In Paul WE (ed): Fundamental Immunology, New York: Raven Press.

Cooper M, Osmond DG (1986): Ontogeny and differentiation of B lymphocytes. Progress in Immunol 6:17.

Cooper MD, Kearny J, Scher I (1984): B-lymphocytes. In Paul WE (ed): Fundamental Immunology. New York: Raven Press, p 43.

Eisen HN (1980): Immunology. New York: Harper & Row, p 382.

Nossal GJV (1986): The Burnetian legacy: A clonal selectionist looks toward the 1990s. Progress in Immunol 6:6.

Singer A, Shortman K (1986): Ontogeny and differentiation of T lymphocytes. Progress in Immunol 6:59.

REVIEW QUESTIONS

Each question or incomplete statement below (questions 1–3) is followed by several suggested answers or completions. Select the ONE that is BEST in each case.

1. Human T cells can be distinguished from B cells and other cells by
   a) morphologic appearance.
   b) the presence of Fc receptors.
   c) the formation of rosettes with sheep red blood cells.
   d) the presence of cytoplasmic granules.
   e) the presence of Ig surface markers.

2. According to the Clonal Selection Theory,
   a) lymphocytes bear multipotent receptors that become specific after contact with antigen.

b) lymphocytes bear receptors that have genetically determined specificities.
c) macrophages ingest antigens and make RNA copies that are transferred to T cells.
d) virgin B cells acquire specific receptors only after contact with antigen.
e) both B and T cell precursors in the bone marrow already have their specificities fixed.

3. Immature B lymphocytes
   a) produce only μ–chains.
   b) are progenitors of T lymphocytes as well as B lymphocytes.
   c) express both IgM and IgD on their surface.
   d) are at a stage in development where contact with antigen may lead to unresponsiveness.
   e) must go through the thymus to mature.

For each of the incomplete statements below (questions 4–10), ONE or MORE of the completions given is correct. Choose the appropriate answer:
A) if only *1, 2, 3* are correct
B) if only *1 and 3* are correct
C) if only *2 and 4* are correct
D) if only *4* is correct
E) if *all* are correct

4. The thymus is
   1) a lymphoid organ near the cloaca.
   2) where T lymphocytes acquire antigen-specific receptors.
   3) where antibodies to T-dependent antigens are produced.
   4) an organ that is maximally active early in life.

5. Processing in the thymus is *not* necessary for maturation of
   1) suppressor T cells.
   2) B cells.
   3) cytotoxic T cells.
   4) monocytes.

6. In the human thymic cortex may be found
   1) T cells with the T11 marker.
   2) T cells with fully rearranged genes for α and β receptor chains.
   3) thymocytes with no ability to function.
   4) mature cells, bearing T4 and T8 markers.

7. T cells differ from B cells by
   1) their ability to be activated by plant lectins such as phytohemagglutinin.
   2) their lack of antigen-specific receptors.
   3) their inability to mature in the absence of a thymus.
   4) their inability to recirculate after leaving the thymus.

8. Mitogens that stimulate human T cells to proliferate include
   1) phytohemagglutinin.
   2) concanavalin A.
   3) pokeweed mitogen.
   4) lipopolysaccharide.

(*Continued on next page*)

9. The following are markers of B cell populations:
1) rosette formation with antibody-coated sheep red blood cells.
2) presence of membrane-associated T3 complex.
3) presence of membrane-associated IgM.
4) presence of an unrearranged germline configuration of genes for H chains.

10. Macrophages
1) are derived from blood monocytes.
2) have a great diversity of form.
3) are able to ingest and degrade micro-organisms.
4) can process and present antigens to T cells.

ANSWERS TO REVIEW QUESTIONS

1. ***c*** Human T cells have the T-11 marker, which is a receptor for SRBC. The morphology of T and B cells is often indistinguishable, and several other types of cell also have Fc receptors.

2. ***b*** The specificity of B and T cells is determined by rearrangement of V region genes which are present in their genome. (a) and (d) are outmoded concepts of the instructional theory in which antigen was supposed to direct the folding of the antibody molecule, while (e) is false because T cell precursors in the bone marrow have not rearranged their genes and acquired specificity until they mature in the thymus.

3. ***d*** Immature B cells are at the stage when they express surface IgM and, at this stage, they are susceptible to induction of tolerance upon contact with antigen. When fully mature, they will express both IgM and IgD.

4. ***C*** 2 and 4 are correct. In the thymus, T cells mature and acquire the receptors. The thymus exhibits most activity in early life and involutes when a full complement of T cells has been put into circulation.

5. ***C*** 2 and 4 are correct. B cells and monocytes are not dependent on the thymus for maturation.

6. ***B*** 1 and 3 are correct. In the thymic cortex, immature thymocytes are found bearing the first marker T-11, and with no antigen-specific receptor or functional ability.

7. ***B*** 1 and 3 are correct. T cells may be activated by phytohemagglutinin while B cells respond to lipopolysaccharide. In contrast to B cells, T cells require the thymus for maturation. Both T cells and B cells have antigen-specific receptors and can circulate.

8. ***A*** 1, 2, and 3 are correct. Lipopolysaccharide is a B-cell mitogen.

9. ***B*** The T3 complex is associated only with T cells, and B cells can be recognized as such only after they rearrange the genes for their H chains and synthesize IgM, which they carry on their surfaces hence 2 and 4 are incorrect. B cells have receptors for Fc as well as surface IgM.

10. ***E*** All answers are characteristics of macrophages.

CHAPTER

10

TRIGGERING THE IMMUNE RESPONSE

INTRODUCTION

Contact with antigen does not invariably lead to formation of antibody. A number of conditions must be met before antibody is produced. In this chapter we describe the conditions that stimulate an immune response, and in Chapter 15 we discuss those that suppress an immune response. Among the important parameters to be considered when an attempt is made to elicit an immune response are the amount of antigen given, the timing of injections, and the route of injection. The immunogenicity of the antigen (i.e. its ability to induce a response) is a function of its "foreignness" to the recipient, its physical form and the use of adjuvant materials that maximize the effect of the antigen on the cells of the immune system. When an immune response is induced, the antibody response to an antigen has certain defined characteristics that are common to all immune responses. Those characteristics are described in the paragraphs that follow.

KINETICS OF THE IMMUNE RESPONSE

The first exposure of an individual to a particular antigen is referred to as the ***priming event*** and the measurable response that ensues is called the ***primary response.*** As shown in Figure 10.1, the primary response may be divided into several phases, as follows:

1. ***Latent or lag phase***. After initial injection of antigen, a significant amount of time elapses before antibody is detectable in the serum. The length of this period is generally 1–2 weeks, depending on the species immunized, the antigen, and the type of adjuvant used. The length of the latent period is also heavily dependent on the sensitivity of the assay used to measure the antibody. The latent period includes the time taken for B cells to make contact with the antigen, to proliferate, to differentiate, and then to secrete antibody in sufficient quantity that it can be detected in the serum. The less sensitive the assay used for detection of antibody, the more antibody will be required for detection and the longer the apparent latent period will be.
2. ***Exponential production phase***. During this phase, the concentration of antibody in the serum increases exponentially.
3. ***Declining phase***. After an interval during which production and degradation of antibody balance each other (***the steady state***), the immune response begins to shut down, and the concentration of antibody in serum declines rapidly.

In this primary response, the first class of antibody detected is generally ***IgM***, which in some instances may be the only class of immunoglobulin that is made. If production of IgG antibody ensues, its appearance is generally accompanied by a rapid cessation of production of IgM (see Fig. 10.1).

SECONDARY RESPONSE

Although production of antibody after a priming contact with antigen may cease entirely within a few weeks (see Fig. 10.1), the immunized individual is left with a cellular memory (i.e. leftover ***memory cells***) of this contact. This memory becomes apparent when a response is induced by a ***second injection*** of antigen. After the second injection, the lag phase is considerably shorter and antibody may appear in less than half the time required for the primary

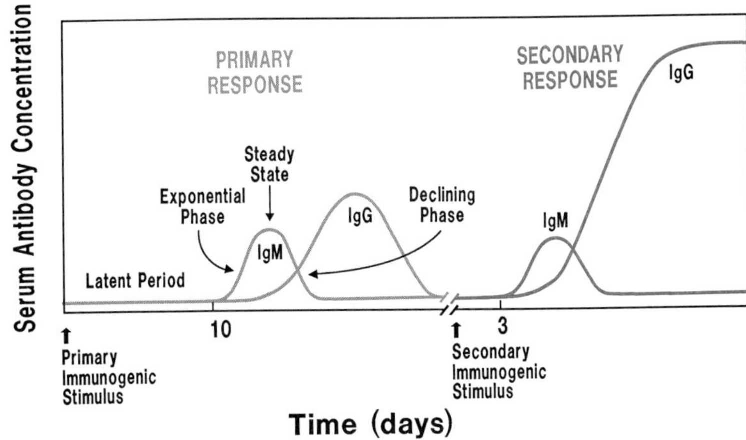

Figure 10.1.
The kinetics of an immune response.

response. The production of antibody is much greater, and higher concentrations of antibody are detectable in the serum. The production of antibody may also continue for a longer period, with persistent levels remaining in serum months, or even years, later.

There is a marked change in the type and quality of antibody produced in the secondary response. There is a ***shift in class response***, with IgG antibodies appearing at higher concentrations, and with greater persistence, than IgM. In addition, a ***maturation*** of the response occurs, such that the average affinity (binding constant) of the antibodies for the antigen increases as the secondary response develops. The driving force for this increase in affinity may be a selection process during which B cells compete with free antibody to capture a decreasing amount of antigen. Thus, only those B cell clones with high-affinity Ig receptors on their surfaces will bind enough antigen to ensure that the B cells are triggered to differentiate into plasma cells. These plasma cells, which arise from preferentially selected B cells, synthesize this antibody with high affinity for antigen.

The capacity to make a secondary or ***anamnestic*** (memory) response may persist for a long time (months in mice; years in humans), and it provides an obvious selective advantage for an individual that survives the first contact with an invading pathogen. Establishment of this memory for generating specific responses is, of course, the purpose of public health immunization programs.

CELLULAR COOPERATION IN THE IMMUNE RESPONSE

Three Types of Cells Are Involved in the Immune Response

Many studies in vivo and in vitro indicate that the central role in the induction of the immune response is played by ***accessory cells*** of the monocyte–macrophage series. After injection of antigen, macrophages in draining lymph nodes and in the spleen trap and concentrate the antigen (see Chapter 2). Studies in vitro have shown that production of antibody involves the formation of clusters of lymphocytes around central macrophages with subsequent, intimate, cytoplasmic contact. Furthermore, if efforts are made to remove the macrophages, the immune response is, in large part, abrogated.

A classic experiment by Claman first demonstrated that ***two types of lymphocytes*** are involved in production of antibody. He studied immune responses in lethally irradiated mice. In such mice, the immune functions destroyed by radiation can be restored by an infusion of spleen cells. When lethally irradiated mice were given cells from the thymus, the mice failed to produce an immune response to antigen. They also failed to produce a response when grafted with bone marrow cells. However, when they were given a mixture of bone marrow and thymus cells, the irradiated mice produced an immune response comparable to the response made possible by infusion with spleen cells. Successful restoration of immune responsiveness by administration of the mixture of bone marrow and thymus cells, showed a requirement for cooperation between at least two distinct populations of lymphocytes, both of which are present in the spleen.

By the use of appropriate cell markers, it was subsequently determined that ***B cells*** from the bone marrow become the actual producers of antibody while ***T cells*** from the thymus are the cooperating "helper" cell type. The nature and essential features of this T-cell–B-cell cooperation were elucidated in another classic series of experiments conducted in 1969 by Mitchison, who used a hapten–carrier system, as described below.

The Carrier Effect

A simple hapten, such as the dinitrophenyl (***DNP***) group, can be used as a primarily technical tool to examine the production of antibody directed against a particular epitope. Thus, it is possible to immunize an animal with DNP attached to one protein carrier and then to look for production of antibody to only the DNP when it is attached to a different carrier. In this way, the difficulty of trying to sort out all the antibodies of different specificities for the many epitopes on the first carrier molecule can be avoided.

The experiment that first exploited this ***hapten–carrier effect*** is shown in Table 10.1. A mouse primed with an injection of DNP_8-BSA (8 molecules of DNP coupled at multiple positions to one molecule of bovine serum albumin carrier) will make a good secondary anti-DNP antibody response if given a second injection of DNP_8-BSA (line 1). If the same mouse is primed with DNP_8-BSA, but given a second injection of DNP_8-OVA (8 molecules of DNP coupled to one molecule of ovalbumin), it fails to make a good anti-DNP antibody response (line 2). In this instance, the second carrier, OVA, is immunologically unrelated to, and non-cross-reactive with, BSA. Its inability to boost the anti-DNP response shows that a secondary response to the hapten requires that the carrier molecule be the same as the one used in the priming injection. The requirement here for identical carrier molecules is an example of the ***carrier effect.***

TABLE 10.1. The Carrier Effect

Primary immunogen	Secondary immunogen	Secondary anti-DNP response
DNP_8-BSA	DNP_8-BSA	++++
DNP_8-BSA	DNP_8-OVA	—
DNP_8-BSA plus OVA	DNP_8-OVA	++++

The critical experiment, on line 3, showed that if the same animal was primed with DNP on the BSA carrier and separately primed with OVA alone, it was then able to mount a secondary anti-DNP response when injected with DNP_8-OVA. Thus, the carrier effect could be overcome by priming with the second carrier and then immunizing with the hapten linked to the second carrier.

From experiments of the type just described, it was concluded that antibody-mediated responses to antigens, such as proteins, require the participation of ***thymus-derived cells.*** Hence, the term ***thymus-dependent antigens*** is associated with proteins in general, since they have multiple but different epitopes on one molecule. Upon primary immunization, T cell clones, recognizing some of the epitopes on the protein carrier, expand. Similarly, clones of

B cells recognizing other epitopes on the antigen (which are analogous to the DNP hapten in the mouse experiments), also expand. When the animal is ***boosted*** (i.e. given a second injection of the same antigen), then the expanded clones of T and B cells cooperate (see Fig. 10.2) to give a ***secondary response***, seen as a heightened production of anti-DNP antibody. If the animal is given a booster injection with the DNP on a different carrier, to which there has been no priming, then there are no expanded clones of T cells specific for epitopes on the heterologous carrier. Therefore, no cooperation with B cells specific for the DNP epitope can occur, and no production of anti-DNP antibody ensues. If the animal is separately primed with the second carrier, however, expanded clones of T cells specific for epitopes on this carrier are available for cooperation with the B cells that are making an anti-DNP response.

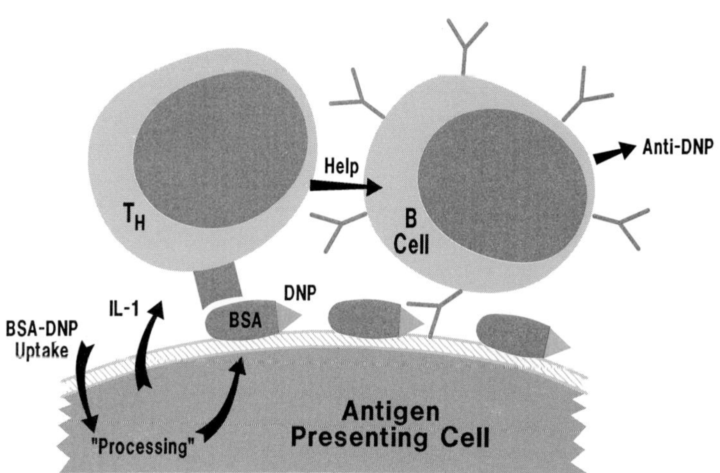

Figure 10.2.
The collaboration between antigen-presenting cell, T cell, and B cell, leading to the synthesis of anti-DNP antibodies.

An important point concerning these experiments is that, while the T cells and B cells could be separately primed by injection with different antigens, a successful secondary response required that the epitopes, for which each type of cell was specific, be given on the ***same molecule***.

A protein antigen, even without added haptenic determinants, has a variety of epitopes towards which T-cell and B-cell clones respond. Since the epitopes to which the T cells are responding and those to which the B cells are responding are on the same molecule, cellular cooperation between B and T cells is assured by the physical bridging between them.

Cell Cooperation Model for Triggering of T and B Cells

In recent years a great deal of effort has been devoted to elucidating the cellular and molecular events involved in triggering B cells to generate antibody. The most widely accepted model involves the following sequence of events:

1. ***Processing of antigen.*** Many phagocytic cells (e.g. neutrophils, Kupffer cells) have the capacity to degrade foreign materials to their constituent building blocks for excretion or re-utilization. The cells that function as accessory cells in the immune response (macrophages, dendritic cells, B cells) have additional characteristics. In these accessory cells, the phagocytosed or pinocytosed antigen is altered, or enzymatically cleaved, to yield peptide fragments that contain the antigenic determinants of these antigens (see Fig. 10.3). In fact, it is possible that differential resistance to enzymatic cleavage may be a property of an antigenic determinant. The antigenic fragments (epitopes) then reappear on the surface of the accessory cells, where they are believed to form, by non-covalent association, an immunogenic complex with the class II MHC (major histocompatibility complex) molecules (termed ***Ia*** in the mouse and ***DR*** in humans), which are also on the surface of this cell. As

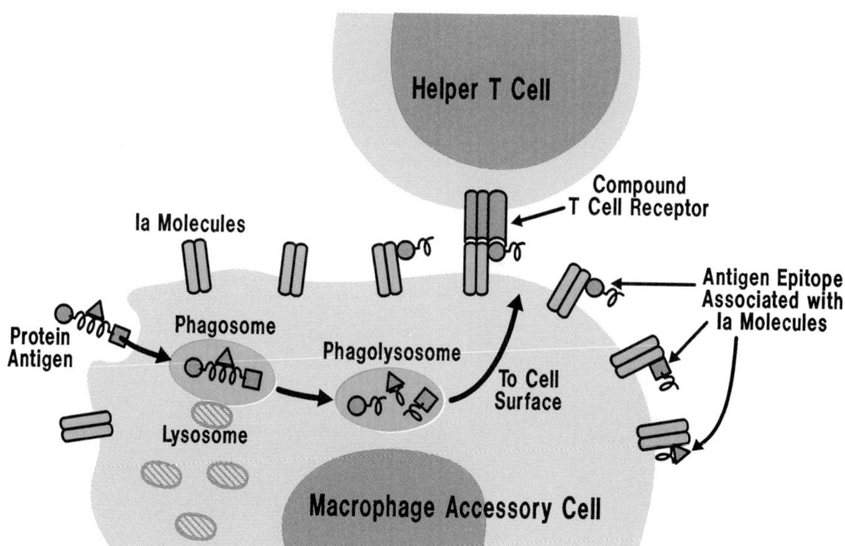

Figure 10.3.
Internalization of antigen by accessory cells, its processing, and the presentation of various epitopes in the context of Ia of the accessory cell, to the T cell receptor.

already mentioned, a prerequisite for an antigen-presenting accessory cell is the presence of class II MHC molecules on its surface. This prerequisite limits the ability to present antigen to ***macrophages, dendritic cells, and B cells***.

2. ***Presentation of antigen***. The complex of the immunogenic epitope and the class II molecule is recognized by the ***compound receptor*** on a specific helper T cell (see Fig. 10.4). This receptor (see Chapter 9) consists of two chains (α and β) that define a ***variable region antigen-combining site (Ti)***, that is associated with a three-chain ***invariant complex (T3)***, which may be involved in transduction of the signal from the Ti receptor to the interior of the cell. In addition, there is another essential molecule ***(T4)*** that is somehow involved in the recognition of the class II MHC glycoprotein associated with the foreign antigenic determinant. Although it still involves some guesswork, a simple model, which includes this complex pattern of receptor-antigen interactions, is shown in Figure 10.4. The class II MHC molecule, complexed with the antigenic fragment, is bound by the Ti receptor and the T4 molecule (which occurs on T cells that recognize antigen, but only when antigen is associated with class II MHC molecules). This requirement for multiple components in functional receptor–ligand binding is unlike that of B cells, which bind free

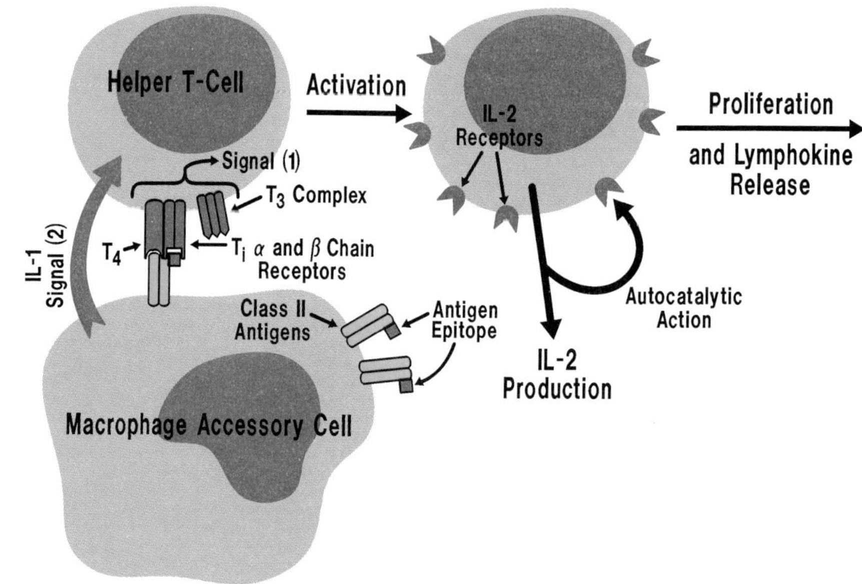

Figure 10.4.
T helper cell activation: the accessory cell presents an epitope to the T cell in the context of Ia (class II) molecules of the presenting cell. The T cell receptor composed of T_4 and T_i (α and β chains) recognizes the Ia and the epitope. This recognition together with the T_3 complex constitute the first signal for the activation of the T helper cell. The second signal is provided by IL-1 released by the accessory cell. T cell activation leads to the appearance of IL-2 receptors which upon binding with IL-2 released by activated T helper cells trigger proliferation and lymphokine release.

antigen by virtue of their immunoglobulin receptors. In effect, the way in which T cells bind antigen provides a useful mechanism for avoiding engagement of T cells by free antigen, which is a role left to antibody.

3. ***Activation of T cells***. Binding by the compound receptor of a T cell to the Ia-antigen complex on the accessory cell constitutes only the first signal for activation of T cells. To complete this process of activation, the accessory cell must deliver a second signal (Fig. 10.4) in the form of the ***lymphokine interleukin-1 (IL-1).*** This small protein (molecular weight 15,000 daltons), which is produced by macrophages, has a variety of other important functions in the body, such as producing fever and causing the release of several so-called acute-phase proteins from the liver. The probable consequence of T-cell contact with IL-1 is the induction, on the surface of the T cell, of specific receptors for another important molecule, ***interleukin-2 (IL-2).*** Having received the two signals (i.e. Ia-antigen complex and IL-1), the helper T cell undergoes activation and engages in several activities, which include the release of IL-2 and a whole battery of soluble substances, the ***lymphokines***, some of which are very important for the ***triggering of B cells***. The interleukin-2 released serves to stimulate T cells that carry receptors for IL-2 to proliferate in an autocatalytic fashion, which magnifies the response initiated by the original T cell that responded to antigen on the accessory cell.

4. ***Activation of B cells***. The next step in the cooperative process leading to production of antibody involves the actual triggering of the B cell. While the events associated with processing and presentation of antigen to T cells have been taking place, the relevant B cells have also been engaged in binding the same antigen directly via the receptors—i.e. immunoglobulins—on their surfaces.

Much more is known about the structure, synthesis and location of the receptors on B cells than about analogous structures on T cells. The B cell receptors are representative immunoglobulin molecules whose Fc domains are anchored in the lipid membrane. They are free to move about in the plane of the membrane much as icebergs move at sea. When they are cross-linked by binding to an antigen that has several identical determinants on the same molecule, they undergo a characteristic pattern of reaction (see Fig. 10.5). First the receptors aggregate into small ***patches***. Then, in an energy-requiring reaction, the patches tend to aggregate over one pole of the cell and form a ***cap***. Finally the cap of aggregated receptors enters the cell by ***endocytosis,*** leaving the surface of the B cell devoid of receptors (immunoglobulin molecules) until new ones are synthesized and put on the surface.

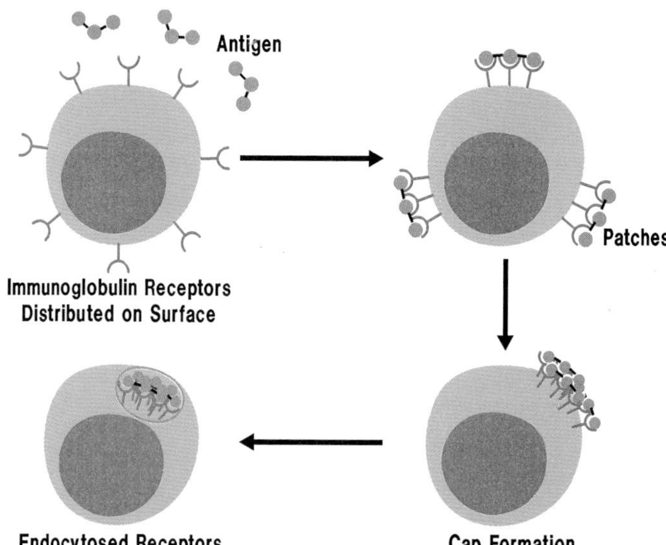

Figure 10.5.
The activation of B cell by antigen, leading to patching, capping, and endocytosis of the antigen-receptors complex.

Originally, it was thought that interaction of antigen with immunoglobulin to cross-link the immunoglobulins was the only signal required for activation of B cells. Subsequently, however, it was determined that (1) most antigens, including proteins, have only one of each antigenic determinant (epitope) per molecule and therefore cannot, by themselves, cross-link the receptors; 2) with such antigens, help from T cells is required to stimulate the B cell to proliferate and differentiate to form clones of antibody-producing plasma cells.

It appears that activation of B cells requires a sequence of signaling events, the first of which is the ***cross-linking*** of the immunoglobulins on the surface of the B cells. Cross-linking alone, however, leads only to a low level of proliferation, without consequent production of antibody. The next stage involves the ***soluble factors*** produced by the activated helper T cells in the process described above. The first lymphokine involved is called ***B-cell growth factor (BCGF),*** and it stimulates the B cell to which antigen is bound to proliferate to a greater extent. Finally, a third signal, also released by the helper T cell, and called ***B-cell differentiation factor (BCDF),*** induces the newly dividing B cells to differentiate into plasma cells and to produce antibody for export.

A composite diagram of this entire process in the response to BSA-DNP is shown in Figure 10.6. Some coordination of these complex events is necessary for the full response to antigens that requires help from T cells. However, it is believed to be unlikely that all three types of cell (T, B and accessory cell) are present at the same time and in the same location, as shown in the diagram. Although the exact sequence of events is unknown, it is likely that activation of T cells occurs first, and that the released lymphokines can subsequently trigger a B cell, which may not be in direct contact.

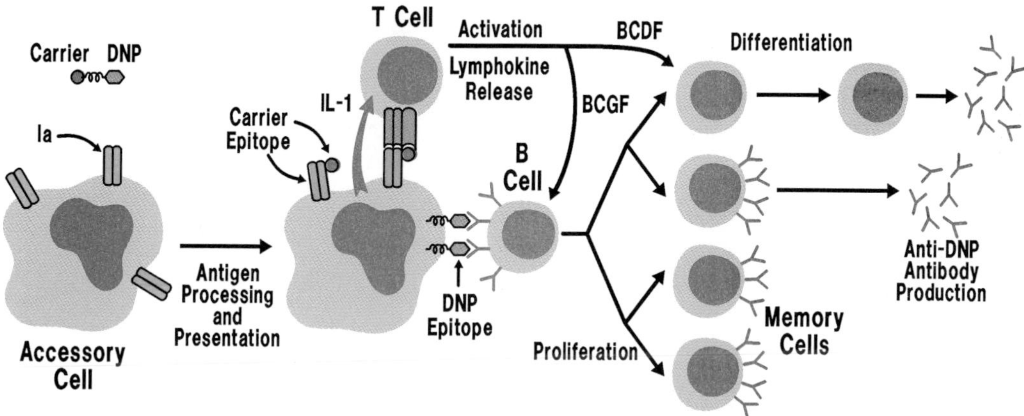

Figure 10.6.
The cellular immune response to BSA-DNP. The carrier is presented to the helper cell in the context of class II molecules, activating the T helper cell to release lymphokines which in turn activate the B cell which recognizes the hapten on the surface of the antigen presenting cell, leading to the synthesis of antibodies to DNP as well as to the generation of DNP memory B cells.

The sequence of events just described need not be the only pathway for production of antibody. In fact, it has recently been shown that, in secondary responses, where both T-cell and B-cell clones have been expanded, direct and very efficient cooperation can be achieved between B and T cells, without involvement of other accessory cells. While not normally phagocytic, B cells have been shown to have the ability to efficiently capture antigen by binding it to their specific immunoglobulin receptors, to internalize and degrade the immunoglobulin–antigen complexes, and then to re-express fragments of the antigen on their surfaces in association with class II MHC molecules (which B cells possess in large quantities). This mode of presentation, apparently, does not require the production of IL-1 (which B cells do not produce) or, alternatively, IL-1 is present in sufficient quantity after having been produced by neighboring accessory cells after their interaction with T cells.

T-INDEPENDENT RESPONSES

While the majority of antigens involved in immune responses are of the type that requires help by T cells in order to provoke a response—i.e. they are (***T-dependent antigens***)—a few antigens are capable of activating B cells to produce antibody in the absence of T cells or helper factors from T cells (see Chapter 3). These antigens, referred to as ***T-independent antigens***, share a number of common properties, in particular, 1) they are ***large polymeric molecules*** with multiple, repeating, antigenic determinants—for example, polysaccharides—2) they frequently have some poorly defined ***mitogenic properties***; i.e. at high concentrations they are able, in a non-specific fashion, to activate B cell clones to produce antibody. Such antigens are called ***polyclonal activators***.

The combination of these properties is apparently sufficient to allow these T-independent antigens (such as ***lipopolysaccharide, dextran,*** and ***ficoll***) to trigger a subset of B cells and to initiate production of antibody (see Fig. 10.7).

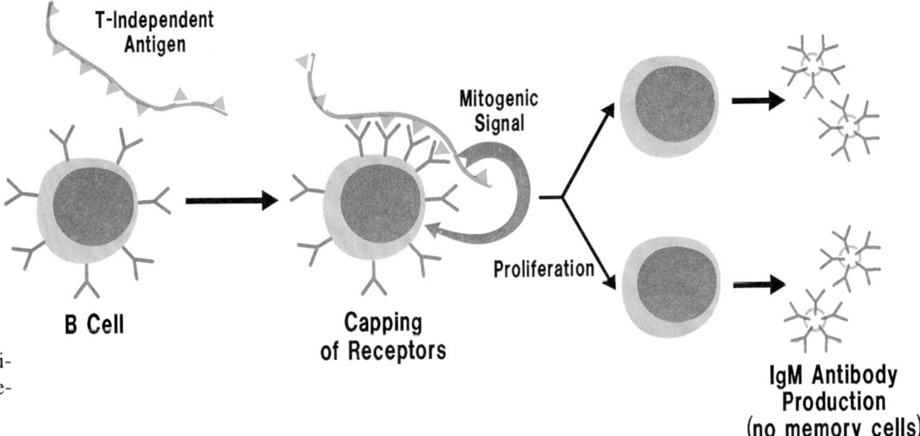

Figure 10.7.
The induction of IgM antibody synthesis by a T-independent antigen.

There are, however, two important differences in the nature of these T-independent responses. Unlike T-dependent responses, they generate primarily ***IgM*** and they ***do not give rise to memory***. In other words, a second injection of a T-independent antigen leads to the same level of production of IgM as the first, with no increase in level, speed of onset, or class switch. Despite the lack of a major role for T cells in these responses, macrophage-like accessory cells are still required, although their exact role in triggering T-independent responses is unknown.

SUMMARY

1. A second exposure to antigen produces a faster response and a higher level of production of antibody than the first exposure. These effects are attributable to the expansion of the specific T- and B-cell clones that follows the first exposure to antigen.

2. In thymus-dependent responses, antigen is generally first processed by accessory cells and is then presented to specific T cells.

3. These cells respond by proliferation and by release of soluble lymphokines which, in turn, stimulate B cells, that also recognize the antigen to undergo proliferation and then to differentiate into plasma cells.

4. The T and B cells may respond to different epitopes on the antigen but for cell cooperation to occur it is necessary that both the epitope to which the T cell responds and the one to which the B cell responds be on the same molecule.

5. Some antigens, such as polysaccharides which have many identical epitopes on each molecule, are capable of triggering B cells without significant help from T cells. These so-called, thymus-independent responses involve predominantly the production of IgM and do not include the development of immunologic memory.

REFERENCES

Howard M, Paul WE (1983): Regulation of B cell growth and differentiation by soluble factors. Ann Rev Immunol 1:307.

Paul WE, Herzenberg LA (1986): B cell subsets and B cell activation. Progress in Immunol 6:335.

Singer A, Hodes R (1983): Mechanisms of T cell–B cell interaction. Annu Rev Immunol 1:211.

Unanue ER (1984): Antigen-presenting function of the macrophage. Annu Rev Immunol 2:395.

Wagner H, Tada T (1986): T cell subsets and T cell activation. Progress in Immunol 6:385.

REVIEW QUESTIONS

Each of the questions or incomplete state ments below is followed by several suggested answers or completions. Select ONE that is BEST in each case.

1. A rabbit has been immunized with DNP_8-BSA. If you wish to induce an anamnestic (secondary) response to DNP_8-OVA a month later, you should
   a) passively administer anti-DNP antibody prior to challenge with DNP_8-OVA.
   b) immunize with OVA one week after immunization with DNP_8-BSA.
   c) boost with DNP one week before challenge with DNP_8-OVA.
   d) transfuse lymphocytes from another rabbit immunized with BSA before challenge with DNP_8-OVA.
   e) irradiate rabbit prior to challenge with DNP_8-OVA.

2. Helper T cells do *not* induce
   a) proliferation of B cells.
   b) differentiation of B cells into plasma cells.
   c) expansion of the pool of memory B cells.
   d) V,J joining in light chains.
   e) immunoglobulin class switch.

For each of the incomplete statements below, ONE or MORE of the completions given is correct. Choose the appropriate answer:
A) if only *1, 2, 3* are correct
B) if only *1 and 3* are correct
C) if only *2 and 4* are correct
D) if only *4* is correct
E) if *all* are correct

3. The secondary antibody response differs from the primary response by having
   1) a shorter latent period.
   2) a longer duration of production of antibody.
   3) a greater quantity of antibody produced.
   4) primarily IgM antibody produced.

4. The following statements concerning T-cell–B-cell cooperation are true:
   1) helper T cells produce soluble factors that induce B cells and T cells to proliferate.
   2) helper T cells recognize carrier determinants which may differ from the determinants, recognized by the B cells.
   3) helper T cells can recognize antigen only when it is presented in association with a class II MHC molecule.

4) helper T cells must be in direct contact with B cells to induce them to proliferate.

5. Roles played by macrophages in immune responses include
   1) phagocytosis and digestion of antigens.
   2) optimal presentation of antigen to B cells.
   3) optimal presentation of antigens to T cells.
   4) release of lymphokines, which increase production of class II MHC molecules.

6. The following statement(s) concerning activation of B cells is/are true:
   1) thymus-independent antigens activate B cells directly to produce both IgM and IgG antibody.
   2) most protein antigens require helper T cells to induce production of antibody by B cells.
   3) optimal collaboration between T and B cells does not require MHC recognition.
   4) when B cells proliferate, some differentiate into plasma cells while others remain as memory B cells.

7. Receptors on T cells differ from receptors of B cells in
   1) having their specificity determined by V-region genes.
   2) requiring other membrane proteins for triggering.
   3) being clonally distributed.
   4) seeing antigen only when associated with Ia molecules.

8. Lyt-1^+ L3T4^+ cells of the mouse
   1) can help B cells make antibody.
   2) can process and present antigen.
   3) can amplify activities of T cells.
   4) can release IL-1.

9. Concerning the nature of antigens, which of the following statements is (are) correct:
   1) T cells recognize the hapten, whereas B cells recognize the carrier.
   2) T-dependent antigens are usually proteins.
   3) B cells are unable, under any circumstances, to present antigen directly to T cells.
   4) processing of antigen by macrophages is an important event in triggering of the immune response.

10. In a response by B cells to thymus-dependent antigen, it is proposed that
   1) helper T cells recognize the antigen in association with Ia molecules on a macrophage.
   2) both carrier and haptenic determinants have to be present on the same molecule for effective cooperation between B cells.
   3) helper T cells produce the lymphokines needed for the B cells to produce the various classes of immunoglobulin.
   4) helper T cells may respond to the same antigen and Ia molecules on both the macrophage and the B cell.

(Continued on next page)

ANSWERS TO REVIEW QUESTIONS

1. ***b*** Because of the carrier effect, a secondary response to the hapten (DNP) on the heterologous carrier (OVA) will result only if the rabbit is primed with OVA some weeks before challenge with DNP_8-OVA.

2. ***d*** All statements are true except "V,J joining in light chains"; the joining of V,J genes occurs in B cells prior to any contact with antigen.

3. ***A*** All statements are characteristic of the secondary response except 4, since production of IgG supersedes production of IgM in the secondary response.

4. ***A*** All properties are characteristic of cooperation between T and B cells except 4, since the helper effect is a function of soluble mediators (BCGF, BCDF) which work at some distance, without cell–cell contact being required.

5. ***B*** Macrophages process antigens (1) and present them to T cells (3) but B cells may react directly with antigen (2), and it is the T cells, not the macrophages that secrete lymphokines, which stimulate production of Ia.

6. ***C*** (1) is false because T-independent antigens produce primarily IgM antibody and collaboration between T and B cells does require recognition by the T-cell of MHC class II antigens in association with the foreign epitope. Hence (3) is also false.

7. ***C*** Both (2) and (4) are true while (1) and (3) are false, since receptors on both B and T cells have specificity-determining V region genes, and each T cell or its clone bears a single specificity.

8. ***B*** The Lyt-1^+ L3T4 markers define a subset of helper T cells in mice. These cells participate in the activation of B cells for production of antibody and also amplify other activities of T cells by release of IL-2.

9. ***C*** Proteins are typical T-dependent antigens that require processing by macrophages for effective presentation. B cells are also able to present these antigens.

10. ***E*** All are correct statements concerning a response of a B cell to a T-dependent antigen.

CHAPTER

11

GENETIC CONTROL OF THE IMMUNE RESPONSE

INTRODUCTION

The search for genes that control the capacity of an animal to make a particular immune response has continued for decades. Given the complexity of the steps involved in such a response, it is obvious that regulatory mechanisms can operate at several levels. This chapter deals primarily with responses that are controlled by loci within the major histocompatibility complex (MHC). Major advances in this field have been made possible by use of genetically inbred strains of animals, immunized with antigens of defined structures and with few antigenic determinants (e.g. synthetic polypeptides composed of 2, 3 or 4 different amino acids).

Using such synthetic polypeptides, Benacerraf (a Nobel prize winner) found that guinea pigs immunized with a DNP conjugate of the homopolymer poly-L-lysine fell into two categories: ***responders and non-responders.*** The responders developed both antibody and delayed hypersensitivity (a T-cell–

mediated response) to the antigen while the non-responders developed neither antibody nor delayed hypersensitivity. Selective inbreeding of the guinea pigs demonstrated that the response to this synthetic antigen is controlled by a ***single dominant gene***. McDevitt then demonstrated that inbred strains of mice segregate similarly into groups of responders and non-responders after immunization with simple, structurally defined polypeptide antigens. The genes controlling these responses are called ***immune response (Ir) genes,*** and they are linked to the ***major histocompatibility complex*** (the ***H-2 complex*** of the mouse and the ***HLA complex*** in humans). In this chapter, we shall discuss the significance of this linkage and its molecular basis.

GENERAL FEATURES

Responses under the control of the ***immune response gene,*** linked to the ***major histocompatibility complex (MHC)***, have several features in common.

1. In general, the immune responses under control of the Ir gene are directed against antigens with few antigenic determinants (epitopes), the structures of which are simple and well defined. The response to each determinant on an antigen is made by clones of particular B and T cells. Thus, it is apparent that response to a complex antigen with many epitopes involves many different clones of cells. If any of the clones are under control of the Ir gene (for example, as non-responders), then the absence of a response by those clones will go undetected because of the response of all the other clones, which are controlled by Ir genes, which confer responder status. Thus, the effects of Ir genes can be seen best when the complexity of the immune response is limited by the presence of only a few determinants on the antigen.

2. All the antigens against which the responses are controlled by Ir genes are ***thymus-dependent;*** in fact, such control operates at the level of the T cell response.

3. Control by Ir genes has a finely tuned specificity: it does not represent a generalized immune incompetence. Thus, a strain of mice unresponsive to ***bovine*** insulin may respond to ***porcine*** insulin while another strain may do the reverse.

4. Control by Ir genes is not always qualitative. Thus, apparent non-responders may generate a response at a low level. Such responses frequently include synthesis of IgM (i.e. they are thymus-independent).

5. In most cases where responsiveness or non-responsiveness has been traced to a single dominant gene, this gene maps to the major histocompatibility complex (MHC).

Regulation of immune responses has been shown to occur through either helper or suppressor effects. An animal that is genetically a non-responder may therefore either ***lack appropriate helper T cells*** or it may have an active mechanism for ***suppressing T cells***. The Ir genes may therefore be represented as response genes or suppressor genes. Although the relationship between the two types of gene is unknown, they are genetically very similar and may represent separate pathways in a single response.

Other genes have been discovered which control a general immunity to a whole infectious agent (e.g. *Leishmania* or *Salmonella*), or to an antigen like the sheep red blood cell. Frequently, the control exhibited by these genes is at the level of the macrophages, and it involves either the intracellular viability of the parasite or the ability of the macrophages to digest the particular antigen. These genes are, in general, not linked to the MHC and will not be discussed further here.

ORGANIZATION AND STRUCTURE OF THE MAJOR HISTOCOMPATIBILITY COMPLEX

Originally, as its name implies, the MHC was recognized by the influence it exerted on the survival of grafts between species (see Chapter 18). The MHC controls the synthesis of cell surface antigens, which provoke intense immunologic responses when the antigens on the donor's cells differ from the antigens on the recipient's cells. All higher organisms possess these antigens, and within each species, they are highly ***polymorphic,*** a result of the existence of multiple alleles (i.e. alternative forms of the gene) at each locus. Polymorphism accounts for the great antigenic disparity among members of an outbred species (e.g. humans), with the consequent rejection of grafts by members of that species unless donor and recipient are monozygotic twins.

Since it is unlikely that a system as complex as the MHC evolved merely to thwart the efforts of transplant surgeons, its natural function became a focus of scientific investigation. Only recently did the mystery begin to unfold, and we now know that the MHC plays an essential role in the recognition of and response to foreign antigens (see Chapter 10).

The two best studied MHC are the murine histocompatibility complex, ***H-2,*** and the human complex, ***HLA.*** The chromosomal organization of the various loci that comprise these MHC complexes is shown in Figure 11.1A and B. Each locus controls the synthesis of a different set of proteins that have different structures, functions, and cellular locations. The proteins whose properties have been elucidated are classified as described in the following sections.

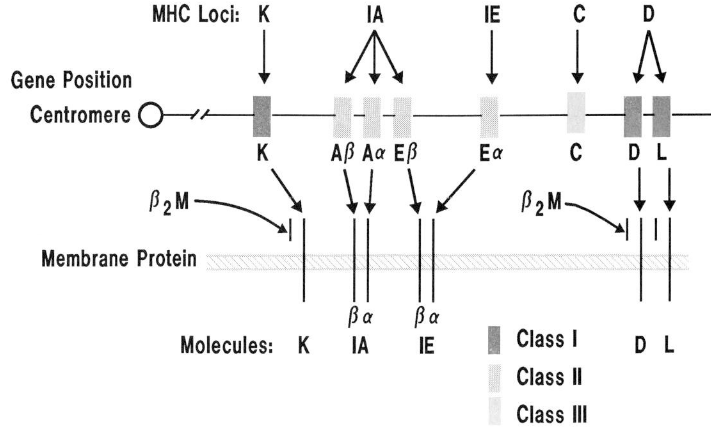

Figure 11.1A.
The major histocompatibility complex (H-2) of the mouse.

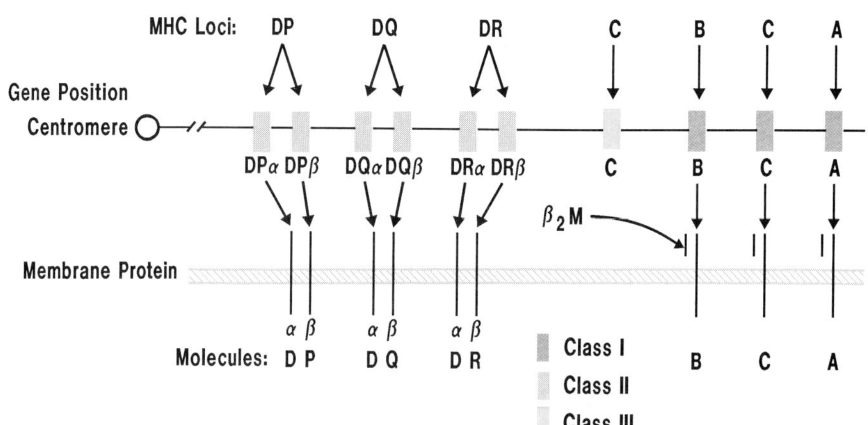

Figure 11.1B.
The major histocompatibility complex (HLA) of the human.

Class I Antigens

Class I antigens, the classic transplantation antigens, were the first to be recognized because of their potency in ***provoking an antibody response***. They consist of a polypeptide chain (molecular weight approximately 43,000 daltons), which always associates non-covalently with an invariant small polypeptide called ***β_2-microglobulin*** (molecular weight 12,000 daltons), which is encoded on another chromosome (see Fig. 11.2). In humans, there are three loci (A,B,C) which code for these class I molecules. The mouse also has three loci (K,D,L) which occupy somewhat different chromosomal positions (see Figure 11.1). There is a high degree of homology between the antigens encoded by the murine K, D and L loci and the human HLA–A, B and C loci, indicating a common ancestral origin. As indicated in Figure 11.2, these antigens are transmembrane proteins and are found on the surface of all nucleated cells. Because the antigens are expressed ***co-dominantly,*** a human that is heterozygous for the A locus (e.g. A10, A3) has two types of A molecules on all its cells, one representative of each allele.

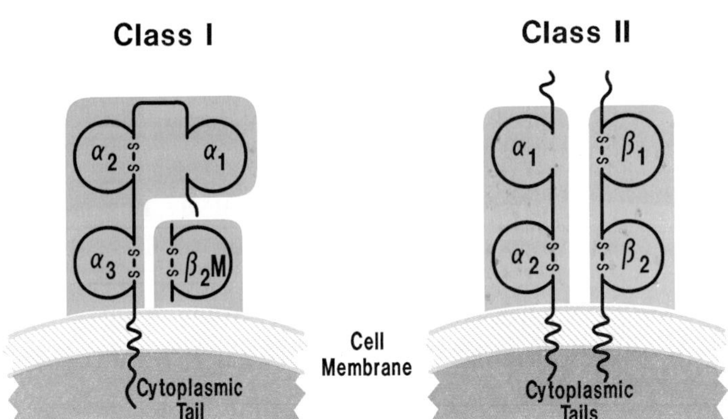

Figure 11.2.
Class I and Class II molecules.

Class II Antigens

Class II antigens are characterized by their ability to ***stimulate lymphocytes*** from genetically different individuals (the mixed lymphocyte response; see Chapter 18). The genetic loci encoding these antigens (called the ***I region*** in mice and the ***D region*** in humans) regulate the production of two polypeptide chains ***(α and β),*** which together make a ***heterodimer transmembrane molecule (Ia in mice, D in humans;*** see Fig. 11.2). The α-chain has a molecular weight of about 33,000 daltons, the β- chain has a molecular weight of about 28,000 daltons. In the mouse, the I region is subdivided into the ***I-A*** and ***I-E*** loci, each of which gives rise to different, but structurally related, heterodimers. Three separate loci ***(DP, DQ, DR)*** of the D region in humans have also been described. Class II molecules have a more limited distribution than class I molecules and, as already described (see Chapter 10), they are found on ***B lymphocytes, macrophages, dendritic cells*** and other accessory cells, such as the ***Langerhans*** cells in the skin.

Class III Antigens

Although their genes are located within the MHC, the class III antigens comprise a group of ***components of complement*** that is not particularly relevant to the control of the immune response. They are proteins found in serum rather than on cells and will not be further discussed here.

ROLE OF MHC IN CONTROL OF THE IMMUNE RESPONSE

Restriction by Class II MHC Molecules

The response of inbred strains of mice to a simple antigen, such as (T,G)-A-L (a polymer of poly-L-lysine, with alanine branches that are tipped with tyrosine and glutamic acid residues), is under the control of a single gene that maps to the ***I-A region*** of the H-2 complex. Thus, all mice carrying the particular allelic form of the ***Ia molecule*** (encoded by I-A) found in the responder strain will be ***responders*** to that antigen. All strains of mice bearing the I-A non-responder allele will be ***non-responders.*** In the case of a different antigen, such as (H,G)-A-L, where histidine replaces tyrosine on the alanine branches of the polymer described above, the responders to (T,G)-A-L may fail to respond to (H,G)-A-L, and vice versa.

This Ir gene was shown not to exert its control at the level of the B cell, since a non-responding mouse could make a satisfactory antibody response to antigen if the antigen was complexed to another carrier molecule which would provide an alternative source of helper T cells. However, these non-responding animals, when immunized with the antigen complexed to another carrier, were unable to mount a T-cell–mediated response in vivo or in vitro when presented with the original antigen. T-cell–mediated responses could be elicited only by the carrier molecule, not by the original antigen. Thus, ***control by the Ir gene operates at the level of the T cells.***

Rosenthal and Shevach, working with guinea pigs, demonstrated that the Ir gene regulates the immune response at the level of ***presentation*** of antigen by the ***accessory cell*** (macrophage) to the T cell (see Chapter 10). They immunized F_1 guinea pigs from a cross between a responder (strain 2) and a non-responder (strain 13) to a given antigen, then looked, in vitro, for proliferative responses to antigen in T cells isolated from these animals. As shown in Table 11.1, macrophages carrying class II antigen from the responder strain (lines 2 and 3) were required for a proliferative response by T cells, while macrophages from a non-responder (line 4) were ineffective, even though they were fully histocompatible with the T cells of the F_1 progeny.

TABLE 11.1. Macrophage Control of Ir Response

Antigen	Source of macrophage	Source of T cells	T-cell response	Conclusion
+	None	Strain 2 × 13	−	Antigen alone not seen without accessory cell
+	Strain 2 × 13	Strain 2 × 13	+	Macrophage required for T-cell response
+	Strain 2	Strain 2 × 13	+	Responder macrophages can present antigen
+	Strain 13	Strain 2 × 13	−	Non-responder macrophages cannot present antigen

When these studies were expanded to include inbred strains of mice, it became possible to use, as the source of macrophages, mice that differed from the donors of T cells only in selected regions of the H-2 complex. Such mice, whose genomes differ at only a single locus, are termed ***congenic.*** Macrophages from mice which differed at any locus except the I locus (IA and IE) could successfully present the antigen to T cells, while macrophages from mice with differences at the I locus were unable to present antigen.

These results are an example of the important phenomenon known as ***MHC restriction,*** and in the particular experiment described above, the responses of the T cells are restricted to class II antigens. In other words, for successful triggering of T cells, the antigen-presenting cell must be identical at the I region (in mice) or at the HLA-D region (in humans) to the T cell that responds to the antigen.

A similar requirement for compatibility of I regions has been demonstrated in the cooperation between T and B cells that is required for production of antibody to hapten-carrier conjugates. T-cells, recognizing the carrier, can cooperate with the B cells, which recognize the hapten, only if they are derived from strains that have ***compatible I regions.*** This requirement for identity of I regions in the T-helper cell and the B cell that it helps is another example of restriction by molecules of the class II MHC.

The cooperative model proposed for the triggering of T cells required for activation of B cells, outlined in Figures 10.2 and 10.5, provides the basis for the regulation of this aspect of the immune response by Ir genes. Helper T cells have receptors capable of recognizing antigen only when that antigen is presented in association with the Ia antigens on the surface of the accessory cells. Thus, T cells can be triggered only by accessory cells that carry the same Ia antigens as the T cell donors themselves, and they can interact only with those B cells that possess the same Ia antigens. The T cells in such a case are said to be ***class II restricted,*** since their receptors will not bind to the antigen when the antigen is associated with an allelic form of the class II MHC molecule. On the basis of this model, several explanations have been proposed for the non-responder status of certain strains or individuals, none of which have been proved convincingly, but all of which may prove to be correct in some circumstances.

Possible Explanations for Non-Responder Status

FAILURE OF THE Ia MOLECULE AND THE PROCESSED ANTIGEN TO ASSOCIATE. It has been shown in several instances that a stable, non-covalently-associated complex can be formed between the isolated Ia molecule of a responder and the processed antigen. A similar association between Ia antigen and processed antigen has not been demonstrated for non-responders. Only strains that make Ia molecules structurally appropriate for such an interaction may be able to act as responders.

In any one individual, there is only a limited number of different Ia molecules, but these molecules must be available for a response by T cells to many different processed antigens. Failure to associate with any epitope on an antigen will result in apparent non-responder status for that particular antigen.

This failure of association is sometimes referred to as a ***presentational defect,*** in what is referred to as the ***''determinant selection''*** model.

ABSENCE OF APPROPRIATE T CELLS. Non-responder status may also be a result of ***absence of T cells*** with receptors specific for the particular complex of antigen and Ia molecule. Absence of such T cells might be due to clonal deletion in ontogeny, if the Ia-antigen complex resembles some "self" antigen so that potentially responsive T cell clones are eliminated. Alternatively, there may be an absence of the V genes required to form a specific receptor. This explanation is often referred to as the ***''hole in the T cell repertoire''*** model.

Restriction by Class I MHC Molecules

In a study of immunity to viral infection, Zinkernagel and Doherty infected one strain of mice with a virus that causes lymphocytic choriomeningitis (LCM). ***T cells*** removed from animals that recovered from this infection could be shown to ***kill*** LCM-infected target cells from the same strain in vitro. These cells were from the Ly-2^+ class of cytotoxic T cells. When infected target cells were chosen from a strain that differed at the H-2 complex, the T cells ***failed*** to kill the target cells (see Fig. 11.3). Use of ***congenic strains*** (strains bred to differ at only one locus of the MHC) then demonstrated that, if the T cells are to kill the target cells, then the target cell and the cytotoxic T cell must have the same class I antigens (encoded by the K or D regions of the MHC). This example of restriction by the MHC involves the ***class I*** antigens required for the functioning of ***cytotoxic T cells.***

THE NATURE OF THE RECOGNITION SYSTEM IN RESPONSES RESTRICTED BY THE CLASS I MHC. While the helper T cell has receptors that recognize antigen in the context of class II molecules, the cytotoxic T cells are adapted for the recognition of foreign antigen in the context of class I MHC molecules (see Fig. 11.4). Another important difference between these two classes of T cells is that cytotoxic T cells are not stimulated to multiply when they come into contact with specific antigen complexed to K or D molecules. The stimulation of proliferation and differentiation requires an additional signal, namely, ***IL-2*** released by the ***helper cells,*** which respond to antigen plus class II MHC products, as noted previously. However, once they become available through proliferation and differentiation, the cytotoxic T cells bind to

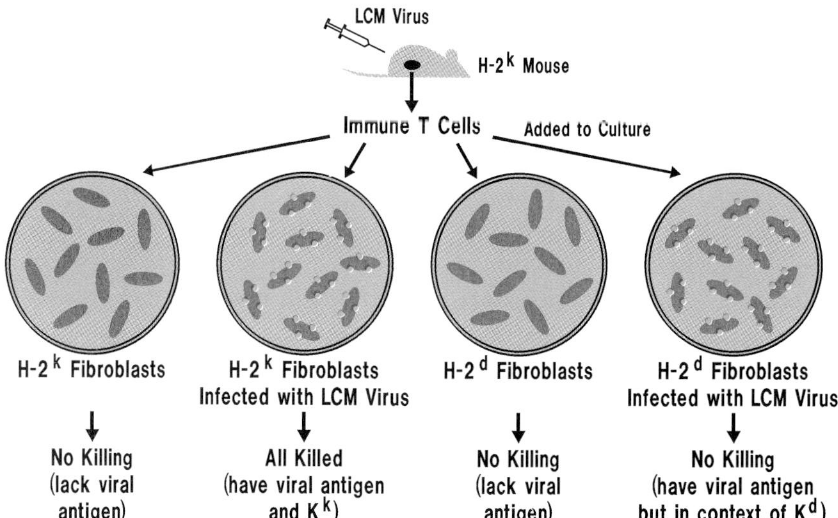

Figure 11.3.
Restriction of cytotoxicity by class I molecules of the MHC.

and kill target cells that have the antigen–class I MHC complex on their surface. The cytotoxic T cells may detach from the target cell to attack additional target cells while the cell that was first attacked dies. Killing is believed to result from the action of cytotoxic substances in the granules of cytotoxic T cells, which produce lesions in the membranes of target cells, similar to those produced by the attack complex (C8,9) of complement (see Chapter 8).

Role of Responses Restricted by the MHC in Immunity

A reasonable hypothesis can be proposed to explain the evolution of the two types of response by T cells that are restricted by the MHC. B cells are generally sessile and, after stimulation by antigen, they establish themselves in lymph nodes and spleen. However, the antibodies that are made by B cells can operate at great distances from them, and can bind free antigens and pathogens in the blood, or other body fluids, to facilitate their elimination. Although similar to antibodies, the receptors on the T cells are not secreted, but the T cell itself is a highly motile cell, circulating through all areas of the body. T cells release their short-range, nonspecific effector molecules only onto, or near the surface of, the cells that carry the specific antigen–MHC molecule

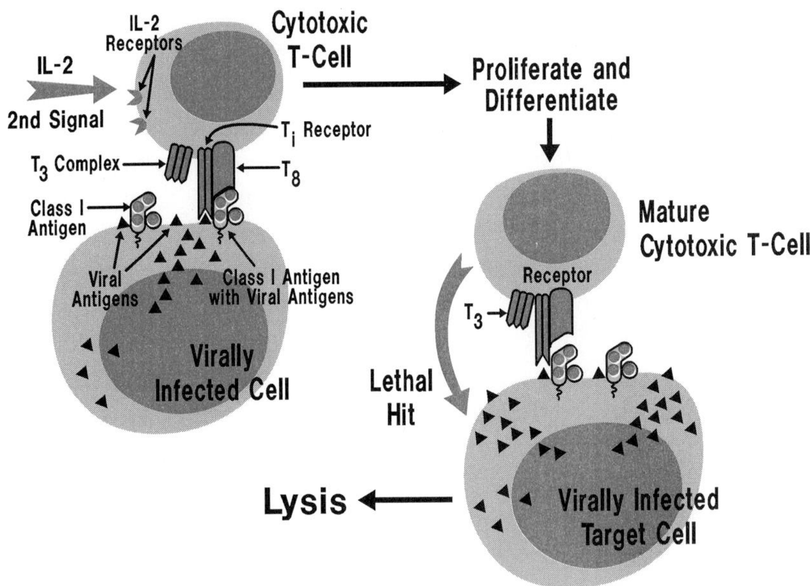

Figure 11.4.
A diagram of the activation of cytotoxic T cells leading to target cell lysis. Viral antigen on the membrane of the infected cell on the left is presented to the cytotoxic T cell receptor (T_8, T_i) in the context of class I molecules. The receptor, together with the T_3 complex, constitutes a first signal for T-cell activation, the second signal being provided by IL-2. Proliferation and differentiation generate mature cytotoxic T cells, which recognize the viral antigen in the context of the same class I molecules as those that initiated the response.

complex with which they react. In the case of B cells, reaction with T cells promotes the activation of B cells to produce antibody. In the case of macrophages, reaction with the effector molecules released by T cells have very important consequences for the macrophages themselves, and for the many types of obligate, intracellular parasites that may live inside them (see Chapter 14). In the case of all other nucleated cells that carry products of the class I MHC, the macromolecules released by cytotoxic T cells produce lesions in cell membranes that result in lysis and death of the target cells.

The immune system thus appears to have evolved at least three different strategies for combining specificity with effector function. All three strategies make use of the rearrangement of genes for the generation of a wide range of specificities. In antibodies, the biologic effector function contained in the Fc domains is united, in the same molecule, with the specificity of the site in the V region, which recognizes and combines with antigen. In the two types of responses by T cells described here, specific recognition of antigen by the mobile T cell results in local release of nonspecific effector factors that can either activate target cells or kill them.

Association of Disease With MHC Type

In humans, HLA-linked Ir genes map to a region within the MHC that is analogous to those regions in mice and guinea pigs. Since immunization of humans with defined antigens and planned, genetic, inbreeding experiments cannot be performed, the analysis of these genes in humans is much more difficult than in other animals. Nevertheless, the association of susceptibility to disease with mutations in the MHC is best analyzed in humans. For example, it has been recognized for many years that individuals with certain allelic HLA genes have a higher risk of contracting certain diseases. Of the various loci in the human HLA complex, association with disease occurs in the following order: alleles of the D locus > B locus > A locus (see Table 11.2 for some examples).

One of the most dramatic examples of all HLA-associated diseases is ***ankylosing spondylitis*** (an inflammatory disease that leads to stiffening of the vertebral joints of the spine). Over 90% of people with the disease carry one particular HLA allele (the B27 allele) but not everyone carrying the B27 allele gets the disease, indicating the need for some other factor.

TABLE 11.2. Association of HLA Types and Disease

Disease	HLA allele	Relative risk factor*
Hashimoto's thyroiditis	DR 5	3
Rheumatoid arthritis	DR 4	6
Dermatitis herpetiformis	DR 3	56
Goodpasture's syndrome	DR 2	13
Multiple sclerosis	DR 2	5
Ankylosing spondylitis	B 27	87
Reiter's disease	B 27	37
Postgonococcal arthritis	B 27	14
Psoriasis vulgaris	C 6	13
Myasthenia gravis	B 8	4

*The risk of contracting the disease for an individual who possesses the HLA marker compared with the risk of an individual who does not.

POSSIBLE EXPLANATIONS OF ASSOCIATION OF DISEASE WITH THE MHC. For almost all known cases of association of a disease with a particular HLA genotype, the explanation is complicated by the fact that the causative agent is unknown. Many of the diseases appear to have an immunologic component, probably of autoimmune origin, and many are also suspected of being of viral origin. The following hypotheses have been proposed to account for these associations:

1. MHC molecules serve as ***receptors*** for the attachment and entry of pathogens into the cell. Thus, individuals with a certain HLA type could be more susceptible to an infection by a particular virus that uses that HLA molecule as a receptor.

2. Serendipitous ***resemblance*** between the antigenic determinants of the pathogen and the MHC molecule of the host (molecular mimicry) may either prevent an immune response, because the pathogen is seen as "self" and no response is made, or, in the event of an immune response to the pathogen, lead to destruction of tissue in an autoimmune reaction.

3. Since antigens are recognized in combination with products of the MHC, it is possible that the antigens of some pathogens, in combination with particular molecules of the MHC, cannot be recognized by T cells. Such a combination would thus be ignored by the host and slip through a ***"hole in the repertoire"*** of the host's T cells.

4. It is possible that an allele in the MHC itself is not responsible for the disease, but rather that some other ***genetic locus closely linked to the MHC*** causes the disease.

Whatever the explanation for the association between HLA and disease, there is great practical value in studying it to identify individuals at risk, to make more precise diagnoses, and to predict the course of the disease.

SUMMARY

1. Several genes, operating at the level of various cellular and molecular processes, control the capacity of an animal to make an immune response. The processes controlled by the MHC are of prime importance.

2. Two major categories of antigen are encoded by the MHC: class I antigens consist of a single polypeptide chain associated with the β_2M molecule on the surface of all nucleated cells; class II molecules consist of two polypeptide chains and are present only on certain cells, such as macrophages and B cells.

3. Class II molecules are involved in the triggering of helper T cells for release of lymphokines. Receptors on these T cells respond to foreign antigen

only when it is presented by accessory cells in conjunction with one of the class II molecules on the surface of the accessory cell. The T cells are said, therefore, to be I region (mice) or HLA-D region-restricted (human), since they require accessory cells with identical I or HLA-D regions for restimulation by antigen.

4. Cytotoxic T cells have receptors that recognize foreign antigen only in the context of class I products of the MHC. Cytotoxic T cells require helper T cells that have responded to the antigens associated with class II molecules, and that produce the IL-2 required for stimulation of proliferation and differentiation of cytotoxic T cells. However, once cytoxic T cells become available, they can respond directly to and kill target cells, which carry the foreign antigen and the same class I molecules on their surface as those on the cytotoxic T cells.

5. Many human diseases are associated with particular variants of the MHC and the exact relationship between the variants and disease processes are of great interest.

REFERENCES

Benjamin DC, Berzofsky JA, East IJ, Gurd FRN, Hannum C, Leach SJ, Margoliash E, Michael JG, Miller A, Prager EM, Reichlin M, Sercarz EE, Smith-Gill SJ, Todd PE, Wilson AC (1984): The antigenic structure of protein, a reappraisal. Annu Rev Immunol 2:67.

Janeway CA (1983): Immune response genes, the problem of the non-responder. J Mol Cell Immunol 1:15.

Klein J, Berzofsky JA (1986): Antigen presentation and processing. Progress in Immunol 6:211.

Klein J, Figueroa K, Nagy ZA (1983): Genetics of the major histocompatibility complex. Annu Rev Immunol 1:119.

Schwartz RH (1985): T lymphocyte recognition of antigen in association with gene products of the MHC. Annu Rev Immunol 3:237.

REVIEW QUESTIONS

Each question or incomplete statement below (questions 1 and 2) is followed by several suggested answers or completions. Select ONE that is BEST in each case.

1. The major histocompatibility complex HLA genes can be described as all of the following *except*
   a) autosomal.
   b) X-linked.
   c) co-dominant.
   d) polymorphic.
   e) located on same chromosome.

2. Certain HLA genes are linked to diseases such as ankylosing spondylitis. This linkage has all the following characteristics, *except*
   a) it is primarily related to the D and B loci.
   b) it may be the result of closely linked immune response genes.
   c) it may be the result of cross-reactivity between alloantigen and infectious agent.
   d) it carries no increased risk for a specific disease for those individuals with the gene.
   e) it may code for a molecule that serves as an attachment site for an infectious agent.

For each incomplete statement below (questions 3–10), ONE or MORE of the completions given is correct. Choose the appropriate answer:
A) if only *1, 2, 3* are correct
B) if only *1 and 3* are correct
C) if only *2 and 4* are correct
D) if only *4* is correct
E) if *all* are correct

3. The D region of the human MHC contains loci that code for
   1) alloantigens found on the surface of macrophages and B cells.
   2) antigen-specific receptors on T cells.
   3) gene products that control the magnitude of the immune response.
   4) β_2-microglobulin.

4. Immune response genes are characterized by
   1) control of the general level of response to all antigens in an individual animal.
   2) inheritance in association with genes of the MHC.
   3) expression of the responder trait in 50% of the offspring of a homozygous

(*Continued on next page*)

responder male and a homozygous non-responder female.
4) operation at the level of presentation of antigen by macrophage to a T cell.

5. Class I and class II MHC proteins share the following features:
1) they are both integral membrane proteins.
2) they both serve to restrict responses of T cells.
3) they are both co-dominantly expressed on cells.
4) they are both expressed on all nucleated cells.

6. A particular mouse may fail to make antibody to an antigen such as poly-glutamic-alanine-tyrosine (GAT) because
1) it lacks the appropriate molecule of the I-A or I-E type.
2) its macrophages cannot digest the antigen.
3) it does not have T cells in its repertoire that are capable of recognizing GAT.
4) it lacks the appropriate K or D molecules.

7. Cytotoxic T cells that destroy virally infected cells
1) release IL-2.
2) bear phenotypic markers on their surface that differ from those of helper T cells.
3) operate only when they can recognize antibody by virtue of their Fc receptors.
4) recognize viral antigen in association with class I proteins of the MHC on the cell surface.

8. T4-positive and T8-positive T cells in humans differ in
1) function.
2) restriction elements encoded by the MHC.
3) production of B cell-activating lymphokines.
4) proliferative response to IL-2.

9. Immunization with vaccinia virus of the F_1 generation from a cross between animals of strains A and B should result in the generation of cytotoxic T cells capable of lysing virally infected target cells from
1) mice of strain A.
2) all strains of mice.
3) $(AxB)F_1$ mice.
4) only female mice of strain A.

10. The K and D loci of the mouse H-2 complex include genes that
1) exhibit co-dominance in heterozygotes.
2) control serologically detectable cell surface antigens.
3) regulate interactions between cytotoxic T cells and target cells.
4) control expression of the components of complement.

ANSWERS TO REVIEW QUESTIONS

1. ***b*** HLA is on chromosome 6, not on the X-chromosome, and has all the other features listed.

2. ***d*** HLA-linked diseases are associated with an elevated risk factor for that disease in individuals with the gene.

3. ***B*** Only (1) and (3) are correct. The genes for receptors on T cells and for β_2-microglobulin are not encoded in the MHC.

4. ***C*** (2) and (4) are correct. Control by immune response genes can be determined only for simple epitopes, not for all complex antigens; thus (1) is incorrect. (3) is also incorrect since all F_1 offspring would be responders in co-dominant inheritance of traits for products of the I region.

5. ***A*** Only (4) is incorrect since class II antigens are expressed on a restricted population of cells (macrophages, dendritic cells, B cells, and some T cells, in humans) while class I antigens are expressed on all nucleated cells.

6. ***B*** Non-responder status for an antigen with a limited array of epitopes may be due to a "presentational defect" (1) or a "hole in the T cell repertoire" (3). There is no evidence that non-responder macrophages fail to process antigens such as GAT, and K or D molecules are not involved in synthesis of antibody. Thus, (2) and (4) are incorrect.

7. ***C*** (1) is incorrect because helper T cells produce IL-2, and (3) is incorrect because antibody is not involved in the function of cytotoxic T cells.

8. ***A*** $T4^+$ cells are helper cells (or involved in delayed type hypersensitivity; see Chapter 14), restricted by class II molecules of the MHC, and they produce several lymphokines, while T8-positive cells have cytotoxic or suppressor function, are restricted by class I molecules of the MHC, and do not induce B cell-activation. (4) is incorrect because both $T4^+$ and $T8^+$ cells proliferate in response to IL-2, which is synthesized by the $T4^+$ cells.

9. ***B*** Cytotoxic T cells will be specific for virally infected cells that have only A or B class I MHC antigens on their surface. There is no preference for female target cells.

10. ***A*** All are correct statements about the K and D loci except (4). Components of mouse complement are encoded by an adjacent, but different, locus.

CHAPTER

12

IMMUNOLOGIC DISORDERS

INTRODUCTION

The immune response is mediated predominantly by B lymphocytes (and antibody), T lymphocytes, phagocytic cells, and complement. The interaction of these components is tightly regulated in a variety of ways to ensure optimal function. Disorders in the development and differentiation of the cells, in the synthesis of their products, or in the regulation of these processes may lead to immunologic disorders that range in severity from mild to fatal. Some disorders are a result of a deficiency in the production or function of one or more of the components of the immune response; others result from the unregulated overproduction of such components. In this chapter, several of the most important disorders of the immune system are described, beginning with disorders that result from immune deficiencies, and concluding with a short description of some of the neoplastic disorders that result in the uncontrolled proliferation of immunocytes and the appearance, in serum, of high concentrations of their products.

IMMUNE DEFICIENCY DISORDERS

Immune deficiency disorders are associated with a deficiency or malfunction of one or more of the major aspects of the immune response, namely, 1) ***B-cell,*** or antibody-mediated, immunity; 2) ***T-cell***-mediated immunity; 3) immunity mediated by the action of ***phagocytic*** cells; and 4) immunity associated with the activation of serum ***complement.***

People with immunodeficiency always suffer from recurrent infections. Thus, an immune deficiency disorder should always be considered a possibility in a patient with recurrent infections. As we shall see, the various disorders have their own particular characteristics and can be diagnosed by specific laboratory tests. The types of infection that occur as a result of an immune deficiency often facilitate the diagnosis of the deficiency. For example, recurrent bacterial otitis media and pneumonia are common in individuals with B-cell (antibody) deficiency; increased susceptibility to fungal, protozoan, and viral infections is common in individuals with deficiencies in T cells and cell-mediated immunity; systemic infections with bacteria, which are normally of low virulence, superficial skin infections, or infections with pyogenic organisms suggest deficiencies in phagocytic cells or their products; and recurrent infections with pyogenic microorganisms are associated with deficiencies in the complement system (Table 12.1).

TABLE 12.1. Four Major Levels of Immune Disorders

Disorder	Associated disease
Deficiency	
B lymphocytes, or antibody deficiency	Recurrent bacterial infections—e.g. otitis media, recurrent pneumonia
T lymphocyte deficiency	Increased susceptibility to viral, fungal, and protozoal infections
Phagocytic cell deficiency	Systemic infections with bacteria of usually low virulence; infections with pyogenic bacteria
Complement components	Bacterial infections, autoimmunity
Unregulated excess	
B lymphocytes	Monoclonal gammopathies
T lymphocytes	Excess of suppressor cells contributes to infections and lymphoproliferative disorders
Phagocytic cells	Hypersensitivity; some autoimmune diseases
Complement components	Angioneurotic edema due to absence of C1 esterase inhibitor

Immune deficiency diseases are frequently divided into two major categories: 1) ***primary immune deficiency diseases,*** which may be hereditary or acquired, and in which the immune deficiency is the cause of a disease, 2) and ***secondary immune deficiency diseases,*** in which the immune deficiency is a result of other disease(s).

PRIMARY IMMUNODEFICIENCY DISEASES

Immunodeficiency Diseases Associated With B Cells or Antibody

Immune deficiency diseases that are associated with deficiencies in B cells or antibody (Table 12.2) stem from disorders that range from defects in development of B cells and the complete absence of all classes of immunoglobulins to deficiencies in a single class or subclass of immunoglobulin. The severity of the disorder determines the degree of severity of the resulting disease. Thus, individuals who lack all classes of immunoglobulins suffer much more from bacterial infections than those who lack only a certain class or subclass of immunoglobulin.

Laboratory tests for disorders of B cells or antibody immunodeficiency include analysis of the number and function of B cells and immunoelectrophoretic and quantitative evaluations to determine the presence and levels of the various classes and subclasses of immunoglobulin. These tests are usually prescribed for patients who are suspected of having immunodeficiency disorders because they suffer from recurrent or chronic infections.

TABLE 12.2. Immune Deficiency Disorders Associated With B or T Lymphocytes

1. B-cell or antibody immunodeficiency disorders
   a. X-linked hypogammaglobulinemia
   b. Transient hypogammaglobulinemia
   c. Common variable hypogammaglobulinemia
   d. Selective Ig deficiencies
2. T-cell immunodeficiency disorders
   a. Congenital thymic aplasia (DiGeorge syndrome)
   b. Chronic mucocutaneous candidiasis
3. B- and T-cell immunodeficiency disorders
   a. Severe combined immunodeficiency disorder
4. Diseases associated with other abnormalities
   a. Wiskott-Aldrich syndrome
   b. Ataxia telangiectasia
   c. Acquired immune deficiency syndrome (AIDS)

It is important to note that, while the complete absence of immunoglobulin is referred to as ***agammaglobulinemia,*** the deficiency is almost always incomplete, and low levels of Ig (mainly IgG) are present. This condition is therefore more correctly referred to as ***hypogammaglobulinemia***, but often the terms agammaglobulinemia and hypogammaglobulinemia are used interchangeably.

X-LINKED HYPOGAMMAGLOBULINEMIA. This disorder, described in 1952 by Bruton, is also called ***Bruton's agammaglobulinemia.*** The disorder is X-linked, occurring only in ***male infants.*** It is expressed at approximately 5–6 months of age when the infant loses the maternally derived IgG that had passed through the placenta. At that age, the infant with X-linked hypogammaglobulinemia begins to suffer from repeated ***bacterial infections.*** The disease is relatively rare (approximately 1/100,000). Analysis of the infant's serum immunoglobulins reveals severe depression in levels or virtual ***absence of all classes of Ig.*** In spite of the involvement of all classes of Ig, the disorder is still referred to as agammaglobulinemia, with the incorrect implication that the deficiency is only in gammaglobulin or IgG.

Analysis of the blood, bone marrow, spleen, or lymph nodes reveals an ***absence of B cells,*** which, together with the complete ***absence of plasma cells,*** explains the depressed levels of Ig.

The major defect in X-linked agammaglobulinemia is the inability of pre-B cells, which are present at normal levels in these infants, to develop into mature B cells.

Infants with X-linked agammaglobulinemia suffer from recurrent ***bacterial*** otitis media, bronchitis, septicemia, pneumonia, arthritis, meningitis, and dermatitis. The most common etiologic agents are *Hemophilus influenzae* and *Streptococcus pneumoniae*. Frequently, patients with this disorder suffer from malabsorption syndrome due to infestation of the gastrointestinal tract with *Giardia lamblia*. Infections that occur in infants with X-linked agammaglobulinemia do not respond well to antibiotics. Consequently, treatment consists of periodic ***passive administration of IgG,*** which seems to be effective in varying degrees.

Although replacement of IgG has maintained several patients for 20–30 years, the prognosis for patients with X-linked agammaglobulinemia is poor, as chronic lung disease often supervenes.

TRANSIENT HYPOGAMMAGLOBULINEMIA. At approximately 5–6 months of age, the concentration of maternal IgG that has been passively transferred through the placenta falls to its lowest level, and the level of IgG synthesized by the infant then begins to rise. Occasionally, an infant may fail to synthesize appropriate amounts of IgG, even when levels of IgM or IgA appear normal. The absence of IgG appears to be due to the ***immaturity of helper T cells,*** which are essential for synthesis of IgG, and it results in a disorder known as ***transient hypogammaglobulinemia.*** Excess suppressor cells have also been found in a few patients. The disorder may persist from a few months to as long as 2 years.

Transient hypogammaglobulinemia is not sex-linked; it can easily be distinguished from the X-linked disease, in which there is an almost complete absence of all classes of IgG, and of B lymphocytes, from the blood.

If a patient with transient hypogammaglobulinemia does not have severe recurrent infections, passive administration of immune serum globulin is not necessary or advisable, especially if the levels of IgM and IgA are not depressed. However, such treatment may be warranted if the infant suffers from severe recurrent infections.

COMMON VARIABLE HYPOGAMMAGLOBULINEMIA. The cause of this disorder, which affects both males and females, is unknown. The onset may occur at any age, with a somewhat higher frequency of onset between the ages of 15 and 35. Affected patients suffer from an increased susceptibility to infection with ***pyogenic bacteria,*** there is also a high incidence of ***autoimmune diseases*** associated with this disorder.

As with patients with X-linked hypogammaglobulinemia, the level of immunoglobulins of all classes is greatly depressed. However, unlike patients with X-linked hypogammaglobulinemia, patients with common variable hypogammaglobulinemia have B cells, but their ***B cells fail to mature into antibody-secreting cells.*** The defect in B cells is not found uniformly in all patients, and there appears to be a heterogeneity in the nature of the defect that ranges from absence of proliferation of B cells and of response to antigen to normal proliferation of B cells but secretion of only IgM. A few patients have an excess of suppressor T-cell activity which impairs the responses of B cells.

The treatment of common variable hypogammaglobulinemia depends on the severity of the disease. For severe disease, accompanied by many recurrent or chronic infections, treatment with immune serum globulin is indicated.

The prognosis for treated patients with this disorder is only fair, but some patients can survive to age 70 or 80. Women with this disease have normal pregnancies, although of course, no maternal IgG is transferred to the fetus (unless the mother receives globulin).

SELECTIVE IMMUNOGLOBULIN DEFICIENCIES. There are several immunodeficiency syndromes that are associated with the selective deficiency of a certain class or subclass of immunoglobulins. Some such deficiencies are accompanied by compensatory elevated levels of other isotypes, as exemplified by the increased levels of IgM levels in cases of IgG or IgA deficiency.

Selective ***IgA deficiency*** is the most common immunodeficiency disorder in this category, with an incidence of approximately 1/800. The cause of IgA deficiency is not known, but it appears to be associated with a decreased release of the IgA synthesized by B lymphocytes.

Patients with this disorder may suffer from recurrent sinopulmonary, viral, or bacterial infections. Increased incidence of celiac disease has been noted in patients with selective IgA deficiency. Paradoxically, some people with IgA deficiency remain generally healthy.

Treatment of symptomatic patients with IgA deficiency consists of administration of wide-spectrum antibiotics. Therapy with immune serum globulin is contraindicated because serum contains only low levels of IgA. Furthermore, the patients may make IgG or IgE antibodies to the IgA in the immune serum. In general, however, the prognosis is good, with many patients surviving to old age.

There are other disorders that result from selective deficiencies in immunoglobulin isotypes. An example is IgM deficiency, a rare disorder, in which patients suffer from recurrent and severe infections with polysaccharide-encapsulated organisms, such as pneumonococci and *Hemophilus influenzae.* Selective deficiencies in subclasses of IgG have been described but are very rare.

Immunodeficiency Disorders Associated With T Cells

Patients with T-cell–deficiency diseases (Tables 12.1, 12.2) are extremely susceptible to ***viral, fungal,*** and ***protozoal*** infections. Moreover, because T-cells participate in the antibody response to thymus-dependent antigens, patients with T-cell deficiency exhibit various defects in the production of antibody after immunization or exposure to many microorganisms. Consequently, patients with T-cell deficiency suffer from diseases against which the body is normally protected by both T cells and B cells.

CONGENITAL THYMIC APLASIA (DiGEORGE SYNDROME). The DiGeorge syndrome is the most important of the T-cell–deficiency diseases. The disease results from a defect in the embryonic development of the ***third***

and fourth pharyngeal pouch, which takes place during approximately the 12th week of gestation. Both the thymus and the parathyroids fail to develop, with consequent ***thymic aplasia*** and ***hypoparathyroidism.*** The newborns suffer from hypocalcemia during the first 24 hours of life, as well as from a variety of other congenital disorders, for example, of the heart and kidneys. The DiGeorge syndrome is not hereditary.

Babies with DiGeorge syndrome suffer from recurrent or chronic infections with ***viruses, bacteria, fungi,*** and ***protozoa.*** They have either no T cells or very few T cells in the blood, lymph nodes or spleen. The few T lymphocytes that are present have a decreased ability to form rosettes with sheep red blood cells (see Chapter 9), indicating developmental abnormalities involving cell surface antigens. These abnormalities are also expressed by the inability of the T cells to respond to mitogens such as concanavalin A and phytohemagglutinin.

Although the B cells, plasma cells, and levels of serum immunoglobulins of patients with DiGeorge syndrome may be normal, many patients fail to produce an antibody response after immunization. Most notably, the IgG response, which requires helper T cells, is absent.

Treatment for DiGeorge syndrome consists of transplantation of fetal thymus. In many cases, the treatment brings about the appearance of T cells within a week after transplantation and may lead to permanent reconstitution of T-cell–mediated immunity. The fetal thymus used for transplantation should not be older than 14 weeks of gestation, to avoid ***graft versus host (GVH)*** reactions, which would occur if mature thymocytes were transferred from the donor into an immunoincompetent host. Donor fetal thymus of less than 14 weeks of gestation provides a sufficient number of thymic epithelial cells to permit successful development of T cells from precursors of bone marrow in the recipient.

The prognosis for untreated patients is poor, but transplantation of fetal thymus has resulted in prolonged survival of patients with DiGeorge syndrome. Other disorders associated with the syndrome (such as congenital heart disorders), however, must also be dealt with, and these can complicate both the treatment and prognosis.

CHRONIC MUCOCUTANEOUS CANDIDIASIS. Chronic mucocutaneous candidiasis, an infection of skin and mucous membranes by a ***fungus*** that is normally present but non-pathogenic (*Candida albicans*), is a poorly defined collection of syndromes associated with a ***selective defect in the functioning of T cells.*** Patients with this disorder have normal T-cell–mediated immunity to microorganisms, other than *Candida* and normal B-cell–mediated immunity to all microorganisms including *Candida* (against which the patients mount a normal antibody response). This disorder affects both males and females, and there is some evidence that it may be inherited. Children are particularly affected. There is additional morbidity associated with this disorder because patients with chronic mucocutaneous candidiasis also suffer from various endocrine dysfunctions such as adrenal or parathyroid deficiencies.

Treatment of candidiasis consists of the administration of anti-fungal agents. However, the general prognosis for the disease is guarded.

Severe Combined Immunodeficiency Diseases

Combined immunodeficiency diseases result from defects in both T cells and B cells. Individuals with severe combined immunodeficiency disease are susceptible to ***viral, bacterial, fungal,*** and ***protozoal*** infections, most notably, cytomegalovirus, *Pneumocystis carinii,* and *Candida*. Symptoms begin in early infancy and untreated patients seldom survive beyond their first year. However, infants with this disorder can be cured by transplantation of bone marrow (see below).

The disease is inherited as an ***X-linked*** recessive or an autosomal recessive trait (the latter formerly known as ***Swiss-type agammaglobulinemia***). Patients with this deficiency may exhibit a complete absence of T and B cells, expressed by a marked ***lymphopenia.*** Consequently all the normal ***functions of T and B cells are absent.*** It must be emphasized that patients with severe combined immunodeficiency disease should not be vaccinated with attenuated live microorganisms. Vaccination could have disastrous results, since the patient is unable to mount an immune response against the inoculated microorganism.

A variant of severe combined immunodeficiency disease that is present in about 50% of patients with the autosomal recessive, inherited form of the disease, is associated with a deficiency in the enzyme ***adenosine deaminase.*** The enzyme is absent from all the patient's cells. However, its absence from lymphoid cells is particularly harmful to these cells since toxic amounts of adenosine triphosphate (ATP) and deoxyATP accumulate within them.

Early diagnosis is very important if treatment is to be initiated before the appearance of irreversible complications. Treatment consists of transplantation with histocompatible bone marrow. In cases where histocompatible bone marrow is not available, transplantation of fetal liver or fetal thymus has been reported to result in improvement.

In addition to the immunodeficiency diseases already described, there are several that are associated with other abnormalities. One such abnormality is ***ataxia telangiectasia,*** a disease in which neurologic symptoms (staggering gait) and abnormal, spider-like vascular dilation (telangiectasia) accompany the immunological disorders (lymphopenia and depressed levels of IgA, IgE, and, sometimes, IgG).

Another immunodeficiency disease, ***Wiskott-Aldrich syndrome,*** affects patients early in life and is associated with thrombocytopenia, eczema, and recurrent infections. The patients suffer from bleeding, due to thrombocytopenia, as well as from recurrent bacterial infections that cause otitis media, meningitis and pneumonia as a result of low levels of serum IgM. These disorders are probably associated with the peculiar inability of these patients to respond to polysaccharide antigens. Additionally, they may have a defective DNA repair mechanism and a particular susceptibility to leukemia.

Phagocytic Dysfunctions

The immunodeficiency disorders discussed so far involve defects in the functions or products of T cells, B cells, or both. Polymorphonuclear leukocytes and monocytes also play an important role in both innate and acquired immunity. They act either alone or in concert with lymphocytes and their products to bring about the destruction of pathogenic microorganisms. Defects in the activity of these cells may lead to diseases of phagocytic dysfunction.

Phagocytic dysfunction may be caused by ***extrinsic factors,*** such as deficiency of antibodies, complement components, or the lymphokines, which activate the phagocytic cells. It may also be caused by ***defects in the metabolic pathways*** of the phagocytic cells, pathways that are essential for the killing of the pathogen. Such deficiences include reduced or absent levels of normal glucose-6-phosphate dehydrogenase, myeloperoxidase, alkaline phosphatase; abnormal functions of microtubules; low levels of lysosomal enzymes ***(Chédiak-Higashi syndrome);*** and others. An important disease associated with a deficiency of NADPH oxidase or NADH oxidase is ***chronic granulomatous disease.***

Chronic granulomatous disease is inherited as an X-linked disorder or as an autosomal recessive disorder. Symptoms begin to appear during the first two years of life. Patients suffer from a greatly enhanced susceptibility to infection with organisms that are normally of low virulence such as *Staphylococcus epidermidis*, *Serratia marcescens* and *Aspergillus*. Frequent abnormalities include lymphadenopathy, hepatosplenomegaly, and chronic draining lymph nodes. Chronic and acute infections occur in lymph nodes, skin, intestinal tract, liver, and bone.

Normally, phagocytosis activates membrane-bound NADPH oxidase, which is required to generate intracellular peroxidase. In patients with chronic granulomatous disease, however, deficiency in NADPH oxidase or NADH oxidase precludes the generation of peroxidase, which is required for the killing of ingested intracellular organisms.

Treatment consists of aggressive therapy with wide spectrum antibiotics and with antifungal agents. Prognosis is poor, although recently the mortality rate has been reduced by early diagnosis and aggressive therapy.

Diseases Due to Abnormalities in the Complement System

Complement components are important in the killing of bacteria, in opsonization, and in chemotaxis (see Chapter 8), and they may also play a role in the prevention of autoimmune diseases by participating in the elimination of antigen–antibody complexes. Thus, deficiencies in complement components may result in a variety of effects, ranging from ***recurrent bacterial infections*** to increased susceptibility to ***autoimmune diseases.*** Excess of a given component of complement or the absence of an appropriate inhibitor of the component may also result in disorders of varying severity.

Particular genetic defects have been shown to be associated with most of the individual components of complement. The defects are inherited as autosomal recessive traits, with heterozygous individuals having half the normal level of a given component of the complement system. The following is a brief outline of complement disorders.

C1q, r, s DEFICIENCIES. Deficiencies in C1q, r, s have been reported in association with ***autoimmune diseases,*** predominantly in patients with syndromes that resemble ***systemic lupus erythematosus (SLE).*** These patients have increased susceptibility to ***bacterial*** infections.

An important disorder associated with C1 is ***hereditary angioneurotic edema.*** Patients with this disease lack a functional ***inhibitor of C1 esterase.*** The absence of this inhibitor leaves the action of C1 on C4 or C2 uncontrolled, generating multiple copies of a fragment which, in turn, is activated by plasmin to yield a vasoactive peptide. Patients with a deficiency in the inhibitor of C1 esterase suffer from local ***edema*** in various organs, which may become life-threatening when it occurs in the larynx and obstructs the passage of air.

Recently, it has been shown that two steroid drugs (danazol and oxymetholone) induce the synthesis of a functional inhibitor of C1 esterase in patients with angioneurotic edema.

C4 DEFICIENCY. Deficiency in C4 has been observed in a few patients with SLE.

C2 DEFICIENCY. Deficiency in C2 is the most common deficiency of complement components, and it has been found to occur in asymptomatic individuals, as well as in individuals with SLE.

C3 DEFICIENCY. Patients with a deficiency in C3 experience recurrent bacterial infections. In some patients, the deficiency is also associated with chronic glomerulonephritis.

C5–C8 DEFICIENCIES. Patients with deficiencies in complement components C5 through C8 have a tendency to increased infections, most notably to recurrent infections with *Neisseria*.

C9 DEFICIENCY. Deficiency in C9 is very rare and has been described for one individual only. Surprisingly, this individual had no history of recurrent infections. However, bacterial lysis may occur, albeit slowly, in the presence of C8 and the absence of C9 (see Chapter 8).

SECONDARY IMMUNODEFICIENCY DISEASES

In contrast to primary immunodeficiency diseases, in which there are hereditary or acquired defects in B or T lymphocytes, phagocytic cells or complement, secondary immunodeficiency diseases are those in which the deficiency is secondary to other disease states and generates further complications. Secondary immune deficiency diseases may result from the loss of T or B lymphocytes or their functions due to illnesses like leukemia, or to other disease states that affect the components of the immune system.

By far the most common cause of immunodeficiency disorders in developed countries is secondary to the use of ***chemotherapeutic agents*** in cancer therapy. Many of these agents are toxic to bone marrow cells and to T and B lymphocytes. Also, the deliberate ***immunosuppression*** induced during organ transplantation, in order to avoid immunological rejection, constitutes a nonspecific immunosuppression. Secondary immunodeficiencies are associated with overwhelming infections by bacteria. These infections are often refractory to antibiotic therapy and are often fatal.

Acquired Immunodeficiency Syndrome (AIDS)

An immune deficiency disease that has become the focus of much publicity and concern is ***acquired immunodeficiency syndrome (AIDS).*** As of 1986, approximately 90% of the cases in the United States have been diagnosed in sexually active, male homosexuals in large cities, but it is clear that the infection is spreading into the heterosexual population. In parts of Africa, the incidence among the general population is much higher than in the United States, and both heterosexual males and females are affected. In the United States, cases have been reported in hemophiliacs and other individuals who have received blood transfusions or who have been users of intravenous drugs. The epidemiology of the disease led to the hypothesis and subsequent proof that AIDS is caused by a virus. Human lymphotropic virus (HTLV III) (now called HIV for human immunodeficiency virus) has been isolated from patients with AIDS. Furthermore, over 80% of patients with AIDS have antibodies to HIV. It is now known that the virus attaches to the T4 marker on $T4^+$ helper cells and kills them. AIDS patients therefore develop abnormally low ratios of helper cells (T4) to suppressor T cells (T8).

Patients with AIDS have normally functioning B cells, and normal or even increased levels of serum immunoglobulins. The immune deficiency is attributed to the ***loss in helper T cells.*** The patients suffer from severe infections by opportunistic organisms, which become pathogenic in the absence of T-cell–mediated immunity. The pathogens include ***viruses, fungi*** and ***parasites.*** Patients with AIDS also exhibit a pronounced susceptibility to ***Kaposi's sarcoma*** (a rare skin cancer) and ***lymphomas.*** These tumors spread with unusual virulence in patients with AIDS and often result in rapid death.

GAMMOPATHIES

There are several neoplastic diseases that involve abnormal proliferation of B cells and plasma cells, the two types of cell that produce antibodies. These diseases are associated with an excessive production of whole immunoglobulins or of immunoglobulin chains. Because the synthesis of these immunoglobulins takes place in clones that arise from a single cell, the synthesized immunoglobulins are referred to as ***monoclonal immunoglobulins,*** and the disorders are referred to as ***monoclonal gammopathies.***

There are three principal monoclonal gammopathies: multiple myeloma, macroglobulinemia, and heavy chain disease. A brief description of these diseases follows.

1. ***Multiple myeloma.*** Multiple myeloma is the most common of the malignant monoclonal gammopathies and results from a malignant proliferation of plasma cells. The disease is associated with the synthesis of large amounts of ***M proteins*** (monoclonal immunoglobulins) of any given isotype, with either κ or λ light chains. Multiple myeloma may also be associated with the occurrence of large amounts of free κ- or free λ-chains in the serum or the urine (these proteins are called ***Bence-Jones proteins).***

Multiple myeloma may involve multiple organ systems (e.g. the skeletal system, the nervous system, the bone marrow, and the kidneys), predominantly as a result of the infiltration of malignant plasma cells into the organ. X-rays of the skeletal system may show many, well demarcated, osteolytic lesions around such infiltrates.

Patients with multiple myeloma suffer from a suppression of the synthesis of normal antibodies and are, consequently, susceptible to recurrent bacterial and viral infections.

2. ***Macroglobulinemia.*** This disease, also referred to as ***Waldenström's macroglobulinemia,*** is associated with the synthesis and release of large amounts of ***IgM.*** The concentration of this macroglobulin in the serum can result in an increased viscosity of the serum which may, in turn, lead to slower blood flow, thromboses, disorders of the central nervous system, and bleeding. In addition to the overproduction of IgM, the disease is often characterized by decreased synthesis of other immunoglobulins, leading to ***hypogammaglobulinemia*** with all its harmful consequences.

3. ***Heavy chain disease.*** This disease is characterized by the appearance in the serum and urine, of large amounts of a monoclonal protein with a molecular weight of approximately 55,000 daltons, similar in composition to the Fc fragment of IgG or IgA or IgM.

Patients with this rare disease have recurrent bacterial infections, enlargement of the lymphoid organs, and anemias. The most frequent causes of death are recurrent infections, which proceed unchecked because of impairment of antibody synthesis.

Treatment of monoclonal gammapathies involves the reduction and elimination of the malignant cells that produce the proteins. Depending on the disease, this therapy usually includes local irradiation and/or cytotoxic chemotherapy with a variety of cytotoxic drugs.

SUMMARY

1. Immune deficiency disorders are called *primary* when the deficiency is the cause of a disease, and *secondary* when deficiency is a result of other diseases.

2. Immune deficiency diseases may be due to disorders in the development or function of B cells, T cells, phagocytic cells or components of complement, as shown in Tables 12.1, 12.2.

3. Immune deficiency disorders frequently predispose patients to recurrent infections. The association of various infections with deficiencies in B cells, T cells, phagocytes, or components of complement is shown in Table 12.1.

4. Whereas immune deficiencies constitute one aspect of disorders of the immune system, another aspect of such disorders is the unregulated proliferation of B lymphocytes, T lymphocytes, phagocytes, and their products, or the unregulated activation of components of the complement system.

REFERENCES

Ammann AJ (1977): T cell and B cell immunodeficiency disorders. Pediatr Clin North Am 24: 293.

Ammann AJ (1984): Immunodeficiency diseases. In Stites DP, Stobo JD, Fudenberg HH, Wells JV (eds): Basic and Clinical Immunology, Ed., 5. Los Altos, California: Lange Medical Publications.

Chandra RK (ed) (1984): Primary and Secondary Immunodeficiency Disorders. New York: Churchill Livingstone.

Church JA, Schlegel RJ (1985): Immune deficiency disorders. In Bellanti JA (ed): Immunology III. Philadelphia: W.B. Saunders.

Gallo RC, Gelfand EW (1986): Congenital and acquired immunodeficiencies. Progress in Immunol 6:537.

Gelfand EW, Dosch H (eds) (1980): Biological Basis of Immunodeficiency, New York: Raven Press.

REVIEW QUESTIONS

For questions 1–5, select the ONE BEST answer or completion in each case:

1. An eight-month-old baby has a history of a repeated succession of gram-positive bacterial infections. The most probable cause for this condition is that
   a) the mother did not confer sufficient immunity upon the baby in utero.
   b) the baby suffers from erythroblastosis fetalis (hemolytic disease of the newborn).
   c) the baby is hypogammaglobulinemic.
   d) the baby is allergic to the mother's milk.
   e) all of the above.

2. A 50-year-old worker at an atomic plant who previously had a sample of his own bone marrow cryopreserved, was accidentally exposed to a minimal lethal dose of radiation. He was subsequently transplanted with his own bone marrow. This individual can expect
   a) to have recurrent bacterial infections.
   b) to have serious fungal infections due to deficiency in cell-mediated immunity.
   c) to respond with antibodies to thymus-independent antigens only.
   d) all of the above.
   e) none of the above.

3. Which of the following immune deficiency disorders is associated exclusively with an abnormality of the humoral immune response?
   a) X-linked hypogammaglobulinemia (Bruton's disease).
   b) DiGeorge syndrome.
   c) Wiskott-Aldrich syndrome.
   d) chronic mucocutaneous candidiasis.
   e) hereditary angioneurotic edema.

4. A sharp increase in levels of IgM, with a spike in the IgM region seen in the electrophoretic pattern of serum proteins, is an indication of
   a) IgA or IgG deficiency.
   b) multiple myeloma.
   c) macroglobulinemia.
   d) hypogammaglobulinemia.
   e) severe fungal infections.

5. Patients with DiGeorge syndrome may fail to produce IgG in response to immunization with T-dependent antigens because
   a) they have decreased numbers of B cells, which produce IgG.
   b) they have increased numbers of suppressor T cells.
   c) they have decreased numbers of helper T cells.

(*Continued on next page*)

d) they have abnormal antigen-presenting cells.
e) they cannot produce IgM during primary responses.

For questions 6–8, ONE or MORE of the completions given is correct. Choose the appropriate answer:
A) if only *1, 2, 3* are correct
B) if only *1 and 3* are correct
C) if only *2 and 4* are correct
D) if only *4* is correct
E) if *all* are correct

6. Immunodeficiency disease can result from
   1) a developmental defect of T lymphocytes.
   2) a developmental defect of bone marrow stem cells.
   3) a defect in phagocyte function.
   4) a defect in complement function.

7. A nine-month-old baby was vaccinated against smallpox with attenuated smallpox virus. He developed a progressive necrotic lesion of the skin, muscles and subcutaneous tissue at the site of inoculation. The vaccination reaction resulted from
   1) B lymphocyte-deficiency.
   2) reaction to the adjuvant.
   3) complement-deficiency.
   4) T cell-deficiency.

8. The most common clinical consequence(s) of C3 deficiency is (are)
   1) increased incidence of tumors.
   2) increased susceptibility to viral infections.
   3) increased susceptibility to fungal infections.
   4) increased susceptibility to bacterial infections.

ANSWERS TO REVIEW QUESTIONS

1. ***c*** The baby is probably hypogammaglobulinemic. Hypogammaglobulinemia leads to recurrent bacterial infections. Viral and fungal infections are controlled by cell-mediated immunity, which is normal in hypogammaglobulinemic individuals. Answer a is incorrect because the mother's IgG, which passed through the placenta, would have a half-life of 23 days, and would therefore not be expected to remain in the baby's circulation for 8 months. At this age any Ig present in the baby's circulation is synthesized by the baby. Answer b is irrelevant since erythroblastosis fetalis is caused by the destruction of the newborn's Rh^+ erythro-

cytes by the Rh^- mother's antibodies to Rh antigen. Answer d is incorrect since, even if allergic to the mother's milk, the baby should not suffer from increased frequency of bacterial infections.

2. ***e*** The autologous bone marrow cells, which contain stem cells, will replicate, differentiate, and repopulate the hematopoietic–reticuloendothelial system, rendering the individual immunologically normal. As such, the individual is not expected to have bacterial, viral, or fungal infections or to respond to antigens differently from a normal individual.

3. ***a*** The only immune deficiency disorder that is associated with an abnormality exclusively of the humoral response is Bruton's hypogammaglobulinemia or X-linked hypogammaglobulinemia. DiGeorge syndrome results from a thymic aplasia, where there is a deficiency in T cells that may influence the IgG responses, which require helper cells. Wiscott-Aldrich syndrome is associated with several abnormalities. Chronic mucocutaneous candidiasis is a poorly defined collection of syndromes associated with a selective defect in the functioning of T cells. Hereditary angioneurotic edema is associated with a deficiency of the inhibitor of C1 esterase.

4. ***b*** This pattern is characteristic of multiple myeloma (IgM myeloma). Multiple myeloma may be recognized by the synthesis of large amounts of homogeneous antibody of any one isotype. Although patients with multiple myeloma may suffer from a decreased synthesis of other Ig isotypes, the electrophoretic pattern is not necessarily an indication of deficiency in IgA or IgG.

5. ***c*** Patients with DiGeorge syndrome have a decreased number of T cells—in particular, helper T cells, which are essential for the IgG response to T-dependent antigens. These patients have normally functioning B cells and are capable of responding to T-independent antigens, or with only IgM responses (primary responses) to T-dependent antigens.

6. ***E*** All are correct. Immunodeficiency disorders may result from defects in the development of bone marrow stem cells into lymphocytes and other cells that participate in the immune response. They can also result from defects in phagocyte functions, which are important in phagocytosis and presentation of antigen. Immunodeficiency disorders may also result from defects in complement function—an absence or malfunction of one or more of the complement components, their activators, or regulators of the complement system.

7. ***D*** Only 4 is correct. T-cell deficiency would result in the absence of the crucial immunological defenses against viral infection, i.e. cell-mediated immunity. Cell-mediated immunity plays a major role in immunity to viral infec-

(Continued on next page)

tions, much greater than the roles of antibodies or complement. In fact, individuals with impaired T-cell–mediated immunity should not be vaccinated with live smallpox which, even if attenuated, may cause a serious infection.

8. ***D*** Only 4 is correct. Deficiency in C3 is associated with increased susceptibility to bacterial infections, since C3 plays an important role in the destruction of bacteria and their increased opsonization, by participating in the classical and the alternative pathways of complement activation. Cell-mediated immunity (CMI) is generally more important in the resistance of the host to viral and fungal infections. Also, in general, CMI is considered to be more important than complement in the resistance of the host to tumors.

CHAPTER

13

HYPERSENSITIVITY REACTIONS

INTRODUCTION

Under some circumstances, ***immunity,*** rather than providing protection, produces damaging and sometimes fatal results. Such deleterious reactions are known collectively as ***hypersensitivity*** reactions, but it should be remembered that they differ from protective immune reactions only in that they are damaging to the host. The cellular and molecular mechanisms of the two types of reaction are virtually identical.

Hypersensitivity reactions were divided into four classes, designated type I–type IV, by Gell and Coombs:

Type I. Anaphylactic reactions are mediated by IgE antibodies, which bind to receptors on ***mast cells.*** When cross-linked by antigens, the IgE antibodies trigger the mast cells to release several pharmacologically active agents that are responsible for the characteristic symptoms of anaphylaxis. Reactions are rapid, occurring within minutes after exposure to antigen.

Type II. Cytolytic or cytotoxic reactions occur when ***IgM*** or ***IgG*** antibodies bind to antigen on the surface of cells and activate the complement cascade, which culminates in destruction of the cells.

Type III. Immune complex reactions occur when aggregates of antigen and IgM or IgG antibody accumulate in the circulation or in tissue and activate the complement cascade. Granulocytes are attracted to the site, and damage results from the release of lytic enzymes from their granules. Reactions occur within hours of exposure to antigen.

Type IV. Cell-mediated immunity (CMI) reaction—also called ***delayed-type hypersensitivity (DTH),*** or the ***tuberculin reaction***—is mediated by T cells rather than by antibody. Upon activation, the T cells release lymphokines that cause accumulation and activation of macrophages, which, in turn, cause local damage. This type of reaction has a delayed onset and may occur 1–2 days after exposure to antigen.

This chapter deals with antibody-mediated hypersensitivity; cell-mediated immunity (type IV) is discussed in Chapter 14.

TYPE I—ANAPHYLACTIC SENSITIVITY

The term ***anaphylaxis*** was coined by Portier and Richet, who studied the effects of the toxin from a Mediterranean anemone on dogs. Several weeks after an initial administration of the toxin, a second dose was given to determine if the dogs had developed a resistance to it. Some of the dogs, rather than showing increased resistance to the effects of the toxin, experienced, within minutes of receiving the dose, excessive salivation, defecation, difficulty in respiration, paralysis of the hind limbs, and death. Portier and Richet named this phenomenon ***anaphylaxis,*** from the Greek *ana,* which means "away from," and *phylaxis,* which means "protection." The term is the antithesis of the phenomenon of ***prophylaxis.*** Subsequent studies revealed that anaphylaxis is the result of increased sensitivity rather than decreased resistance to the toxin. The discovery of anaphylaxis provided the first example of the ability of the immune system to cause harm.

There is evidence to suggest that type I sensitivity originated as a means of ridding the body of certain parasites, particularly worms. Nevertheless, most of our understanding of the basic mechanisms of this response comes from studies of its pathologic consequences.

The sequence of events involved in the development of anaphylactic sensitivity can be divided into several phases, as follows: 1) the ***sensitization phase,*** during which IgE antibody is produced and binds to specific receptors on mast cells and basophils; 2) the ***activation phase,*** during which re-exposure to antigen triggers the mast cells to respond by release of the contents of their granules; and 3) the ***effector phase,*** during which a complex response (anaphylaxis) occurs as a result of the effects of the many pharmacologically active agents released by the mast cells and basophils.

Sensitization Phase

All normal individuals can make IgE antibody specific for a variety of antigens when the antigen is introduced parenterally in the appropriate manner. Approximately 50% of the population generates an IgE response to antigens that are encountered only on mucosal surfaces, such as the lining of the nose and lungs and the conjunctiva of the eyes. However, only 10% of the general population develops hay fever after repeated exposure to a plethora of airborne antigens (called ***allergens*** by allergists) such as plant pollens, mold spores and animal danders. Allergists frequently use the archaic term ***atopy*** to refer to this syndrome and the term ***atopic*** to describe affected patients. Since all members of a given population have roughly the same quantitative contact with any particular allergen, such as ragweed pollen, it is unclear why a clinically significant response is made by only a small proportion of the population. It has been suggested that the response is under the control of ***immune response (Ir) genes*** (since familial tendencies are seen) and that differences in mucosal permeability may restrict the effects of antigens lodging on the surface, but the actual reasons remain to be identified.

Once adequate exposure to the allergen has been achieved by repeated mucosal contact, ingestion, or parenteral injection, and IgE antibody has been produced, then an individual is considered to be sensitized. IgE antibody is made in very small amounts (its concentration in the blood is the lowest of all immunoglobulins) and very rapidly becomes attached to mast cells as it circulates past them. Mast cells (and basophils) have specific receptors on their cell membranes that bind the Fc portion of IgE molecules with very high affinity. Once they are bound to a mast cell, the IgE molecules persist for weeks, and the particular mast cell will remain "sensitized" as long as enough antibody remains attached to trigger the activation of the cell when it comes into contact with antigen.

Sensitization may also be effected passively by the transfer of serum that contains IgE antibody to a specific antigen. A procedure known as the ***Prausnitz-Küstner (P-K)*** test used to be performed as a test for the antibodies responsible for anaphylactic reactions. In the P-K test serum from an allergic individual was injected into the skin of a normal person. After a lag period of

1–2 days, during which the locally injected antibody diffused toward neighboring mast cells and became bound to them, the site of injection was said to be sensitized, and it showed an urticarial reaction after injection into it, of the antigen to which the donor was allergic. Such a reaction in passively sensitized animals is called ***passive cutaneous anaphylaxis (PCA).***

Activation Phase

The anaphylactic reaction itself may be triggered by injection of the specific antigen into the skin of a sensitized individual. The response called "wheal and flare" is characterized by ***erythema*** (redness due to dilation of blood vessels) and ***edema*** (swelling produced by release of serum into tissue). The anaphylactic reaction is the most rapid of all hypersensitivity reactions and reaches its peak within 10–15 minutes; then it fades without leaving any residual damage.

The local reaction observed when an allergic patient is tested or challenged by intradermal injection of a battery of potential antigens is called ***cutaneous anaphylaxis.*** The size of the response to any given allergen is roughly indicative of the degree of sensitivity to that particular substance. In addition, if the clinical history of symptoms correlates well with the time of contact with the antigen, then the cutaneous anaphylactic response may be taken as strong evidence that the symptoms (e.g. sneezing, itchy eyes) are attributable to the allergens of the particular plant pollen or animal dander that engendered the skin response. Other more quantitative tests are used as well (see below).

Mast cells, the main effectors of type I responses, are a ubiquitous family of cells generally found around blood vessels in the connective tissue, in the lining of the gut, and in the lungs. They are large, mononuclear cells, heavily granulated and deeply stained by basic dyes such as toluidine blue (see Fig. 13.1). In some species, a circulating, polymorphonuclear granulated cell, called a ***basophil,*** also takes part in type I responses, and functions in much the same way as the tissue-based mast cells. The relationship between these two types of cell and the existence of a common precursor, as suggested by their similar appearance and function, are unknown. The binding of IgE molecules to the specific receptors on mast cells and basophils prepares those cells for reaction when antigen appears, but otherwise, it does not seem to affect these cells.

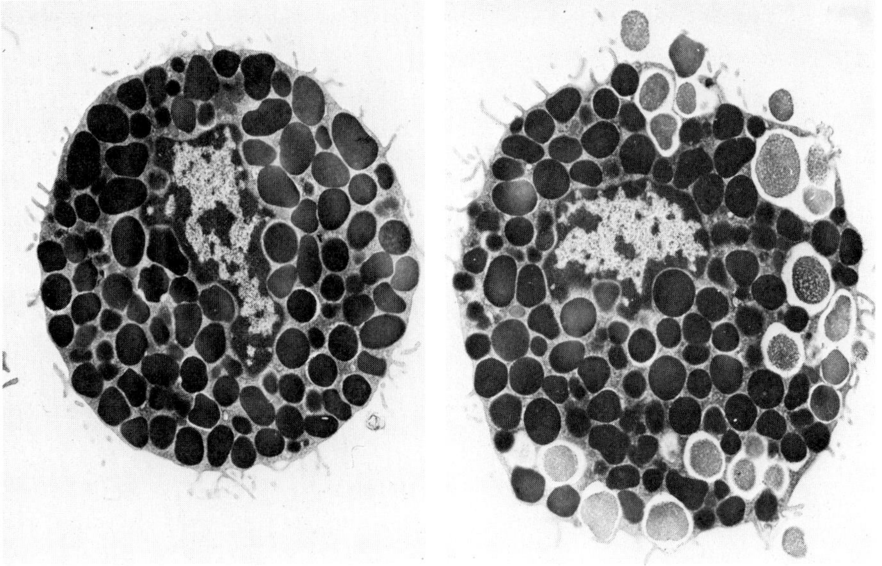

Figure 13.1.
Electron micrograph of a normal mast cell illustrating the large monocyte-like nucleus and the electron-dense granules. On the right, a mast cell has been triggered and is beginning to release the contents of its granules, as seen by their decrease in opacity and the formation of vacuoles connecting with the exterior. (Photos courtesy of Dr. T. Theoharides, Tufts Medical School.)

Triggering of the mast cell to release its granules and their pharmacologically active contents requires that at least two of the receptors for the Fc portion of the IgE molecules be bridged together in a stable configuration. In the simplest and immunologically most relevant manner, this linkage is accomplished by a multivalent antigen that can bind a different molecule of IgE to each of several epitopes on its surface, thus cross-linking them and effectively triggering the cell to respond (see Fig. 13.2). This linking of receptors may also be accomplished in other, experimentally useful ways, such as by addition of an antibody that is specific for IgE molecules, or for the IgE receptor molecules on the surface of mast cells, or even by use of dimers or aggregates of IgE (see Fig. 13.2).

The triggering of a mast cell by the bridging of its receptors initiates a rapid and complex series of events which, because of the ease with which its outcome can be measured, has served as a model for the study of activation of cells in general. Among the rapid changes known to occur are changes in membrane fluidity, which result from methylation of phospholipids and are followed by an influx of Ca^{2+} ions. At about this stage, energy generated by

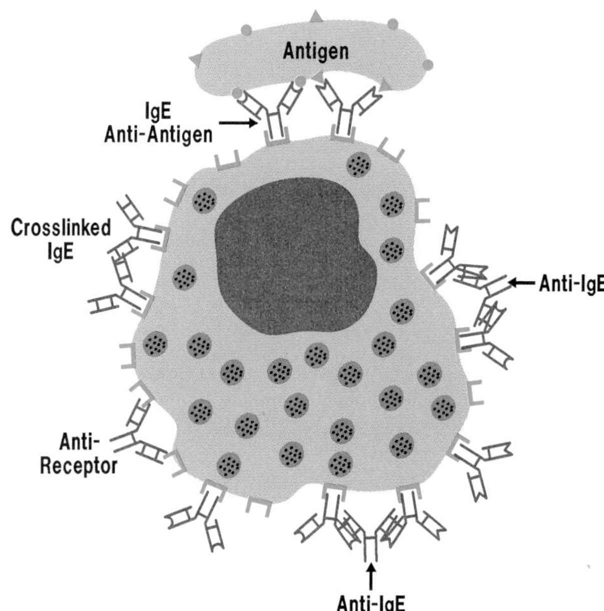

Figure 13.2.
Various modes of cross-linking receptors leading to mast cell activation and degranulation.

glycolysis is required, and certain enzymes are activated that allow the movement of the granules to the cell surface. The intracellular levels of cyclic adenosine monophosphate ***(cAMP)*** and cyclic guanosine monophosphate ***(cGMP)*** are known to affect subsequent events and are important in the regulation of those events. In general, an increase in intracellular cAMP at this stage will slow, or even stop, the process of degranulation. Thus, activation of ***adenylate cyclase,*** the enzyme that converts adenosine triphosphate (ATP) to cAMP, provides an important mechanism for controlling anaphylactic events, as is discussed in more detail later.

As a very rapid consequence of this series of events, the granules are moved, probably by microfilaments, to the cell surface, where their membranes fuse with the cell membrane and all the contents are released to the exterior (see Fig. 13.1). Depending on the extent of cross-linking on the cell surface, any cell can release some or all of its granules. Furthermore, this explosive release of granules is physiologic and does not imply lysis and death of the cell. In fact, the degranulated cells regenerate and, once the contents of the granules have been synthesized, the cells are ready to resume their function.

Effector Phase

The symptoms of anaphylaxis are entirely attributable to the pharmacologically active materials released by the activated mast cells. It is helpful to consider these mediators in two major categories (Table 13.1). One category consists of ***preformed mediators,*** which are stored in the granules by electrostatic attraction to a matrix protein and are released as a result of the influx of ions, primarily Na^+. The other category consists of ***substances synthesized de novo,*** in part from membrane lipids, and released during the anaphylactic response. Only the most important members of each category are considered in detail here.

TABLE 13.1. Mediators Released During Mast Cell Activation

Mediator	Structure	Function
A. *Preformed*		
Histamine	β-Imidazol-ethylamine (mol wt 111)	Increase vascular permeability; constrict smooth muscle
Serotonin	5-Hydroxytryptamine (mol wt 176)	Increase vascular permeability
Eosinophil chemotactic factor of anaphylaxis (ECF-A)	Tetrapeptides	Chemotactic attraction of eosinophils
Heparin	Acid proteoglycan (mol wt >500,000)	Inhibit coagulation of blood
B. *Newly synthesized*		
Slow reacting substance of anaphylaxis (SRS-A)	Cysteine peptide complexed to leukotrienes	Contraction of bronchiole; increased vascular permeability
Platelet-activating factor (PAF)	Lipid (?) (mol wt 400)	Platelet aggregation and release of histamine

HISTAMINE. Histamine is formed in the cell by decarboxylation of the amino acid histidine, and it is stored bound by electrostatic interaction to an acid matrix protein called ***heparin.*** When released, histamine binds rapidly to a variety of cells via two major types of receptor, ***H1 and H2,*** which have different distribution in tissue and which mediate different effects. When histamine binds to H1 receptors on smooth muscles it causes constriction;

when it binds to H1 receptors on endothelial cells it causes separations at their junctions, resulting in ***vascular permeability.*** H2 receptors are also involved in increased vascular permeability, as well as in the release of acid from stomach mucosa. All these effects are responsible for some of the major signs in systemic anaphylaxis—difficulty in breathing or asphyxiation due to ***constriction of smooth muscle*** around the bronchi in the lung, and a ***drop in blood pressure*** that results from extravasation of fluid into tissue spaces as the ***permeability of blood vessels increases***. H1 receptors are blocked by ***antihistamines***, such as benadryl, by direct competition, and when these drugs are given soon enough they can counteract the effects of histamine (blockage of H2 receptors requires other drugs, such as cimetidine). However, some time after the introduction of antihistamines, it was noted that they were ineffective in controlling constriction of smooth muscles that was slower in onset and more persistent than that produced by histamine. This observation led to the discovery of SRS-A, the slow-reacting substance of anaphylaxis (see below).

SEROTONIN. Serotonin is present in the mast cells of only certain species, such as rodents. Its effects are similar to those of histamine, in that it causes ***constriction of smooth muscle*** and ***increases vascular permeability.***

EOSINOPHILIC CHEMOTACTIC FACTOR OF ANAPHYLAXIS (ECF-A). Eosinophilic chemotactic factor is a set of ***peptides*** that produces a chemotactic gradient capable of attracting ***eosinophils*** to the site of release of these peptides. In anaphylactic reactions the eosinophils appear to serve as a belated indicator of the presence of IgE-mediated reactions; they may also release arylsulfatase and histaminase, which affect mediators of the hypersensitivity reaction. They have an additional function in parasitic worm infections that is discussed later in this chapter.

HEPARIN. Heparin is an ***acidic proteoglycan*** that constitutes the matrix of the granule, and to which basic mediators, such as histamine and serotonin, are bound. Its acidic nature accounts for the metachromatic (high-staining) properties of the mast cell when basic dyes such as toluidine blue are applied to it. Release of heparin causes ***inhibition of coagulation,*** which may be of some use in the subsequent recovery of the mast cell, but it is not involved in the symptoms of anaphylaxis.

SLOW-REACTING SUBSTANCE OF ANAPHYLAXIS. When a preparation of smooth muscle, such as a guinea pig uterine horn, is treated with histamine, rapid contraction occurs. The contraction is the basis of a sensitive bioassay for histamine, the ***Schultz-Dale reaction***. When the histamine is washed out, rapid relaxation occurs. Addition of an antihistamine to the assay inhibits the contraction effect of histamine, but if the supernatant solution from a preparation of activated mast cells is also included in the assay, the immediate contraction effect of histamine does not occur, but, instead, a slower prolonged contraction results, and it cannot easily be reversed by washing.

This observation led to the discovery of the ***slow-reacting substance of anaphylaxis (SRS-A),*** which is so potent and is present in such low concentration that its chemical structure defied analysis for many years. It is now known to consist of a set of peptides which are coupled to a metabolite of arachadonic acid called ***leukotrienes***. The leukotrienes have been named LTB4, LTC4, and LTD4 and, in minute amounts, they cause ***prolonged constriction of smooth muscle.*** They are considered to be the cause of much antihistamine-resistant asthma in humans.

PLATELET-ACTIVATING FACTOR. Platelet-activating factor (PAF) induces platelets to aggregate and release their contents of mediators, which include histamine and, in some species, serotonin. Activation of platelets may also induce release of metabolites of arachadonic acid, thus augmenting effects generated by mast cells.

Clinical Aspects of Type I Hypersensitivity

To summarize all the events that follow the release of the mediators of the anaphylactic response, we can describe a typical sequence of events. Contact with antigen causes cross-linking of IgE receptors on mast cells. The cross-linking induces each mast cell to release its contents of mediators. Probably the first mediator to act would be histamine (or serotonin in some species), which would induce dilation of blood vessels (flush) and an increase in their permeability (edema) if release of histamine occurred locally—for example, as a result of an intradermal injection. If release of histamine occurred systemically, as a result of the widespread dispersion of antigen, then much more severe consequences would ensue. This could include difficulty in breathing because of constriction of bronchiolar muscles, to uterine cramps, or to involuntary urination and defecation. In addition, widespread vascular permeability could produce a massive loss of fluid into tissue spaces and a collapse of blood pressure.

These life-threatening systemic problems are most effectively treated by the prompt administration of ***epinephrine,*** which directly reverses the effects of histamine by relaxing smooth muscle and decreasing vascular permeability. At this point, however, the effects of leukotrienes and various prostaglandins might become apparent, and a persistent, antihistamine-resistant asthma might appear. Eosinophilia might also be a symptom, indicating an IgE-mediated response.

If the causative agent of the response were one of many worm parasites, an additional series of events might occur. In such a case, the effects of increased permeability due to histamine serve to bring serum components, which include IgG autibody, to the site of worm infestation. The IgG antibody binds to the surface of the worm and attracts the eosinophils, which have migrated to the area as a result of the chemotactic effects of the ***eosinophilic chemotactic factor (ECF-A).*** The eosinophils then bind to the IgG-coated worm, by virtue of their membrane receptors for Fc, and release the contents of their granules (Fig. 13.3). The major constitutent of the contents of these granules is a very ***basic protein,*** which coats the surface of the worm and

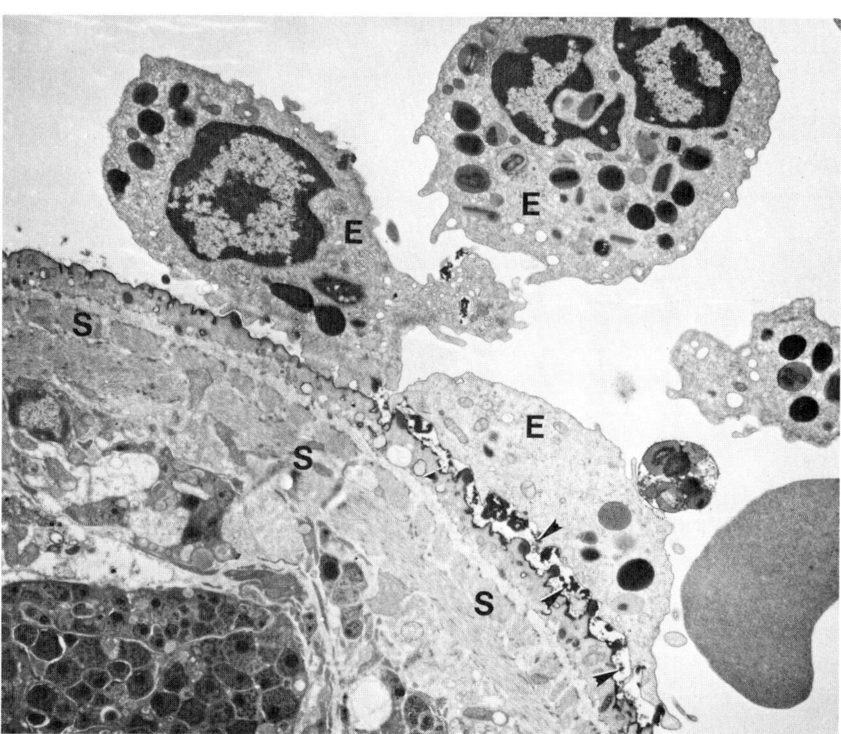

Figure 13.3.
Electron micrograph (× 6,000) of eosinophils (E) adhering to an Ab-coated schistosomulum (S). The cell on the left has not yet degranulated, but the one on the right has discharged electron-dense material (arrows), which can be seen between the cell and the worm. (Photo courtesy of Dr. J. Caulfield, Harvard Medical School.)

leads, in some unknown way, to the death of the worm and its eventual expulsion. Thus, all components of the type I reaction combine to perform this protective function.

The symptoms of anaphylaxis seen in systemic reactions vary widely with the species observed, although the basic mechanisms are the same. Guinea pigs, for example, die from asphyxiation produced by histamine-induced constriction of bronchioles, whereas dogs suffer from a pooling of the blood in the intestine and liver, vomiting, and diarrhea. Humans are confronted with three different possibilities of a lethal outcome: a) asphyxiation from laryngeal edema, b) suffocation from bronchiolar constriction, or c) loss of adequate blood pressure from overwhelming peripheral edema.

Intervention

ENVIRONMENTAL INTERVENTION. In some cases, the easiest treatment for allergy is avoidance. Thus, if the offending allergen is cat dander, the best advice to the patient (but advice that, surprisingly, is followed quite infrequently) is to get rid of the cat. If some pollens are the cause of the reaction, it may be possible for the patient to go to pollen-free areas during the season when the offending plant is pollinating. Masks and air filters also have a useful role to play, but usually avoidance is difficult for the general, atopic population.

PHARMACOLOGIC INTERVENTION. Modern pharmaceutical chemistry has provided a host of drugs that are more or less effective at various stages in the evolution of the anaphylactic reaction. In brief, these drugs include: 1) ***cromolyn sodium,*** which stabilizes membranes and decreases or preventsmast cell degranulation when inhaled before antigen exposure; 2) ***corticosteroids,*** especially when topically applied, which block the metabolic pathwayto arachadonic acid, and have general, anti-inflammatory effects and preventlate phase reactions; 3) ***antihistamines*** which compete with histamine for receptorsites,therebydecreasingorpreventingimmediatesymptomssuchassneezing, itching, and runny nose; and 4) ***epinephrine,*** which relaxes smooth muscle and constricts dilated blood vessels, reversing the effects of histamine.

IMMUNOLOGIC INTERVENTION. One form of intervention is injection therapy or ***hyposensitization.*** For many years, allergists have practiced a form of therapy whereby they inject patients, over an extended period, with increasing doses of the antigen to which they are sensitive. The improvement in symptoms noted in some patients has been ascribed to several different factors. The most popular rationale is based on the observation that such injections serve to increase the synthesis of IgG antibody specific for the allergen. Such antibody presumably binds to the allergen as it penetrates mucosal membranes and removes the allergen before it has a chance to react with the IgE antibody on the surface of mast cells. Thus, the term ***blocking antibody*** has become associated with this IgG, and there is a rough correlation between titers of this IgG antibody and clinical improvement.

Other findings during hyposensitization include an initial increase in levels of IgE antibody, followed by a prolonged decrease upon continued therapy. This decrease has been linked to a decrease in intensity of symptoms and is attributed either to induction of ***tolerance*** or of ***suppressor T cells*** (see Chapter 15). After repeated, subclinical doses of the antigen, there is also a progressive decrease in the sensitivity of mast cells and basophils to triggering by antigen. It is likely that the explanation for the apparent benefits of this therapy encompasses more than one of these demonstrable effects. Whatever the reason, this form of therapy is generally more successful in dealing with allergens that enter the circulation directly, such as bee sting venom, than for those allergens contacted via mucosal surfaces, such as pollen.

Hyposensitization therapy should be distinguished from ***desensitization***. Occasionally, a patient must be treated promptly with a substance to which he or she is allergic, for example, when horse anti-venom serum for treatment of a rattlesnake bite is given to someone who is sensitive to the horse serum antigens. The sensitive patient must then be given increasingly large doses of the horse anti-venom over a short period of time (hours), each dose being below the level that will precipitate a serious, systemic reaction. During this time, sufficient horse antigens are given to trigger enough sub-lethal discharges from mast cells that a therapeutic dose of antitoxin can be given without danger of inducing fatal anaphylaxis. The risk of severe reactions may also be reduced by prior administration of antihistamines and steroids. Such preliminary treatment causes a more-or-less temporary period of unreactivity during which, presumably, the available supply of IgE-sensitized mast cells is used up. In time, recovery of mast cells and new synthesis of IgE antibody lead to a restoration of the original sensitivity if the horse antigens in the antiserum are no longer administered.

In a clinical setting, the degree of sensitivity to a particular allergen is usually determined by a history and by the size of skin test reactions. A more quantitative assay is now available in the laboratory. Known as the ***radioallergosorbent (RAST) test***, this procedure (see Chapter 7) involves covalent coupling of the allergen to an insoluble matrix, such as paper discs or beads.

The prepared matrix is then dipped into a sample of the patient's serum and allowed to bind any antibody that is specific for the allergen. Then, after the disk is washed, a radiolabeled antibody specific for IgE is added. The amount of radioactivity bound is a measure of the amount of specific IgE antibody in the serum sample (see Fig. 7.15).

MODIFIED ALLERGENS. Experiments in animals have demonstrated that administration of a ***chemically altered allergen*** (e.g. ragweed pollen denatured by urea or coupled to polyethylene glycol) will suppress a primary or established IgE response. The mechanism appears to involve stimulation of ***suppressor T cells*** that are both antigen-specific and isotype-specific. The modified allergens do not combine with pre-existing IgE antibodies and, therefore, they do not trigger anaphylactic responses. Use of such modified allergens ***(allergoids)*** seems to offer a promising approach to treatment of allergy.

TYPE II—CYTOTOXIC REACTIONS

Introduction

In this form of hypersensitivity, binding of antibody directly to an antigen on the surface of a cell produces damage to that cell through a variety of mechanisms. These mechanisms involve either the complete complement sequence and eventual lysis of the cell or opsonic effects mediated by receptors for Fc or C3b, which lead to phagocytosis and destruction of the cell by macrophages and neutrophils.

Transfusion Reactions

The simplest form of cytotoxic reaction is seen after transfusion of ABO incompatible blood (see Chapter 17). As an example: people with type O blood have, in their circulation, as a consequence of lifelong exposure to antigens on bacteria, vegetables, etc., IgM anti-A and anti-B antibodies which react with the A and B blood group substances. If such a person were to be inappropriately transfused with a unit of packed type A red cells, the immediate consequences could be disastrous. Because there is a considerable amount of IgM anti-A antibody in this person's circulation, all the transfused type A red cells will bind some antibody. Because of the efficiency of IgM antibody in fixing complement (a single IgM molecule is sufficient to activate many complement molecules), and because of the absence of repair mechanisms, red cells will be lysed intravascularly by the destructive action of the complex of C5, 6, 7, 8, 9 on their membranes. The individual is then faced with the risk of kidney damage from blockage by large quantities of red cell membrane, plus the possible toxic effects from the release of the heme complex.

Rh Incompatibility Reaction

A somewhat similar mechanism is exemplified by the ***Rhesus (Rh) incompatibility reaction*** seen in infants born of parents with Rh-incompatible blood groups (see Chapter 17). In the simplest case, an Rh^+ child born to an Rh^- mother, releases some of its red cells into the mother's circulation sometime around birth. Only if the mother is thereby sufficiently immunized to produce anti-Rh IgG antibody will subsequent Rh^+ children be at risk, since, as stated in Chapter 5, only IgG antibody is capable of crossing the placenta.

When the anti-Rh IgG antibodies have crossed the placenta, they bind to the Rh antigen on the red cells of the fetus. Because the density of Rh antigen on the surface of red blood cells is low, these antibodies usually fail to agglutinate or lyse the cells directly. However, the antibody-coated cells are readily destroyed by the opsonic effect of the Fc portions of the IgG, which interact with the receptors for Fc on the phagocytic cells of the reticuloendothelial system. The result is progressive destruction of the fetal or newborn red cells, with the pathological consequences that come from decreased transport of oxygen and result in jaundice from the products of the breakdown of hemoglobin. Until fairly recently, replacement transfusion was frequently required to save these infants from lasting damage.

A very simple prophylactic measure is now used to avoid these disastrous consequences. In cases of Rh-incompatible matings, the mother is given an injection of anti-Rh antibody ***(Rhogam)*** shortly after the birth of her Rh^+ child. This passively administered antibody serves to remove the child's Rh^+ red cells from the mother's circulation before they have been able to immunize her. Thus, when the passive antibody has been removed, the mother remains an immunologic virgin, able to carry another child without possible disastrous consequences.

Autoimmune Hemolytic Anemia

As a consequence of certain infectious diseases, or for other, still unknown reasons, some people produce an antibody reactive against their own red cells. This antibody, on reacting with the red cells, shortens their life-span by mechanisms that involve hemolysis or phagocytosis via receptors for Fc and C3b and that lead to progressive anemia if the production of new red cells cannot keep pace with destruction. Occasionally, the antibody only binds effectively at lower temperatures ***(cold agglutination),*** in which case lowering of the body temperature, and particularly the temperature of the arms and legs, leads to effective antibody-binding and destruction of the red cells.

Drug-Induced Reactions

In some people, some drugs act as haptens and combine with circulating blood constituents to induce antibody formation. When antibody and the cell that carries the drug are present together, cytotoxic damage results. The type of pathologic injury depends on the type of cell that binds the drug. Thus, for example, Sedormid (a sedative) binds to platelets and the resulting antibody directed against it causes lysis of the platelets and ***thrombocytopenia*** (low blood platelet count). This disorder, in turn, can give rise to ***purpura*** (bleeding) which is the main problem in thrombocytopenic purpura. Withdrawal of the offending drug leads to a cessation of symptoms.

Other drugs, such as chloramphenicol (an antibiotic), may bind to white cells; phenacetin (an analgesic) and chlorpromazine (a tranquilizer) may bind to red cells. The consequences of an immune response to these drugs can lead to an ***agranulocytosis*** (decrease in granulocytes) in the case of white cells and a ***hemolytic anemia*** in the case of red cells. Damage to the target cell in these examples may be mediated by either of the two mechanisms described above: by cytolysis via the complement pathway or by destruction of cells by phagocytosis mediated by receptors for Fc or C3b.

TYPE III—IMMUNE COMPLEX REACTIONS

Introduction

In 1903, a French scientist named Arthus immunized rabbits with horse serum by repeated intradermal injection. After several weeks, he noted that each succeeding injection produced an increasingly severe reaction at the site of inoculation. At first a mild ***erythema*** (redness) and ***edema*** (accumulation of fluid) was noticed within 2–4 hours of injection. These reactions subsided without consequence by the following day, but subsequent injections produced larger edematous responses, and by the fifth or sixth inoculation the lesions became hemorrhagic with ***necrosis*** and were slow to heal. This phenomenon, known as the ***Arthus reaction,*** is the prototype of all immune complex reactions or reactions mediated by aggregates of antibody and antigen.

A second type of immune complex reaction is called ***serum sickness***. This term derives from observations made at the turn of the century by Von Pirquet and Schick of the consequence of the treatment of certain infectious diseases, such as diphtheria and tetanus, with antisera made in horses. It was well known that the pathologic consequences of infection by both the Corynebacterium and the Clostridium organisms were due to the secretion of exotoxins that are extremely damaging to host cells. The bacteria themselves are relatively noninvasive and of little consequence. Hence, the strategy that evolved to treat these diseases was to neutralize the toxins rapidly, before quantities large enough to kill the host became fixed in tissues. Since active immunization required several weeks before useful levels of antibody were produced, it was necessary to inject large amounts of a preformed, antitoxin antibody as soon as the disease was diagnosed, in order to prevent death by toxin. Horses, being readily available, easily immunized, and capable of yielding large quantities of useful antisera, were the animals of choice for the production of antitoxin. Today, we know that the administration of large quantities of heterologous serum causes the recipient to synthesize antibodies to the heterologous Ig and leads to serum sickness.

The Arthus Reaction

The Arthus reaction usually requires relatively large amounts of antibody and antigen and, hence, is demonstrated most readily in rabbits, which can be induced by immunization to make large quantities of IgG. However, similar reactions are seen in many species including humans.

Antigen injected intradermally in an immune animal diffuses towards blood vessels which contain the circulating antibody. When antigen and antibody meet, at the appropriate concentrations, in or near vessel walls (venules), they form ***insoluble antigen–antibody complexes*** and accumulate (see Fig. 13.4), much as they would on a gel diffusion (Ouchterlony) plate (see Chapter 7). When the aggregates become large enough, the adjacent Fc regions of the IgG molecules bind the first component of complement and begin the ***activation of the complement cascade*** (see Chapter 8). The formation of ***C3a and C5a (anaphylotoxins)*** causes an increased local permeability of blood vessels, with leakage of fluid from the vessels (edema). Other components are chemotactic and attract ***neutrophils,*** and these neutrophils, together with ***platelets,*** begin to

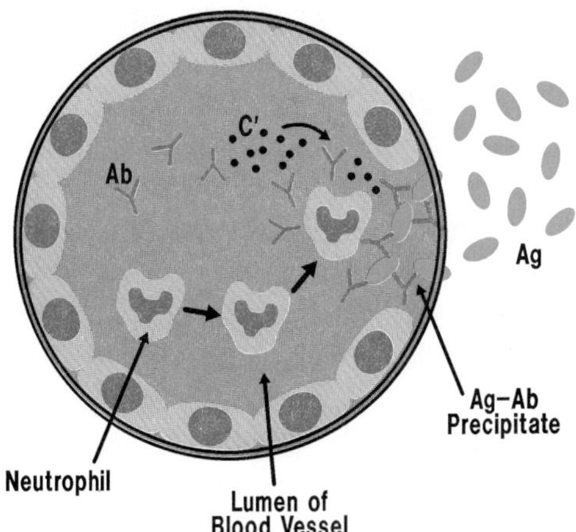

Figure 13.4.
A schematic representation of the Arthus reaction.

pile up at the site of the reaction. Eventually, stasis of blood flow and complete blockage of the blood vessel occurs. The activated neutrophils phagocytize the immune complexes and, together with the clumped platelets, release a complex array of ***proteases, collagenases,*** and ***vasoactive substances.*** The end result is rupture of the vessel wall and ***hemorrhage,*** accompanied by ***necrosis*** of local tissue.

The experimental proof of this course of events involves the demonstration, by use of fluorescent antibodies, that antigen, antibody, and various complement components can all be detected at the site of damage to the vessel wall. The requirement for complement and granulocytes together was shown in experiments in which animals depleted of complement ***(by cobra venom factor)*** or of neutrophils (by specific anti-polymorphonuclear cell serum) formed aggregates of antigen and antibody, but did not produce the characteristic Arthus reactions.

While it is the prototype for type III immune aggregate reactions, the Arthus reaction is clinically the least commonly seen. Nevertheless, it best illustrates the underlying mechanism of immune aggregate reactions.

Serum Sickness

The strategy of passive immunization for treatment of diseases whose effects were due to production of toxins worked very well and was widely used until universal immunization of children became standard practice. However, some recipients of therapy with horse antisera, while spared the bacteriologic disease and the effect of the toxin, developed undesirable reactions. About 1–2 weeks after receiving the horse serum they developed fever and itchy, edematous rashes over parts of their bodies, painful swollen joints and enlarged lymph nodes. Occasionally their urine was found to contain red cells and albumin, a sign of inflammation in the glomerular apparatus of the kidney. In time, all these symptoms subsided with little residual damage, but a repeat injection of horse serum could induce much more severe symptoms and even death. While this sequence of events, as we shall see, can be induced by many other types of antigens, it still bears the name ***"serum sickness."***

The mechanism of the type of reaction typified by serum sickness is best understood by reference to the animal model that was instrumental in its clarification. In this model, a rabbit is injected with a large amount of a foreign protein, such as bovine serum albumin (BSA). After equilibration in the body fluid spaces, the protein begins to disappear at a rate characteristic of normal, biodegradative processes (Fig. 13.5). After about 8–10 days, there is a sudden

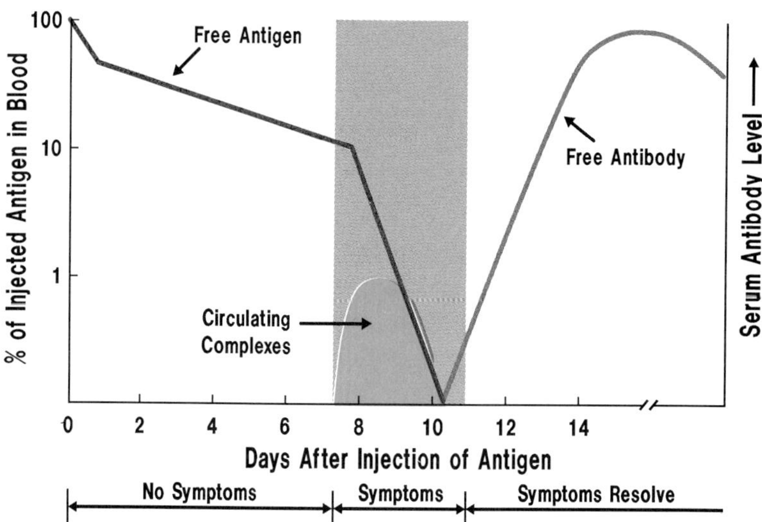

Figure 13.5.
The relationship between circulating antigen-antibody complexes and serum sickness.

change in the rate of disappearance, and the residual free protein is completely cleared from the circulation. This event, termed ***immune elimination***, is soon followed by the appearance of free circulating antibodies to BSA. It is during the period that corresponds with the onset of rapid disappearance of antigen and ends with the rise in the level of free antibody that the symptoms of serum sickness appear. At the same time, there is a drop in the normal level of complement activity in the serum.

These changes were explained by the discovery, in the circulating blood, of soluble complexes of the antigen BSA and antibodies to BSA. With the onset of production of antibody, the first complexes formed are those that involve a relatively small amount of antibody and an excess of antigen. Reference to the precipitin curve (see Chapter 7) will show that such complexes are small (of the order of $\boldsymbol{Ag_2Ab}$ or $\boldsymbol{Ag_3Ab_2}$) and soluble. Nevertheless, these complexes are unable to penetrate various tissue barriers, and so they tend to pile up against the basement membrane in glomeruli, in joint synovia, and on the walls of blood vessels. As more antibody is formed, the complexes increase in size and are progressively removed from the circulation, so that the rate of clearance of antigen increases.

An important observation in the rabbit model of serum sickness was that if several rabbits were similarly injected with a large dose of BSA, they tended subsequently to fall into three groups. The first group made no antibody and cleared the antigen at a steady rate with no symptoms of serum sickness. The second group produced copious amounts of antibody, cleared the antigen very rapidly, and had only transient and minimal symptoms. Apparently, large amounts of antibody produce large complexes, which are removed by the macrophages of the reticuloendothelial system and produce few clinical symptoms. It was in the third group, i.e the group that made only small amounts of antibody, that symptoms of serum sickness were most prolonged and most severe. In this group, a chronic disease resulted from the continual production of soluble complexes generated from excess of antigen and low levels of antibody. The continuous pile-up of such complexes on membranes leads to the appearance of so-called ***lumpy-bumpy deposits*** that are visualized by fluorescence microscopy of lesions on glomerular basement membrane lesions (see Fig. 13.6). Once deposited, the complexes behave much as those in the Arthus reaction. Adjacent Fc regions of the IgG molecules bind C1q and initiate the ***complement*** cascade. The chemotactically induced influx of ***granulocytes*** into the lesion is the critical event that leads to the loss of integrity of the basement membrane. As a result of the actions of the degradative enzymes released from the ***lysosomal granules*** of the ***neutrophils,*** the membrane is disrupted and leaks serum and red cells into the urine. The attendant ***necrosis,*** if sufficiently widespread, can jeopardize the entire kidney function.

Similar events may occur in blood vessels of the skin, heart, and lung, as well as in joint synovial spaces. While there tends to be preferential localization of lesions in certain clinical conditions (e.g. in skin, rather than in glomerular basement membrane or joints) the reasons for this preferential localization are not well understood. It may be that the nature of the complexes or of the antigen determine their eventual localization.

An alternative mechanism for generating complexes at a specific site has been described recently. This mechanism involves the nonspecific infiltration of a tissue site by antigen before synthesis of antibody commences. When circulating antibody appears, it binds to the tissue-fixed antigen, thus generating complexes in situ rather than in the circulation. This mechanism may be particularly relevant for certain antigens, such as DNA, which is known to bind preferentially to the collagen of basement membranes. In all other details, however, the consequences are identical whether the complexes are formed locally or in the circulation.

Infection-Associated Immune Complex Disease

In a variety of infections and for as yet unknown reasons, some individuals produce an antibody that cross-reacts with somc constitucnt of normal tissue. Thus, in ***Goodpasture's syndrome,*** for example, ***pulmonary hemorrhage*** and ***glomerulonephritis*** have been shown to be due to an antibody that binds directly to the ***basement membrane,*** fixes complement, and causes membrane damage as a consequence of accumulation of neutrophils and release of degradative enzymes. The only distinction between infection-associated immune complex disease and immune aggregate disease is that microscopic examination of the lesions reveals a linear, ***ribbonlike deposit*** along the basement membrane (see Fig. 13.6), as would be expected if an even carpet of antibody were bound to surface antigens.

Rheumatic fever, a disease that can follow a throat infection with group A streptococci, involves inflammation and damage to heart, joints, and kidneys. A variety of antigens in the cell walls and membranes of streptococci have been shown to be cross-reactive with antigens present in human heart muscle, cartilage, and glomerular basement membrane. It is presumed that antibody to the streptococcal antigens binds to these components of normal tissue and induces inflammatory reactions via a pathway similar to that described above.

In ***rheumatoid arthritis,*** there is evidence for the production of ***rheumatoid factor,*** an IgM autoantibody, that binds to the Fc portion of normal IgG. These immunoglobulin complexes are thought by some investigators to be ultimately responsible for the inflammation of joints and the damage characteristic of this disease.

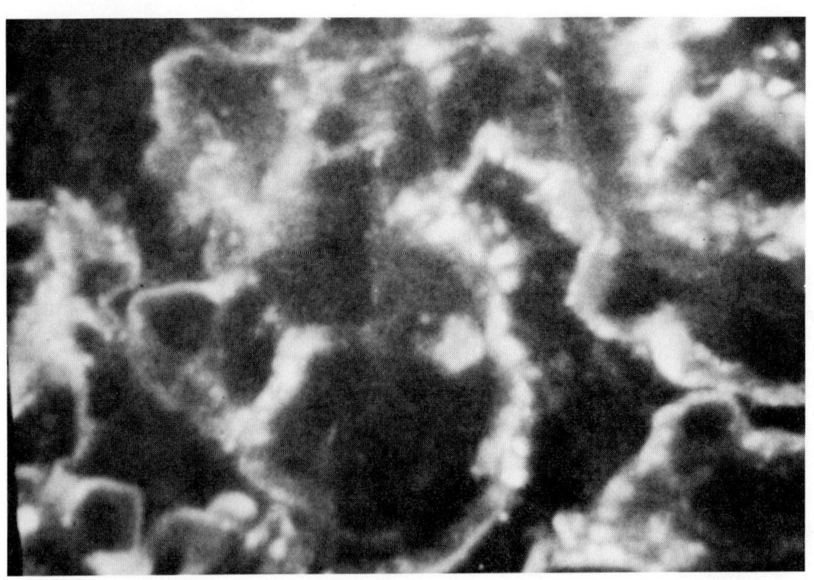

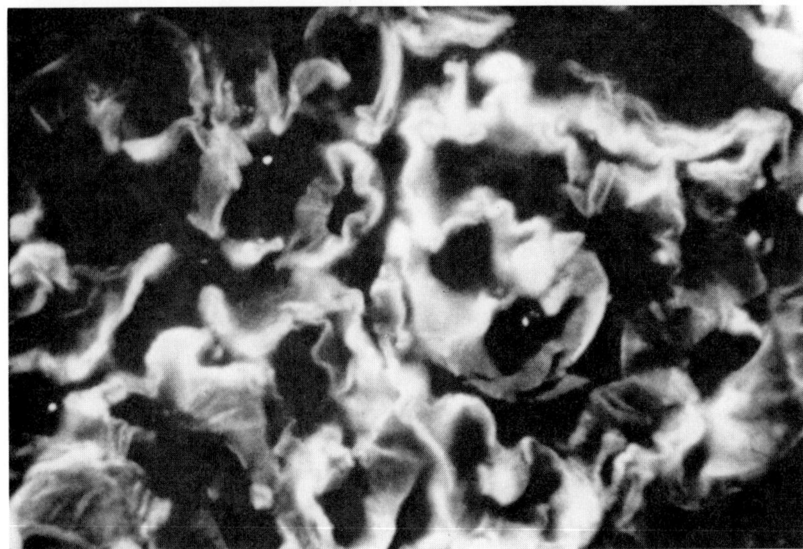

Figure 13.6.
Histology of immune aggregate lesions in kidney glomeruli. On top, the "lumpy-bumpy" deposits produced by a pile-up of antigen–antibody aggregates against basement membrane is revealed by staining with a fluorescent antibody to human IgG. On the bottom, the "ribbonlike" or "linear" deposits, produced by binding of antibody to an antigen present in the basement membrane, is revealed by staining with a fluorescent antibody to human IgG. (Photos courtesy of Dr. A. Ucci, Tufts Medical School.)

In a number of ***infectious diseases*** (malaria, viral infections, leprosy) there may be times during the course of the infection when large amounts of antigen and antibody exist simultaneously and cause the formation of immune aggregates that are deposited in a bewildering variety of locations. Thus, the complex of symptoms may include a component attributable to a type III hypersensitivity reaction.

Occupational Diseases

Farmer's lung is a prototypic form of the class III reactions classified as ***"occupational diseases."*** In sensitive individuals, exposure to mouldy hay leads, within 6–8 hours, to severe respiratory distress or ***pneumonitis.*** It has been shown that affected individuals have made large amounts of IgG antibody specific for the thermophilic actinomycetes that grow on spoiled hay. Inhalation of the bacterial spores leads to a reaction in the lungs that resembles the Arthus reaction seen in skin—namely, the formation of antigen–antibody aggregates and consequent inflammation.

There are many similar pulmonary type III reactions that bear names related to the occupation or causative agent, such as ***Pigeon breeder's disease, Cheese washer's disease, bagassosis*** (bagasse refers to sugar cane fiber), ***Maple bark stripper's disease, Paprika worker's disease,*** and the increasingly rare, ***Thatched roof worker's lung.*** Dirty work environments, involving massive exposure to potentially antigenic material, obviously lend themselves to the development of this form of occupational disease.

SUMMARY

1. *Type I anaphylactic reactions* are mediated by IgE antibodies, which bind to specific receptors on the surface of mast cells and basophils. When these receptors are cross-linked by contact with specific antigen, the cell is triggered to respond by releasing its granules and their contents. The combined pharmacologic effects of the mediators produce the immediate symptoms typical of this response: *increased vascular permeability, constriction of smooth muscles,* and *influx of eosinophils*. Despite the dangerous systemic reactions produced by this mode of immune response, its value probably lies in its ability to provide immunity to parasitic infections.

2. *Type II hypersensitivity reactions* involve damage to target cells and are mediated by antibody through two major pathways. In the first pathway, antibody (usually *IgM,* but also *IgG*) activates the entire *complement* sequence and causes *cell lysis*. In the second pathway, antibody (usually *IgG*) serves to

engage receptors for *Fc on phagocytic* cells and causes destruction of the antibody-coated target. These reactions usually involve circulating blood cells, such as red cells, white cells and platelets, and the consequences are those that would be expected from destruction of the particular type of cell.

3. *Type III immune complex reactions* involve the formation of antigen-antibody complexes that can activate the complement cascade. Release of certain products of the complement sequence (*C3a* and *C5a*) causes a local increase in vessel permeability and permits the release of serum (*edema*) and the chemotactic attraction of *neutrophils*. The neutrophils, in the process of ingesting the immune complexes, release degradative *lysosomal enzymes* that produce the tissue damage characteristic of these reactions. If the site of reaction is a vessel wall, the outcome is *hemorrhage* and *necrosis;* if the site is a glomerular basement membrane, loss of integrity and release of protein and red cells into the urine results; and if the site is a joint meniscus, destruction of synovial membranes and cartilage occurs. Multiple forms of this response exist, depending on the type and location of antigen and the way in which it is brought together with antibody. In all cases, however, the outcome depends on complement and granulocytes as mediators of tissue injury.

REFERENCES

Bellanti JA (ed) (1985): Immunology. Chapter 13. Philadelphia: W.B. Saunders.

Ishizaka T, White JR, Saito H (1986): Biochemical events involved in IgE-dependent mediator release. Progress in Immunol 6:870.

Parker WC (ed) (1980): Clinical Immunology, Vol I, chapters 5 and 6. Philadelphia: W.B. Saunders.

(*Continued on next page*)

REVIEW QUESTIONS

For questions 1–14, choose the ONE BEST answer or completion:

1. Injection therapy (hyposensitization)
   a) is safe if used initially with high concentrations of antigen.
   b) is more effective for symptoms of hay fever than for wasp sting.
   c) directly affects stability of membranes.
   d) is a form of active immunity.
   e) induces large amounts of endogenous antihistamines.

2. Epinephrine
   a) causes bronchodilation.
   b) is effective even after anaphylactic symptoms commence.
   c) relaxes smooth muscle.
   d) decreases vessel permeability.
   e) all of the above.

3. An IgE myeloma protein
   a) can competitively inhibit binding of normal IgE to mast cells.
   b) is the most commonly found form.
   c) will inhibit binding of antigen to IgE antibody.
   d) will spontaneously induce anaphylaxis.
   e) will increase a patient's immediate skin test response to an antigen.

4. The following mechanism(s) may be involved in the clinical efficacy of injection therapy:
   a) enhanced production of IgG, which binds allergen before it reaches mast cells.
   b) enhanced production of suppressor T cells.
   c) decreased sensitivity of mast cells and basophils to degranulation by allergen.
   d) decreased production of IgE antibody.
   e) all of the above.

5. Fatal anaphylaxis in humans and dogs
   a) has identical symptoms.
   b) involves mast cells in humans only.
   c) is very rapid.
   d) has similar target organs.
   e) occurs only in genetically susceptible individuals.

6. Which of the following clinical diseases is most likely to involve a reaction to a hapten in its etiology?
   a) systemic lupus erythematosus.
   b) hemolytic anemia after treatment with penicillin.
   c) rheumatoid arthritis.
   d) farmer's lung.
   e) rejection of kidney graft.

7. In order to prevent hemolytic disease in a newborn with a type O, Rh^- mother and a type AB, Rh^+ father, you would:

a) administer Rhogam to the mother after the birth of her first child.
b) administer Rhogam to her first Rh^+ child.
c) administer Rhogam to each subsequent child.
d) administer Rhogam to the mother after each child.
e) do nothing; there is little danger to any of her children.

8. An IgA antibody to a red cell antigen is unlikely to cause autoimmune hemolytic anemia because
a) it would be made only in the gastrointestinal tract.
b) its Fc region would not bind to receptors for Fc on phagocytic cells.
c) it can fix complement only as far as C 1, 4, 2.
d) it has too low an affinity.
e) it requires a secretory component to work.

9. The glomerular lesions in immune complex disease can be visualized microscopically with a fluorescent antibody against
a) IgG heavy chains.
b) kappa light chains.
c) C1.
d) C3.
e) all of the above.

10. The lesion in immune complex-induced glomerulonephritis
a) is dependent on erythrocytes and complement.
b) results in increased production of urine.
c) requires both complement and neutrophils.
d) is dependent on the presence of macrophages.
e) requires all nine components of complement.

11. Serum sickness occurs only
a) when anti-basement-membrane antibodies are present.
b) in cases of extreme excess of antibody.
c) when IgE antibody is produced.
d) when soluble immune complexes are formed.
e) in the absence of neutrophils.

12. Immune complexes are involved in the pathogenesis of
a) post-streptococcal glomerulonephritis.
b) Pigeon breeder's disease.
c) glomerulonephritis of systemic lupus erythematosus.
d) an edematous hemorrhagic reaction in the skin of a bee keeper, 2 hours after he was stung for the 20th time.
e) all of the above.

13. The Arthus reaction and Farmer's lung *differ* because
a) only the former is due to antigen–antibody complexes.
b) the mode of contact with the antigen is different.
c) only the former requires complement.
d) only the latter can occur in farmers.
e) the reactions in Farmer's lung are much more rapid.

(*Continued on next page*)

14. The final damage to blood vessels in immune-complex–mediated arthritis is due to
    a) lymphokines from T cells.
    b) histamine and SRS-A.
    c) the C5, 6, 7, 8, 9 attack complex.
    d) lysosomal enzymes of polymorphonuclear leukocytes.
    e) cytotoxic T cells.

For questions 15–23, ONE or MORE of the completions given is correct. Choose the appropriate answer:
A) if only *1, 2, 3* are correct
B) if only *1 and 3* are correct
C) if only *2 and 4* are correct
D) if only *4* is correct
E) if *all* are correct

15. Serum sickness is characterized by
    1) deposition of immune complexes in blood vessel walls, when there is a moderate excess of antigen.
    2) phagocytosis of complexes by granulocytes.
    3) consumption of complement.
    4) appearance of symptoms before free antibody can be detected in the circulation.

16. The Arthus reaction involves
    1) lymphocytic infiltrate around veins.
    2) formation of antigen–antibody precipitates on vessel walls.
    3) cross-linking of IgE antibody.
    4) complement fixation.

17. In the Masugi model of autoimmune disease, IgG antibody to rat kidney antigens is produced in rabbits. When this antibody is injected into rats it might be expected to
    1) produce nephrotoxic damage.
    2) produce a linear deposit in the kidney.
    3) induce neutrophils as the predominant cell type in the kidney lesions.
    4) require complement for deposition of antibody in the kidney.

18. Circulating immune complexes are an etiologic factor in the following diseases:
    1) skin lesions of systemic lupus erythematosus.
    2) Farmer's lung.
    3) glomerulonephritis, after treatment with horse anti-tetanus antiserum.
    4) Goodpasture's syndrome.

19. Immediate hypersensitivity skin reactions
    1) usually occur within 15 minutes.
    2) exhibit a raised wheal due to infiltration by mononuclear cells.
    3) exhibit a red flare due to vasodilation.
    4) can be elicited by monovalent haptens.

20. Mast cells
    1) are found circulating in the blood.
    2) release their granules by lysing.
    3) are basophilic after complete degranulation.
    4) are very similar to basophils.

21. Antihistamines
    1) bind to receptors for histamine, thereby preventing the histamine from exerting a pharmacologic effect.
    2) are more effective given before, rather than after, the onset of allergic symptoms.

3) do not influence the activity of leukotrienes.
4) do not affect binding of IgE to mast cells.

22. In the RAST assay for ragweed pollen
1) the patient's serum is first mixed with a radiolabeled anti-IgE.
2) only IgE anti-ragweed antibodies are detected.
3) the patient's serum competitively inhibits binding of the anti-IgE.
4) the allergen is covalently coupled to an insoluble matrix.

23. Antigen interaction with IgE antibody is associated with
1) Prausnitz-Kustner reaction.
2) Schultz-Dale reaction.
3) rhinitis due to ragweed pollen.
4) eosinophilia.

ANSWERS TO REVIEW QUESTIONS

1. ***d*** At least one of the proposed rationales for use of injection therapy involves the production of IgG-blocking antibody induced by active immunization. a,b, and e are false, and there is no basis for c.

2. ***e*** All are effects of epinephrine and make it useful for treatment of acute anaphylactic symptoms.

3. ***a*** IgE is the least common myeloma protein because of the smaller number of precursor B cells for this type of antibody. Production of large amounts of IgE globulin will compete for binding sites on mast cells, preventing specific IgE from binding. c and d are false; the converse of e is true.

4. ***e*** All are considered to be involved to varying degrees in injection therapy.

5. ***c*** Anaphylaxis is very rapid in all species but differs in symptomatology. Anaphylactic sensitivity can be induced in virtually all individuals, but only a proportion becomes sensitized through normal, air-borne contact.

6. ***b*** Penicillin can function as a hapten, binding to red cells and inducing a hemolytic anemia. a, b, and c are examples of immune aggregate (type III) reactions requiring complement and neutrophils for pathologic effects. Graft rejection is primarily T-cell–mediated (type IV).

(Continued on next page)

7. ***e*** Since the mother is type O, she would presumably have circulating antibodies to A and B blood groups. These antibodies should bind to the child's red cells (which would be A^+ or B^+), thus removing them from the circulation and reducing the risk that she would be immunized to the Rh^+ antigen. a or d would be required if, for some reason, she had low circulating isohemagglutinin titers or none at all. Under no circumstances is Rhogam given the child (b, c) since it would reproduce the disease in the child.

8. ***b*** Since phagocytic cells have Fc receptors for IgG, bound IgA would not cause engulfment and damage. a, c, d, e are false.

9. ***e*** The lesions in immune complex disease are dependent on the presence of antigen, antibody, and complement. Hence, all can be demonstrated by immunofluorescence at a lesion: a and b, because they are parts of IgG; c and d, because they are the early components of complement fixed by the immune aggregates.

10. ***c*** Damage by immune complexes requires complement components to attract neurophils, which are the agents responsible for subsequent tissue damage. Lysis by the final sequence of C6, 7, 8, 9 is not required.

11. ***d*** Anti-basement membrane antibodies may produce damage but can be distinguished from serum sickness lesions by their ribbonlike appearance compared to the "lumpy-bumpy" appearance of serum sickness lesions. Excess of antibody would clear antigen rapidly with few lesions. IgE antibody is responsible for anaphylactic reactions and neutrophils are required for the lesions typical of serum sickness.

12. ***e*** All are examples of type III hypersensitivity reactions: a, by production of antibody, which reacts with normal kidney antigen; b, by inhalation of antigens from pigeon droppings; c, by deposition of immune complexes formed by binding of an autoantibody to native DNA; and d is a description of an Arthus reaction in someone who has been immunized by repeated injection of bee venom.

13. ***b*** Both the Arthus reaction and Farmer's lung are examples of immune aggregate reactions that require complement and neutrophils. The former involves antigen injected into the skin, the latter involves inhaled antigen.

14. ***d*** Neither T cells nor mast cells are responsible for the final tissue damage in immune complex disease. Therefore a, b and e are eliminated. The final lytic complex of complement is similarly not involved, since complement activation up to C5 is sufficient to bring in the polymorphonuclear leukocytes, whose lysosomal enzymes cause the tissue damage.

15. ***E*** All are characteristics of serum sickness.

16. ***C*** 1 is characteristic of cell-mediated immunity (type IV) reactions and 3 of anaphylactic (type I) reactions.

17. ***A*** Complement is not required for binding of the injected antibody to the basement membrane, but once antibody is bound, complement is fixed, neutrophils are attracted and kidney damage occurs in the usual pattern for glomerulonephritis. Since the antigen is present on kidney membranes, antibody will form linear arrays.

18. ***B*** Farmer's lung involves formation of local rather than blood-borne antigen–antibody aggregates, and Goodpasture's syndrome is caused by antibody binding to antigen in situ. 1 and 3 have circulating soluble complexes.

19. ***B*** 2 is incorrect because the wheal is due to fluid, and 4 is incorrect because multivalent antigens are required to cross-link IgE molecules.

20. ***D*** Mast cells release granules physiologically and not by lysing, they are basophilic before they degranulate, and they are not found circulating freely.

21. ***E*** All are correct statements.

22. ***C*** The RAST assay measures IgE antibody which is allowed to bind to allergen coupled to an insoluble matrix.

23. ***E*** All involve IgE-mediated responses: 1) in the skin; 2) in an experimental system in vitro; 3) in an atopic nose; and 4) in response to a chronic antigenic challenge (to worm parasites, for example).

CHAPTER

14

DELAYED TYPE HYPERSENSITIVITY: T-CELL–MEDIATED IMMUNITY

INTRODUCTION

In contrast to antibody-mediated immunity, ***cell-mediated immunity (CMI)*** involves those aspects of immune function that are primarily carried out by antigen-specific, thymus-derived lymphocytes (T cells). When activated by contact with an antigen presented by appropriate accessory cells (see Chapter 11), the T cells release soluble mediators called lymphokines, which attract and activate other mononuclear cells such as monocytes, macrophages, and non-immune lymphocytes. This activation is an example of a cascade: the activation of very few, antigen-specific T cells leads to a reaction in which the large majority of the mononuclear cells that are present and responsible for the eventual outcome of the reactions is non-antigen-specific in function. The antigen eliciting this type of response may be foreign tissue (as in allograft reactions), an intracellular parasite (e.g. viruses and mycobacteria), a soluble protein, or one of many chemicals capable of penetrating skin and coupling to body proteins which serve as carriers.

The nomenclature for this type of response has varied over the years, based on historic usage. Originally the response was termed the ***tuberculin reaction,*** from the observation by Koch, in 1890, that people infected with

Mycobacterium tuberculosis gave a positive skin test when injected intradermally with a concentrated lysate of a mycobacterial culture (old tuberculin; OT). Subsequently, the delayed nature of the onset of these responses (days, in contrast to minutes or hours for antibody-mediated responses) has led to their collective designation as ***delayed-type hypersensitivity*** (DTH) reactions. With the discovery that all these reactions are the consequence of an initial response by T cells, they are now classified as examples of T cell–mediated or, more simply, cell-mediated immunity (CMI). According to the Gell and Coombs classification of hypersensitivity reactions, DTH or CMI reactions are classified as type IV reactions. This chapter deals with the nature and underlying mechanisms of these reactions.

GENERAL CHARACTERISTICS

Induction

A period of sensitization (1–2 weeks) after the first contact with antigen is required to permit an increase in the size of the T cell clone(s) specific for the particular antigen. The antigen involved must first be presented in association with the requisite ***class II MHC*** product (***Ia*** antigen in the mouse; ***HLA-D*** in humans) on the surface of an accessory cell. In the case of intracellular parasites that reside in macrophages, this presentation may be a direct consequence of their growth in these cells. Other antigens, such as proteins or viruses growing in MHC class II^- cells, may have to be processed first and then presented by MHC class II^+ accessory cells.

Because T cells are recirculating cells, once induced in adequate numbers they can make their way through lymph nodes to draining lymphatics, into the general circulation via the thoracic duct, and back into lymph via post-capillary venules. Thus, a T cell is eminently capable of contacting antigen at any site in the body, no matter how remote. Upon second contact with antigen, again in association with class II MHC antigens, a series of events is triggered that leads to the outcome characteristic of CMI.

Gross Appearance and Histology

An intradermal injection of antigen in a sensitized animal or person does not lead to an apparent response until some 18–24 hours after challenge. This time course characteristically distinguishes CMI from antibody-mediated reactions, which appear much more quickly (see Chapter 13). After about 18–24 hours, evidence of ***erythema*** (redness) and ***induration*** (raised thickening) appear, reaching maximal levels 24–48 hours after the challenge. The induration can easily be distinguished from edema (fluid) by absence of pitting when pressure is applied. These reactions, even when severe, rarely lead to necrotic damage and resolve slowly.

A biopsy taken early in the reaction would reveal primarily mononuclear cells of the monocyte–macrophage series with a few scattered lymphocytes (see Fig. 14.1). Characteristically, the monocytes appear as a perivascular cuff before extensively invading the site of deposition of antigen. Neutrophils are not a prominent feature of the reaction. Later biopsies show a more complex pattern, with the arrival of B cells and the formation of ***granuloma*** (accumulation of macrophages) in persistent lesions. The hardness or induration is attributable to the deposition of fibrin in the lesion.

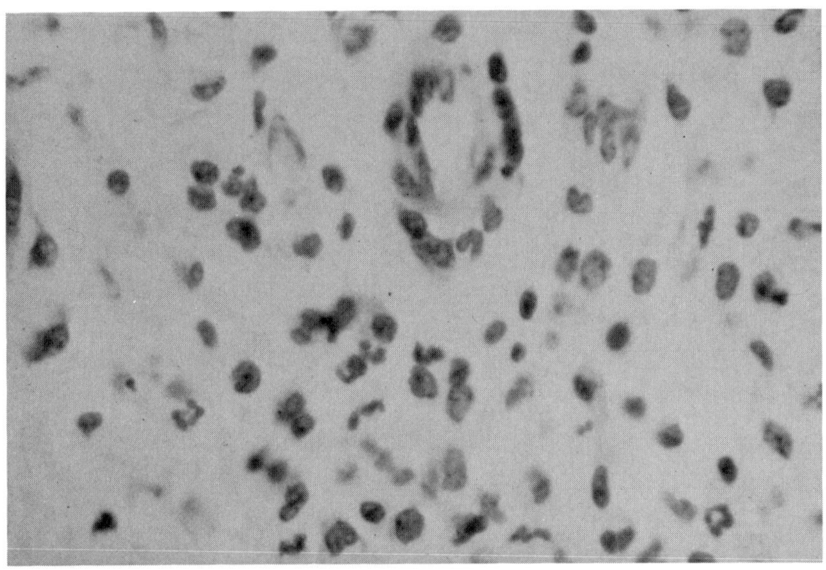

Figure 14.1.
Delayed-type hypersensitivity reaction (DTH), 24 hours after injection of antigen into skin. The infiltrate of mononuclear cells and the appearance of a perivascular cuff can be seen. (Photograph courtesy of Dr. M. Stadecker, Tufts Medical School.)

Mechanism of CMI

The elucidation of the mechanism of CMI resembled the assembly of a jigsaw puzzle. Many separate aspects of CMI, dissected in specialized assays in vitro or in vivo, were finally assembled into the present, reasonably comprehensive picture. As the steps shown in Figure 14.2 are described in the paragraphs that follow, details are given of some of the techniques that are still regarded as important correlates of CMI and are occasionally used to measure it.

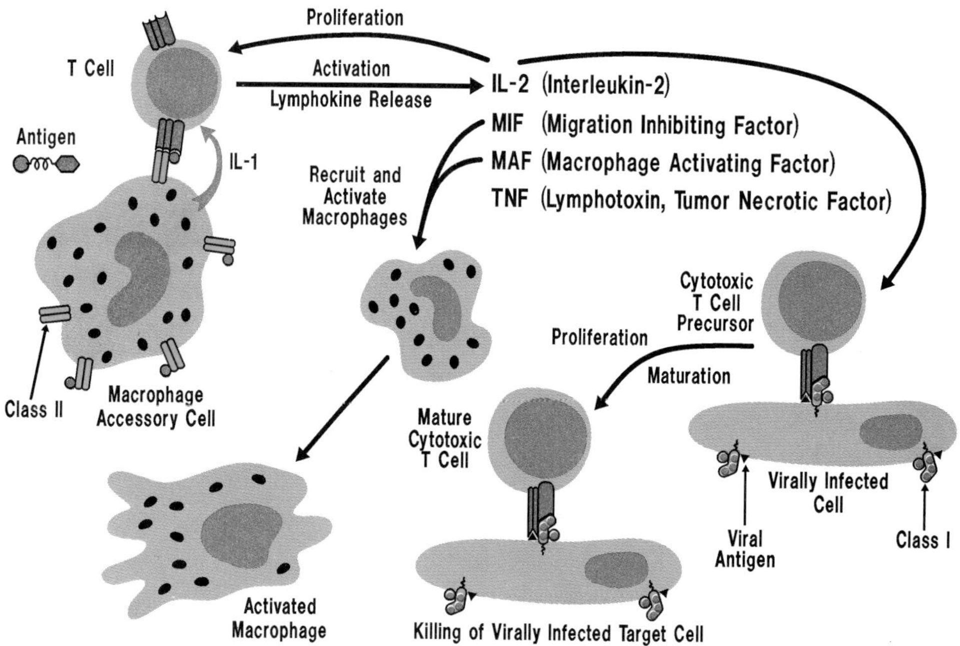

Figure 14.2.
The activation of T cells, leading to the release of lymphokines and to the activation of macrophages and cytotoxic T cells.

PRESENTATION OF ANTIGEN. The recirculating, antigen-specific T cell ($T4^+$ in humans; $L3T4^+$ in mice) comes in contact with antigen presented by an appropriate class II MHC-bearing accessory cell. A second signal (***interleukin-1 IL-1***), secreted or carried by the accessory cells, activates the T cell, whose receptors have bound the antigen–Ia complex. Activation of the T cells may be recognized in several ways: the T cells enlarge, become blastoid, and divide. While these events can be seen by direct visualization, such observations are difficult and tedious. Consequently, direct visualization has been replaced by a widely used assay that measures proliferation of cells. Cells stimulated to divide must synthesize DNA. If they are supplied with a pulse of

^{3}H-labeled thymidine, they will incorporate that radiolabeled material into the newly synthesized DNA, and the cells themselves will become labeled. It is then a simple matter to count the incorporated radioactivity in a given aliquot of cells, and, since incorporation is proportional to DNA synthesis, to determine the extent to which the cells have proliferated. This ***proliferative assay*** is commonly used in vitro as a correlate of CMI and is used to determine the capacity of T cells to respond to antigen, as well as the existing degree of sensitivity to a specific antigen. However, it should be noted that cells other than those responsible for delayed-type hypersensitivity may proliferate and give discordant results.

RELEASE OF LYMPHOKINES. After triggering, and concomitant with proliferation, T cells release an array of lymphokines with a variety of functions. It is not known at this time whether each different function represents the effect of a different mediator or whether, as is quite likely, several different effects studied by different assays are produced by the same factor. The lymphokines include the substances described below.

Macrophage Chemotactic Factor. This factor exerts a positive chemotactic effect on monocytes and macrophages, causing them to migrate to the site of the T cell response, where they are acted on by the other lymphokines.

Migration Inhibiting Factor (MIF). An inhibiting factor released by stimulated T cells acts on blood-borne monocytes to make them sticky and adherent to the endothelial lining of venules. Many monocytes force their way through the endothelial cells into the surrounding tissue (hence the perivascular cuffing in early stages) where their migration is thus inhibited. The manifestation of this phenomenon in vitro can be seen by use of preparations of normal monocytes and macrophages collected in capillary tubes (Fig. 14.3). When these tubes are placed in tissue culture medium on a petri dish, the cells migrate out of the tubes, over the course of 24 hours, producing a fan-like array from the open end of the tube. If a preparation containing MIF (e.g. the supernatant from T cells previously stimulated with specific antigen or with nonspecific mitogens, such as phytohemagglutinin) is added, reduced migration or none at all is observed from the end of the capillary tube, hence the term ***"migration inhibition factor."*** The degree of inhibition is proportional to the amount of MIF released and is often used as a measure of the extent of reaction of T cells.

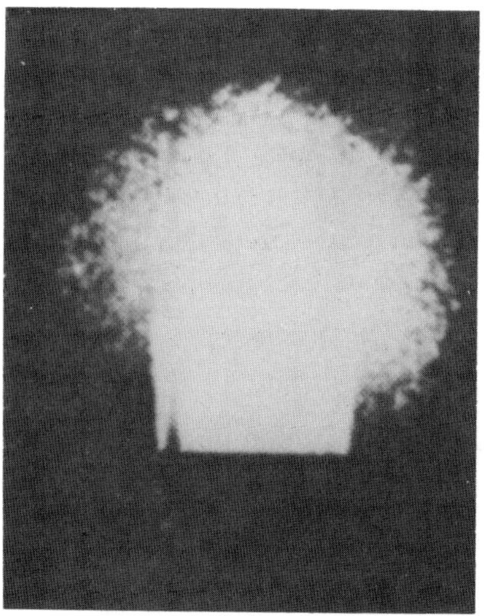

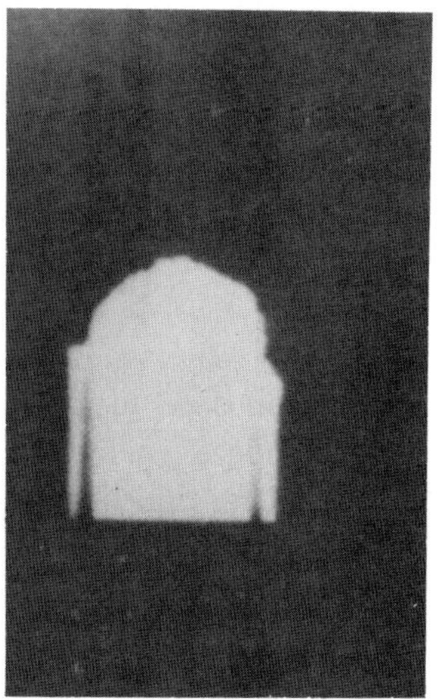

Figure 14.3.
Migration of macrophages out of a capillary tube (left) and its inhibition by macrophage inhibiting factor (MIF) (right).

Macrophage Activating Factor (MAF). An activating factor appears to be the next lymphokine to affect the remaining monocytes, which have migrated to the site of response. It is not a single compound. Its effects include activation of the monocytes so that they mature into macrophages with increased size, content of lysosomal granules, respiratory activity and ability to ingest particles and debris in the area (Fig. 14.4). The activation of these cells increases their ability to ingest and kill bacteria, tumor cells, or obligate intracellular parasites (e.g. *Brucella, Leishmania, Listeria*) that have been growing unchecked in the unstimulated macrophages. Study of activation of macrophages in vitro has demonstrated that many, if not all the changes induced by MAF can be produced by treatment with highly purified ***γ-interferon (γ-IFN),*** produced by activated T cells, or by γ-IFN synthesized by use of recombinant DNA technology. The changes induced by γ-IFN include increased size, lysosomal content, phagocytosis, synthesis of membrane-bound antigens (in particular class II MHC), and the ability to kill ingested organisms. Thus, in addition to its antiviral properties, the activity of γ-IFN can account for most of the MAF activity produced by T cells (although other substances with MAF activity are known). The ability to increase the level of class II MHC antigens on the surfaces of cells other than macrophages is another important property of γ-IFN that may play a critical role in a positive feedback loop of the immune response.

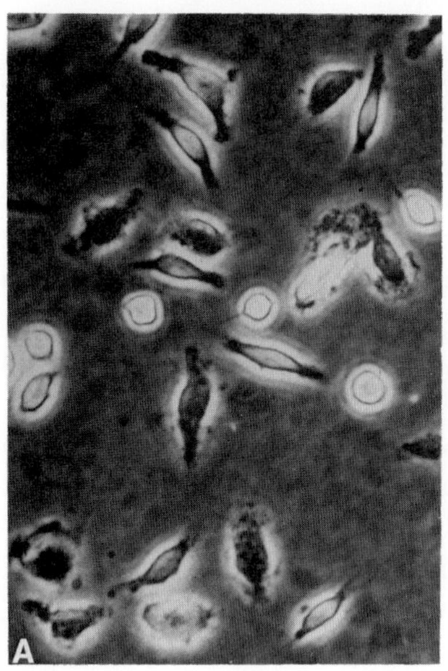

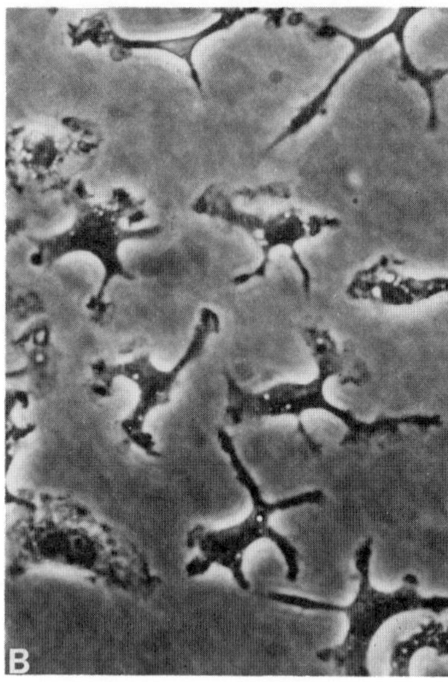

Figure 14.4.
The effect of macrophage activating factor (γ-IFN) on peritoneal macrophages. Figure 14.4A shows normal macrophages in culture as they are just beginning to adhere. Figure 14.4B shows macrophages which, after activation with γ-IFN, have adhered, spread out with the development of numerous pseudopodia, and grown larger. More lysozomal granules are also visible. (Photographs courtesy of Dr. M. Stadecker, Tufts Medical School.)

Lymphotoxin. Lymphotoxin is a recently purified factor with a unique amino acid sequence that has some experimentally defined ability to kill certain tumor cells. It has some sequence homology with ***tumor necrosis factor B (TNF$_B$)*** and may, like TNF_B, have some potential in the treatment of cancer.

Interleukin-2 (IL-2). Interleukin-2 is a major lymphokine released both by the T cells, which participate in CMI, and by the helper T cells involved in production of antibody by B cells. This lymphokine induces proliferation of T cells in an almost autocatalytic fashion (see Chapter 10). It is, moreover, the second signal required to trigger yet another class of T cells, the ***cytotoxic T cells*** ($T8^+$ in humans, Lyt-2^+ in mice), which have receptors that respond to antigen only when it is associated with class I MHC products. Thus, cytotoxic T cells are generated mainly through the T-cell pathway outlined for CMI above. The cytotoxic T cells play a large role in immunity to viral infections, presumably by killing those cells in which the virus is growing. A role for these cells in contact sensitivity (see below), and in rejection of tumors and grafts, has been suggested but has not been proved. Other putative lymphokines with various activities, such as ***leukocyte inhibitory factors (LIF), osteoclast***

activating factor (OAF), skin reactive factor, and ***histamine releasing factor,*** have been described, but neither the identity of the substances involved nor the nature of their possible roles in CMI is clearly understood.

CONSEQUENCES OF CMI. It should be apparent from the above discussion that many of the effector functions in CMI are performed by ***activated macrophages***. In the most favorable circumstances, CMI results in destruction of the organism that elicited the response in the first place. This destruction is believed to result predominantly from ***ingestion*** by macrophages followed by ***degradation*** by ***lysosomal enzymes***, as well as by the by-products of the burst of ***respiratory activity***, such as ***peroxide*** and ***superoxide*** radicals. Foreign tissues, tumor tissue, and soluble or conjugated antigens are dealt with in a similar manner. When ***cytotoxic T cells*** also become involved, the destruction of target cells requires ***direct contact*** with the cells that results in a ***"lethal hit,"*** the mechanism of which is still unknown.

In circumstances where the antigen is readily disposed of, the lesion resolves slowly, with little tissue damage. In some circumstances, however, the antigen is protected and very persistent, for example schistosomal eggs and lipid-encapsulated mycobacteria. In such cases, the response can be prolonged and destructive to the host. Continuous accumulation of macrophages leads to clusters of ***epithelioid cells***, which fuse to form giant cells in ***granulomas***. These granulomas, in turn, can be destructive because of their displacement of normal tissue and can result in ***caseation*** and ***necrosis***. The disease process may then be attributable not so much to the effects of the invading organisms as to the persistent attempts of the host to isolate and contain the parasite by the mechanisms of CMI.

In diseases like smallpox, measles, and herpes, the characteristic skin rashes are largely attributable to the responses of cell-mediated immunity to the virus, with additional destruction attributable to the attack by cytotoxic T cells on the virally infected epithelial cells.

VARIANTS OF DTH

Several known variants of classical DTH or tuberculin reactions have the same basic mechanisms, but they have additional features, and those features are described in the sections that follow.

Contact Sensitivity

Contact sensitivity is a form of DTH in which the target organ is the skin, and the inflammatory response is produced as a result of contact with sensitizing substances on the surface of the skin. The prototype for this form of response is ***poison ivy dermatitis***. The offending substance is ***urushiol***, an oil secreted by the leaves of the poison ivy vine and other, related plants. Urushiol is a mixture of catechols (dihydroxyphenols) with long, hydrocarbon side chains. These features allow it to penetrate the skin by virtue of its lipophilicity (which gives it the ability to dissolve in skin oils and sweat) and its ability to couple covalently (by formation of quinones) to some carrier molecules on cell surfaces. Other contact sensitizers are generally also ***lipid-soluble haptens***. They have a variety of chemical forms, but all have, in common, the ability to ***penetrate skin*** and form ***hapten-carrier conjugates***. Experimentally, chemicals such as 2,4-dinitrochlorobenzene (DNCB) are used to induce contact sensitivity. Since virtually every normal individual is capable of developing hypersensitivity to a test dose of this compound, it is frequently used to assess a patient's potential for T-cell reactivity. Various metals, such as nickel and chromium, which are present in jewelry and clasps of undergarments, are also capable of inducing contact sensitivity, presumably by way of ***chelation*** (ionic interaction) by skin proteins.

The induction of contact sensitivity is thought to proceed via presentation of the offending allergen by ***Langerhans cells,*** which are specialized accessory cells in the skin. It is not yet known whether the sensitizer couples directly to components on the surface of the Langerhans cell or whether it couples first to proteins in serum or tissue that are then taken up by the Langerhans cells. The initial contact results in expansion of the clones of T cells capable of recognizing the specific contact sensitizer. Subsequent contact with the sensitizer triggers a sequence of events analogous to those described for CMI. An additional pathologic component of contact sensitivity reactions in humans is the separation of epithelial cells, ***spongiosis,*** produced by the infiltrating effector cells. This in turn leads to a leakage of fluid and ***blister*** formation.

The commonly performed procedure for testing for the presence of contact sensitivity is the ***patch test*** in which a bit of the suspected antigen is spread on the skin and covered by an occlusive dressing. The appearance 2–3 days later of an area of induration and erythema indicates sensitivity.

Allograft Reaction

Grafts of cells, tissues or organs taken from a ***syngeneic*** donor (a donor of identical genetic composition to the recipient) are readily accepted by the recipient and become vascularized and function normally. If the graft is taken from an ***allogeneic*** donor (a genetically different individual of the same species), it will initially be accepted and become vascularized. However, if the genetic difference is at any of the histocompatability genes, especially those that encode the major histocompatibility complex (MHC), a rejection process ensues whose duration and intensity is related to the degree of incompatibility between donor and recipient (see Chapter 18). The rejection reaction, in general, follows the course described for CMI. After vascularization, there is an initial invasion of the graft by a mixed population of lymphocytes and monocytes through the blood vessel walls. This inflammatory reaction soon leads to destruction of the vessels, quickly followed by necrosis and breakdown of the grafted tissue, which is now deprived of nutrients.

The in vitro correlate of the allograft reaction is the ***one-way mixed lymphocyte reaction*** (***MLR***) (see Chapter 18). Lymphocytes from an individual, when cultured in vitro with irradiated cells from an allogeneic donor, are induced to proliferate, and the degree of proliferation is proportional to the degree of disparity at the MHC between donor and recipient. Since the donor cells are irradiated, they do not proliferate, but they are still able to stimulate the responder cells; hence, the term "one-way reaction."

Graft Versus Host Reaction

When mature, immunocompetent T cells are transfused into an allogeneic recipient that for any reason is unable to reject them, the cells are free to react against the host. They do so by inducing an often fatal, ***graft versus host (GVH) response.*** This response consists of a broad-scale attack on organs and tissues where cells that carry class II MHC products are present. These class II MHC products, in turn, trigger the circulating transfused T cells to respond and induce CMI reactions at multiple sites. Signs of GVH reaction include enlargement of lymph nodes, spleen, and liver; diarrhea; skin rash and hair loss; general weight loss (runting); and death. Death is presumably the outcome of destruction of host cells and tissues, a consequence of an overwhelming CMI response against the many host targets that contain MHC type II antigens.

The graft versus host reaction may occur as a consequence of bone marrow grafts into immunosuppressed hosts or as a consequence of transfusions of fresh whole blood into immunodeficient children or neonates, when care has not been taken to remove all the mature, immunocompetent donor T cells prior to grafting or transfusion. In both instances, normal rejection by the recipient of the transfused lymphocytes is not possible.

Cutaneous Basophil Hypersensitivity (CBH)

An unusual form of delayed reaction has been observed in humans, following repeated intradermal injections of antigen. The response is delayed in onset (usually by about 24 hours) but consists entirely of erythema, without the induration typical of classic, delayed hypersensitivity reactions. When this condition was studied experimentally, it was found that the erythema was attended by a cellular infiltrate, but that the predominant cell type was the ***basophil*** (Fig. 14.5). Studies in guinea pigs showed that the response was primarily mediated by T cells and was subject to the same MHC restrictions as classic T-cell–mediated responses. When classic delayed hypersensitivity was

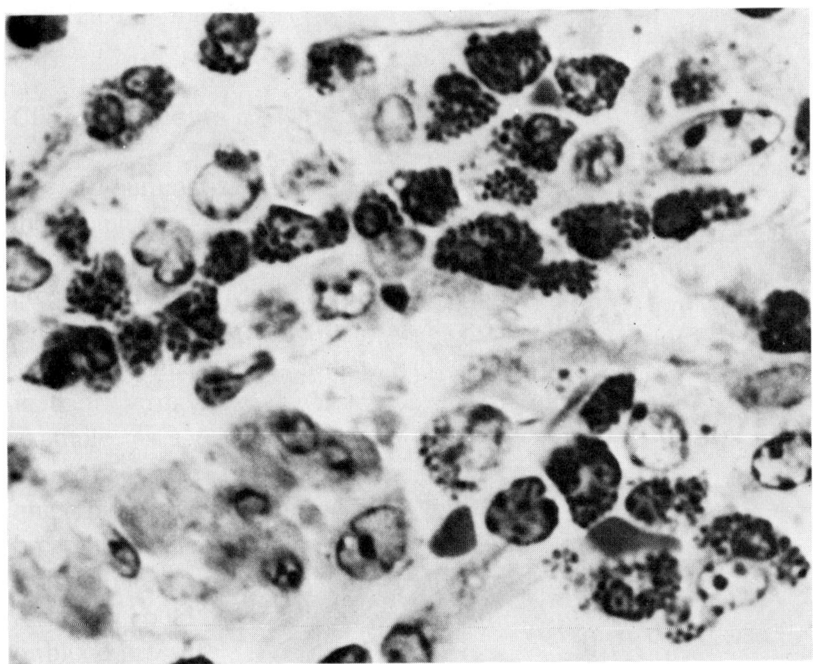

Figure 14.5.
Cutaneous basophil reaction in skin, 24 hours after injection of antigen. Some mononuclear cells are present, but many, heavily granulated basophils, not observed in classical DTH reactions, are seen. (Photograph courtesy of Dr. M. Stadecker, Tufts Medical School.)

present, however, infiltrates of basophils were not seen. Thus, CBH seemed to be a variant of T-cell–mediated responses, but its exact mechanism was unknown. The picture was complicated still further when it was shown that passive transfer of serum could, under some circumstances, evoke a basophil response.

The function of CBH remained a mystery until it was shown that guinea pigs bitten by certain ticks had severe CBH reactions at the site of attachment of the tick. The infiltration of basophils and, presumably, the release of pharmacologically active materials from their granules resulted in death of the tick and its eventual detachment. Thus, CBH may have an important role in certain forms of immunity to parasites. More recently, basophil infiltrates have also been found in cases of contact dermatitis with allergens such as poison ivy, in cases of rejection of renal grafts, and in some forms of conjunctivitis. These observations indicate that basophils may also play a role in some hypersensitivity disease.

SUMMARY

1. All CMI (DTH) responses are T-cell–mediated and may be passively transferred with an appropriate quantity of such cells.

2. CMI responses are initiated by the reaction of specifically sensitized T cells with antigen that is presented in association with MHC type II antigens on accessory cells.

3. The triggering event leads to proliferation of the T cells and the release of several lymphokines, which cause the nonspecific accumulation and activation of monocytes and macrophages. It is the presence and activity of these macrophages that are the major histologic features of CMI and that account for the protective outcome (by ingestion and destruction by released enzymes, or by direct attack on invading cells).

4. CMI is a crucial mode of immunologic reactivity for protection against intracellular parasites, such as viruses, many bacteria, and fungi.

5. In addition to DTH or tuberculin type reactions, contact sensitivity, allograft rejection, and the GVH response represent variants of the basic mechanism of CMI.

REFERENCES

Pick E, Cohen S, Oppenheim J (1979): Biology of the Lymphokines. New York: Academic Press.
Symposium on Cell-Mediated Immunity in Human Disease (1986): Human Pathol 17:2 and 3.
Turk JL (1975): Delayed Hypersensitivity. Amsterdam: North Holland.
Waksman BH (1980): Cellular Hypersensitivity and Immunity, Chapter 7. In Parker C (ed): Clinical Immunology, Vol 1. Philadelphia: W.B. Saunders.

REVIEW QUESTIONS

For questions 1–5, choose the ONE BEST answer.

1. Which of the following does not involve CMI?
   a) contact sensitivity to lipstick.
   b) rejection of a liver graft.
   c) serum sickness.
   d) tuberculin reaction.
   e) immunity to chicken pox.

2. A positive DTH skin reaction involves the interaction of
   a) antigen, complement, and lymphokines.
   b) antigen, antigen-sensitive lymphocytes, and macrophages.
   c) antigen–antibody complexes, complement, and neutrophils.
   d) IgE antibody, antigen, and mast cells.
   e) antigen, macrophages, and complement.

3. Cell-mediated immune responses are
   a) enhanced by depletion of complement.
   b) suppressed by cortisone.
   c) enhanced by depletion of T cells.
   d) suppressed by antihistamine.
   e) enhanced by depletion of macrophages.

4. Four strains of inbred mice (A, B, C, and D) were tested against each other by MLR in vitro. The results are shown below:

	Stimulators			
Responders	A	B	C	D
	cpm of ^{3}H-TdR Incorporated			
A	90	16,200	15,100	15,000
B	16,100	100	17,500	14,900
C	15,200	15,000	150	16,400
D	16,200	17,000	16,400	120

   Which of the following statements is *true*?
   a) all strains are identical at class I MHC loci.
   b) all strains are identical at class II MHC loci.

(Continued on next page)

c) none of these strains is identical at class II MHC loci.
d) strain A is compatible only with strain B.
e) identity cannot be determined since background counts exist.

5. Delayed skin reactions to an intradermal injection of antigen may be markedly decreased by
a) exposure to a high dose of X-irradiation.
b) treatment with antihistamines.
c) treatment with an anti-neutrophil serum.
d) removal of the spleen.
e) decreasing levels of complement.

For questions 6–9, ONE or MORE of the completions given is correct. Choose the appropriate answer:
A) if only *1, 2, 3* are correct
B) if only *1 and 3* are correct
C) if only *2 and 4* are correct
D) if only *4* is correct
E) if *all* are correct

6. Patients with the DiGeorge syndrome (congenital absence of the thymus), who survive beyond infancy, would be incapable of
1) rejecting a bone marrow transplant.
2) mounting a DTH response to dinitrochlorobenzene.
3) resisting intracellular parasites.
4) forming antibody to T-independent antigens.

7. Which of the following statements is (are) characteristic of contact sensitivity?
1) The best therapy is oral administration of the antigen.
2) Patch testing with the allergen is commonly used for diagnosis.
3) Sensitization can be passively transferred with serum from an allergic individual.
4) Some chemicals acting as haptens induce sensitivity by covalently binding to host proteins that act as carriers.

8. Macrophage activation factor (MAF)
1) is synthesized by macrophages.
2) is released as a consequence of antigen- or mitogen-induced activation of lymphocytes.
3) specifically binds to the antigen that induces its release.
4) induces macrophages to ingest and destroy bacteria in a nonspecific fashion.

9. T-cell–mediated immune responses can result in
1) formation of granulomas.
2) runting of an irradiated recipient of a bone marrow graft.
3) rejection of a heart transplant.
4) eczema of the skin in the area of prolonged contact with a rubberized undergarment.

ANSWERS TO REVIEW QUESTIONS

1. ***c*** Serum sickness is an example of those reactions mediated by an antibody–antigen complex that involve components of the complement system and neutrophils. All others involve CMI to a significant extent.

2. ***b*** CMI reactions result from the triggering of T cells by antigen with recruitment of macrophages. Neither antibody, complement, nor mast cells plays a role in this process, although they do play a role in immediate hypersensitivity responses.

3. ***b*** Cortisone has a general anti-inflammatory effect and is also lytic for some T cells. Complement plays no role, and antihistamines have little effect on this type of response. Depletion of T cells or macrophages would suppress, not enhance, this type of response since the response is dependent on these cells.

4. ***c*** Since each strain gives a significantly increased incorporation of thymidine when tested with the other three strains, the only correct conclusion is that none are identical at class II MHC loci, which are the loci that control proliferative responses in vitro.

5. ***a*** High doses of X-irradiation will destroy T cells, which are responsible for initiating the response. Histamine, neutrophils, spleen, and complement do not play a role, and any treatment that affects them would not affect a DTH response.

6. ***A*** Patients with DiGeorge syndrome have congenital thymic aplasia and lack all T cell functions. Since 1, 2, and 3 are all aspects of a CMI response, they would be absent, while formation of antibody against T-independent antigens is dependent on B cells and would still occur in these patients.

7. ***C*** Patch testing consists of application of the offending allergen under an occlusive dressing, and a positive DTH response after 24–48 hours is considered evidence of sensitivity. The allergens involved are those capable of penetrating skin and binding to host carrier proteins. Oral ingestion, which, in certain experimental situations, can be shown to induce suppression after subsequent induction of contact sensitivity,

(*Continued on next page*)

has not been shown to be an effective therapeutic maneuver in humans. Passive transfer of CMI responses is accomplished with T cells, not with serum.

8. ***C*** MAF is released during activation of T cells and induces macrophages to phagocytize and destroy nonspecifically any particles, organisms, or debris in the area.

9. ***E*** All of these effects are manifestations of CMI. Formation of granulomas is characteristic of a chronic DTH reaction, and runting is an end stage of a GVH response induced by immunocompetent T cells in the bone marrow graft. Rejection of the heart is an example of an allograft response. Some of the chemicals used to cure rubber can induce contact sensitivity after prolonged exposure of the skin to them.

CHAPTER

15

CONTROL MECHANISMS IN THE IMMUNE RESPONSE

INTRODUCTION

An understanding of the immune response as a complete physiologic system requires, in addition to an understanding of the "on" signals described in previous chapters, some understanding of the "off" signals as well. It is only with such a complete understanding of the system that it is possible to answer such diverse questions as:

1) Why does the response to any particular antigen not continue to increase in magnitude until it takes over the whole immune apparatus?

2) Why is a fetus, which is an example of an allotransplant, not rejected by a maternal immune response against paternal antigens?

3) Why is the development of an autoimmune response against antigens of our own tissues an exceptional rather than a commonplace event?

In a system as complex as that which produces an immune response, it is to be expected that multiple levels of control exist. This chapter explores several mechanisms that control the immune response.

REGULATION BY ANTIGEN

Not every injection of an antigen results in an immune response. Generation of a response is a highly empirical process, depending on dose, timing, and nature of the antigen involved. In cases where antigens have low intrinsic immunogenicity, ***adjuvants*** that enhance the response in a variety of ways may be used (see Chapter 3). ***Alum precipitates*** provide depots for enhanced phagocytosis and continuous release of antigen, while suspension of the antigen in ***Freund's adjuvant*** allows the antigen to be presented in a slowly dissipating mineral oil emulsion, and at the same time supplies the T-cell–stimulating properties of killed mycobacteria.

Antigens of proven immunogenicity do not provoke an immune response if they fail to reach lymphoid tissues. Thus, lens protein of the eye is immunogenic but is found in a ***privileged site*** inaccessible to lymphocytes. When the lens capsule is traumatized and protein escapes, an immune response may ensue that could damage the other eye. Other antigens, present on certain tumor cells, apparently fail to elicit a response because they are covered with sialic acid residues, which somehow inhibit the interactions required to generate the immune response.

REGULATION BY ANTIBODY

The production of antibody results in a ***feedback inhibition*** of further production of antibody, as already discussed. Thus, appearance of IgG antibody results in a shut-off of synthesis of IgM antibody. The shut-off presumably results because of competition for antigen, and the IgG receptors on B cells represent a more efficient system for capture of antigen, by virtue of an affinity for antigen that is higher than that of IgM receptors. Similarly, as the level of antibody rises, the concentration of antigen declines, and the net affinity of resulting antibody increases as competition for the remaining antigen favors those B cells with high-affinity receptors.

IMMUNOLOGIC TOLERANCE MEDIATED BY ANTIGEN

Immunologic tolerance can only be defined operationally; a definition based on the underlying mechanisms is not possible because the mechanisms are numerous and not all have been definitively established. A reasonable definition of immunologic tolerance would be: "A state of the immune system that, with respect to one or more specific antigenic determinants, is manifested by a diminished or absent capacity to express either cell-mediated or humoral immunity."

Defined in this way, tolerance may be regarded as a concept, the major importance of which is the fact of its ***immunological specificity***. This is because, regardless of its underlying mechanisms, the existence of specific tolerance is the *only* reason that we can exist as individuals, with our own tissues and cells, while responding to everything else that is foreign to us.

Such tolerance of "self" is an evolutionary device that, as long as it remains intact, is a necessity for normal growth, development, and existence. When something occurs to destroy the integrity of self-tolerance (and there are probably various exogenous influences that can precipitate such an event), the consequences may be minimal or catastrophic, depending on the extent to which the integrity of self-tolerance has been destroyed. A variety of disease states, usually referred to as ***autoimmune disorders,*** reflect to a degree the consequences of a ***loss of self-tolerance*** (see Chapter 16). Thus, tolerance of self has evolved as a cardinal feature of the immune system, together with its extreme opposite—namely, the highly specific and normally very effective ability to recognize "non-self."

It is obvious why evolution has favored, and selected for, the development of efficient mechanisms for recognition and elimination of non-self antigens. Such mechanisms provide a defense against all foreign antigens, whether they be infectious agents, toxins, or the tissue antigens that can occur in neoplastically transformed cells.

A clear understanding of the nature of immunological tolerance and how it is regulated is immensely important in the practice of medicine. For example, the control of the rejection of transplants is necessary for future, widespread application of organ transplantation. Furthermore, the prevention or control of many autoimmune disorders and allergic diseases demands a more precise understanding of tolerance. In addition, successful application of immunological control and prevention of malignant neoplasias require the application of techniques that exploit tolerance to eliminate selectively one form of an undesirable immune reaction, which, in fact, may enhance the growth of tumors.

Investigations of the phenomenon of tolerance began with the observations of Owen in 1945 that ***dizygotic cattle twins***, which shared common vascular supplies in utero, developed into erythrocyte ***chimeras;*** that is, each calf possessed a mixture of its own erythrocytes plus those of the twin with which an intrauterine vascular anastomosis had existed.

The study of this accident of nature was extended by the demonstration that such dizygotic cattle twins were mutually tolerant of skin grafts from one another, regardless of differences in sex and color. These observations provided the basis for experiments by Medawar and his collaborators that reproduced natural tolerance in the laboratory and led to a Nobel prize.

Medawar and his colleagues injected ***neonatal*** mice of one strain (A) with viable spleen cells of another strain (CBA). When such mice grew to adulthood, they were tested and found to be specifically tolerant of skin grafts from normally histoincompatible donors of the CBA strain (see Fig. 15.1), even

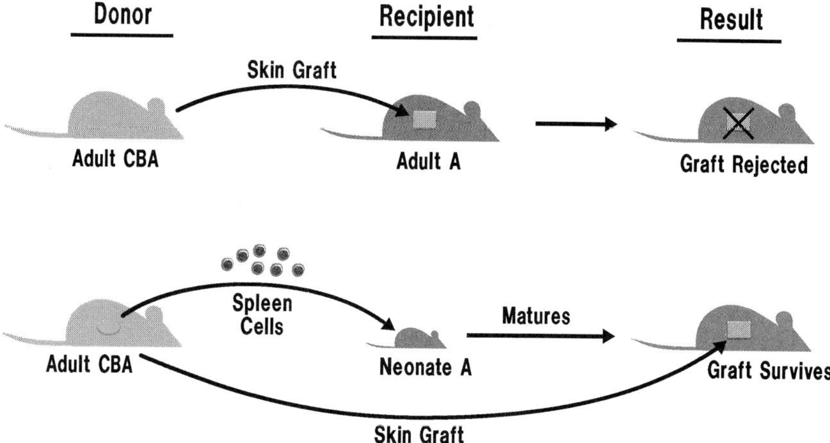

Figure 15.1.
The induction of tolerance to an allograft in a neonatal mouse.

though grafts from a third and different strain were rejected in a normal fashion. A most important observation was that the tolerant state of the injected animals of strain A could be abolished by injection of lymphoid cells from a normal, syngeneic donor of strain A. The abolition of tolerance indicated that the original, induced defect occurred at the level of immunocompetent lymphocytes. Induction of tolerance of this type can also be achieved in ***adult*** animals, if the differences in histocompatibility are weak, and if measures such as prolonged parabiotic union or repeated intravenous injections of cells are employed.

Studies like the ones just described, involving complex transplantation antigens, have been supplemented more recently by studies of acquired tolerance to more defined antigens such as proteins, and methods have been developed to generate tolerance in adult animals to such defined antigens. The use of antigens other than cell-bound transplantation antigens has facilitated investigations into aspects of molecular structure which are crucial to the induction of tolerance. These are described below.

EXPERIMENTAL CONDITIONS FOR INDUCTION OF TOLERANCE

The capacity to induce tolerance experimentally depends upon attention to certain conditions with respect to the animal and the antigen, as follows:

1. ***Maturity*** of the animal is important. As indicated in the description of the pioneering work on tolerance, the state of specific unresponsiveness is most easily obtained in the immunologically immature animal during ***embryonic or neonatal life***. Induction of tolerance is also facilitated under conditions in which the immune systems of adult animals are rendered more or less nonfunctional, for example by ***whole-body X-irradiation*** or by administration of ***immunosuppressive drugs*** such as methotrexate, cyclophosphamide, or 6-mercaptopurine, all of which destroy lymphocytes nonspecifically.

2. The inherent ***immunogenicity*** of the substance being used for induction of tolerance is critically related to the ease of induction of tolerance. For example, a very weak immunogen, such as bovine gamma globulin (BGG), requires a less stringent regimen for induction of tolerance to it in mice than a very strong immunogen, such as hen egg albumin or diphtheria toxoid.

3. The ***form*** of the antigen is also important. BGG in soluble form readily induces tolerance in mice, but if it is given in an adjuvant or in an aggregated form, BGG is immunogenic. If a normally antigenic material is injected in solution in its monomeric form, tolerance rather than immunity will frequently result. This effect is exemplified by the following example: if a suspension of BGG in saline, which is normally immunogenic in rabbits, is subjected to ultracentrifugation, then the supernatant that contains the monomeric BGG is no longer immunogenic but is, in fact, ***tolerogenic,*** while the sediment, which consists of aggregated BGG, is highly immunogenic.

The most likely explanation of these findings is that forms of antigen that are ***not readily phagocytized*** by macrophages are ***more likely to exhibit tolerogenicity*** than immunogenicity. This explanation is supported by the fact that changing the physical state of such tolerogenic substances by heating, which causes aggregation of proteins, or by incorporation into adjuvants converts them to potent immunogens.

4. ***Dosage*** of the substance may be critical. An important observation, first made by Mitchison, is that ***tolerance can be induced by opposite extremes of dosage***. The initial studies, showing that tolerance can be induced in adult animals, were accomplished by the use of relatively large doses of antigen, given repeatedly over long periods of time. Very small doses given similarly were also found to induce tolerance. Intermediate doses resulted in immunity.

5. ***Non-metabolizable substances*** may be tolerogenic. Pneumococcal polysaccharides and synthetic D-polypeptides (made with D rather than L isomers of amino acids) are resistant to enzymatic digestion. These substances are immunogenic when administered in very low quantities (1 μg), but slightly higher doses (10 μg) induce a long-lasting state of specific tolerance. One contributing factor in this case is that, although pneumococcal polysaccharide SIII (for example) is phagocytized, it is not digested and is repeatedly released back into circulation, where it can bind to antibody and prevent its detection in serum.

ROLE OF ACCESSORY CELLS IN TOLERANCE

The following observations led to the conclusion that an ***antigen-processing cell,*** like the macrophages discussed previously, is central to the outcome of the immune response. Generally, if antigen reaches this type of cell, immunity results; ***if the processing cell is bypassed, some form of tolerance is induced***. Thus, destruction of accessory cells by various agents, before antigen is given, leads to tolerance, and tolerance is easily induced in newborns with small or absent populations of accessory cells. Furthermore, differences in the ease with which tolerance can be induced in certain mouse strains reside in the properties of macrophage-like cells.

ROLES OF T AND B LYMPHOCYTES IN TOLERANCE

Soon after the phenomenon of cooperation between T and B cells in humoral immune responses became established, the conceptual and experimental approach to the study of tolerance was reappraised. The immediate questions dealt with the issue of whether the T or the B cells were affected by tolerance-inducing regimens. This issue seems relatively simple but, in fact, the initial studies of this problem resulted in more confusion and controversy than clear-cut answers.

However, the elegant experiments of Chiller and Weigle have provided a much clearer perspective on this matter. They demonstrated 1) that both ***T and B lymphocytes are susceptible*** to induction of tolerance; 2) that the susceptibilities of these two classes of lymphocytes differ considerably, with respect to both the ***dose of antigen*** against which tolerance is induced and the ***time*** required for induction of tolerance; 3) that the ***duration*** of tolerance is significantly ***shorter in B cells*** than in T cells; and finally, 4) that the ***immunological status*** of the whole animal reflects that of the population of T cells in the case of a thymus-dependent antigen.

By transfer of various cell mixtures into irradiated recipients, it was shown that T cells were apparently rendered tolerant very rapidly after injection of antigen (within 24 hours) and that the tolerant state was maintained in T cells for around 100 days (see Fig. 15.2). The population of bone marrow cells also became tolerant, but not until somewhat later (day 10–11) and recovery in this population occurred by day 49. Normal animals injected with the antigen manifested tolerance in parallel with the tolerance of the T–cell population. Therefore, an animal whose population of bone marrow cells had recovered from tolerance by day 60 would, nevertheless, remain functionally unresponsive because of the continued absence of immunocompetent antigen-specific T cells (see Fig. 15.2).

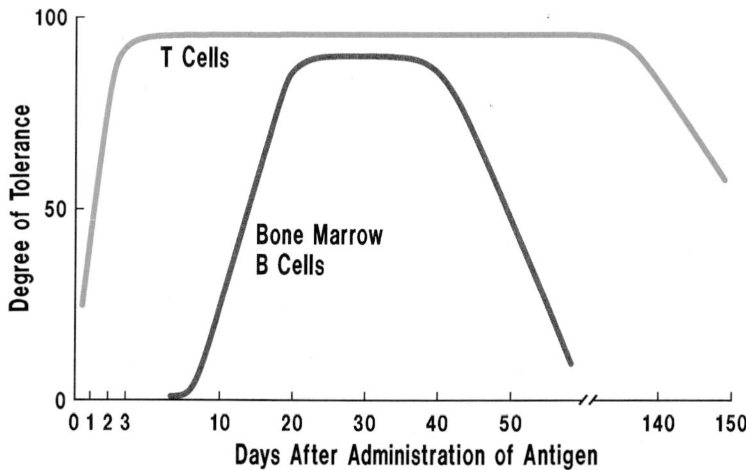

Figure 15.2.
The kinetics of the induction and maintenance of B and T cell tolerance.

The reasons for the different recovery times of T- and B-cell populations lie in the ontogenetic origins of these cells. It may be recalled (Chapter 9) that the thymus is most active after birth and tends to atrophy with maturity. Thus little replacement of T cells occurs in adult animals, and tolerance of T cells would be long lasting. By contrast, bone marrow functions throughout life and constantly provides new B cells to replace those made tolerant.

The essential conclusions from the experiments described above are that T cells become tolerant at lower doses of antigen and remain tolerant for longer periods than B cells. Mitchison's observations on tolerance induced by high and low doses of antigen can now be explained by assuming that tolerance was induced only in T cells by low doses of antigen, while tolerance was induced in both T and B cells by high doses of antigen.

MECHANISMS OF IMMUNOLOGIC TOLERANCE

Elucidation of the cellular and molecular mechanisms involved in immunologic tolerance has been difficult because of the various types of cells involved and the multiple modes of attaining an identical final result—namely, specific unresponsiveness. Nevertheless, considerable progress has been made in sorting out several ways in which tolerance is achieved in each type of cell.

Mechanisms of Unresponsiveness in B Cells

CLONAL ABORTION. When Burnet reviewed Owen's studies on dizygotic cattle twins, he proposed a ***"Theory of Self-Recognition."*** He proposed that if any antigen appears in an animal prior to the maturation of its immune system, then that antigen is identified as self and, henceforth, cannot stimulate an immune response. If an antigen appears later, it is recognized as non-self and is able to trigger a response. Such discrimination could be accomplished by a hypothetical process called ***clonal abortion,*** in which immature lymphocytes that make contact with antigen are aborted, while others survive to generate a response in mature animals. In this way, all self-reactive clones would be eliminated before the immune response matured. Two more recent observations have led to a revival of this concept.

1. B cells, at an early stage in ontogeny (see Chapter 9), when they have only IgM receptors on their surfaces, are very easily rendered tolerant by

contact with antigen. However, when they mature subsequently and reach a stage where IgD receptors are also present, they are more prone to be stimulated.

2. By actually counting all B cells that had receptors for a specific self antigen, Klinman demonstrated that spleens of mature mice contained few or no B cells of that specificity. However, if bone marrow cells from the same mice were allowed to mature in vitro into B cells, many of them had receptors specific for the self antigen. Thus, it appeared that B cells developed from precursors in bone marrow were deleted if they made contact with the self antigen in vivo, but survived in vitro in its absence.

CLONAL DELETION BY RECEPTOR BLOCKADE. As in the study of cooperation between T and B cells, the use of hapten-carrier systems has provided some useful insights into the development of tolerance. A study of the responses of B cells to a hapten showed that ***tolerance by B cells to specific haptens*** could be achieved if: a) the hapten was ***attached to a non-immunogenic carrier***, such as a synthetic D-polypeptide (poly-D-glutamic-D-lysine); b) the hapten was attached to a carrier, which ***could not elicit help*** because it was a protein to which self-tolerance was present (e.g. mouse γ-globulin in the mouse); and c) a large dose of ***hapten on a thymus-independent carrier*** (e.g. polysaccharide) is given in a situation where help from T cells is not available.

A reasonable model to account for these observations suggests that, in the absence of help from T cells, the engagement of a large number of Ig receptors on the B cell by antigen leads to a signal that induces ***tolerance***, which causes either the ***destruction*** or the ***suppression*** of the B cell. Suppression of B cells may involve either the removal of all receptors from the cell by capping and endocytosis or, alternatively, their extensive cross-linking by antigen into some form of ***frozen matrix*** on the surface of the cell. Whatever the actual sequence of events, it is generally reversible at an early stage by addition of appropriate factors from helper T cells. Thus, there exists a subtle balance between the ability of an antigen to turn a B cell on or off.

Mechanisms of Induction of Tolerance in T Cells

CLONAL ABORTION. The absence of functional T cells specific for self antigens suggests the operation of a process similar to that seen for clonal abortion of B cells. However, no formal proof yet exists that an immature T-cell is aborted on contact with a self antigen.

CLONAL DELETION. Most early experiments on the induction of tolerance in adult animals, in which cells or soluble antigens were employed, indicated that the T cells of the tolerant animals were functionally devoid of one specific reactivity but possessed all others. This result implies that, if animals were rendered tolerant to BGG, for example, then their spleen cells could be used to transfer reactivity to many other antigens into irradiated recipients, but the same spleen cells lacked the ability to make a response to BGG. T cells, reactive against BGG, appeared to be functionally absent.

SUPPRESSOR T CELLS. Some early studies showed that mice rendered tolerant to a particular antigen did not demonstrate a restoration of specific immunity after they were grafted with large numbers of normal T cells. This effect remained something of a mystery until Gershon showed that such animals possessed a class of T cells capable of ***actively suppressing the normal T cells***, which were specific for that antigen. He further demonstrated that the passive transfer of the ***Lyt-2***$^{+}$ T cells from such a tolerant animal into a normal recipient prevented the development of immunity to that particular antigen. He called this process ***"infective tolerance."*** In humans, suppressor cells bear the ***T8*** phenotypic marker (Lyt-2 in the mouse) but are not cytotoxic. Thus suppression is not due to cell death.

The phenomenon of active or infectious tolerance as a mechanism of specific unresponsiveness is the subject of intense scrutiny at present. There are well-documented, experimental models in which this process can be demonstrated. The best evidence can be interpreted to mean that certain T cells apparently are capable of specifically suppressing the functional response of other lymphocytes to antigen. There are data suggesting that such suppressor T cells exert their effects primarily on other T lymphocytes, as well as on B lymphocytes by as yet unknown mechanisms. Still under active study, many suggested levels of complexity, as required for the fine tuning of any homeostatic mechanism, are already apparent.

Suppressor cells have been shown to be able to recognize ***antigen epitopes***, or ***allotypic and idiotypic determinants*** on Ig molecules. This characteristic of suppressor cells led Jerne to postulate a ***network theory,*** in which products of V-region genes, present on antibody, and antigen-specific receptors on B cells and T cells, may be recognized as immunogenic in the host and, thus, activate other helper or suppressor T cells, depending on the particular circumstances. These events would lead to complex control loops, which modulate the extent of the immune response. In this model, the loop can be

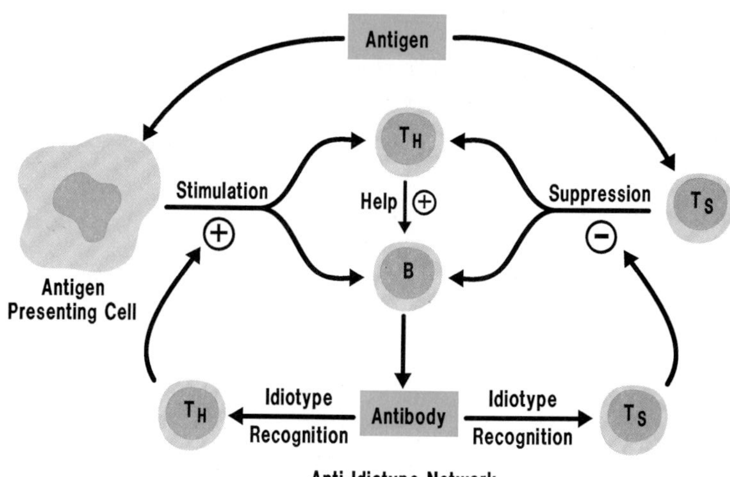

Figure 15.3.
A schematic diagram of regulation of the immune response.

entered and homeostasis perturbed at any point. Thus, introduction of antigen provides only one of the mechanisms by which the system can be driven (Fig. 15.3).

In such complex interacting networks, many opportunities for disruption arise, and a host of diseases have been associated, with greater or lesser degrees of certainty, with defects in these regulatory networks. Such diseases are representative of one of the most exciting areas for clinical research—both because of their frequency, and also because an understanding of a defect can provide the basis for its repair.

SUMMARY

1. In the regulation of the immune response, multiple controls are used to ensure the correct functioning of the system.

2. For successful initiation of a response, antigens must have certain immunogenic properties, such as size, complexity and foreignness, and they must be administered by routes that engage accessory cells.

3. Tolerance, or unresponsiveness, induced by antigen occurs in neonates or adults when methods that bypass the accessory cell are used.

4. Tolerance may be a property of both B cells and T cells. It is more easily induced, and it is induced with lower doses, in T cells. Tolerance in B

cells may involve clonal deletion or clonal abortion, produced by cross-linking of receptors on B cells by antigen, either early in ontogeny or in the absence of help by T cells.

5. Tolerance in T cells is mediated either by clonal deletion or by the appearance of suppressor T cells, which may be antigen-, allotype- or idiotype-specific.

REFERENCES

Green DR, Flood PM, Gershon RR (1983): Immunoregulatory T cell pathways. Annu Rev Immunol 1:439.

Nossal GV (1983): Cellular mechanisms of immunologic tolerance. Annu Rev Immunol 1:33.

REVIEW QUESTIONS

For questions 1–3, choose the ONE correct answer.

1. Immunologic unresponsiveness, induced by immunosuppressive drugs, is different from immunologic tolerance because
   a) only B cells are affected by the drugs.
   b) only T cells are affected by the drugs.
   c) liver enzymes are involved in the former and not in the latter.
   d) drug-induced unresponsiveness is not antigen-specific but tolerance is.
   e) drug-induced unresponsiveness is antigen-specific but tolerance is not.

2. Immunologic tolerance
   a) involves only humoral immunity.
   b) involves only cell-mediated immunity.
   c) may involve only some antigenic determinants on a protein.
   d) is induced with ease in adults.
   e) is best achieved with particulate antigens.

3. All of the following procedures would be likely to induce tolerance to a protein antigen except
   a) intravenous injection of deaggregated protein.
   b) injection of cyclophosphamide with the antigen.
   c) injection of antigen into the fetus in utero.
   d) intravenous injection of small amounts of antigen.
   e) intramuscular injection of the antigen in adjuvant.

For questions 4–10 ONE or MORE of the completions given is correct. Choose the appropriate answer:
A) if only *1, 2, 3* are correct
B) if only *1 and 3* are correct
C) if only *2 and 4* are correct
D) if only *4* is correct
E) if *all* are correct

4. Regulatory elements in the Jerne network hypothesis include
   1) products of V-region genes.
   2) anti-idiotypic suppressor T cells.
   3) T-cell idiotypes.
   4) helper T cells.

5. When a tolerogenic injection of a protein antigen is given to a mouse, it can be determined that
   1) B-cell tolerance is most rapidly induced.
   2) T-cell tolerance is most rapidly induced.
   3) B-cell tolerance can be induced only when low doses are used.
   4) B-cell tolerance is lost as new B cells come from the bone marrow.

6. T suppressor cells
   1) can be induced by helper T cells.
   2) may block the activity of helper T cells.
   3) express T8 antigens in humans.
   4) can prevent delayed-type hypersensitivity.

7. Specific non-responsiveness to self and other antigens may be mediated by
   1) clonal abortion of self-reactive B cells at early stages of maturation.
   2) clonal abortion of self-reactive T cells at early stages of maturation.
   3) idiotype-specific suppressor T cells.
   4) rapid digestion and removal of antigen from the circulation.

8. Consider the following experimental groups of mice:
   Group 1: Mice injected with 2 mg of bovine γ-globulin (BGG) emulsified in Freund's adjuvant.
   Group 2: Mice injected with 0.02 mg of the supernatant after centrifugation of a solution of BGG.
   Transfer of which of the following sets of cells will reconstitute the ability of irradiated mice to respond to an immunogenic injection of BGG?
   1) T cells from group 2 + B cells from group 1.
   2) T cells from group 1 + B cells from group 1.
   3) T cells from group 2 + B cells from group 2.
   4) T cells from group 1 + B cells from group 2.

(Continued on next page)

9. The induction of immunologic tolerance may be facilitated by
   1) the use of high doses of nonmetabolizable antigens.
   2) haptens.
   3) intravenous injection of soluble antigen.
   4) the use of previously immunized animals.

10. The induction of tolerance
    1) is a nonspecific form of unresponsiveness.
    2) may involve suppressor T cells.
    3) can only be achieved in neonates.
    4) can be achieved with high or low doses of soluble antigen.

ANSWERS TO REVIEW QUESTIONS

1. ***d*** Drugs eliminate B and T cells nonspecifically; only antigen-induced tolerance has the elements of specificity.

2. ***c*** Tolerance is achieved in specific clones of B or T cells and may involve only those clones specific for certain epitopes on an antigen and not others.

3. ***e*** Use of adjuvant is designed to achieve immunity and avoid tolerance. All other procedures could induce tolerance.

4. ***E*** All are regulatory or recognition elements in the network. Products of V-region genes (1) would be the idiotypes of receptors on B and T cells.

5. ***C*** T-cell tolerance (2) is most rapidly achieved and lasts longest. As new B cells are produced by the bone marrow, tolerance in this compartment wanes. T-cell tolerance, by contrast, persists because the thymus of an adult no longer actively produces new T cells.

6. ***E*** All are correct attributes of suppressor T cells.

7. ***A*** 1, 2, and 3 are possible mechanisms for inducing or maintaining tolerance. Removal of antigen from circulation (4), if anything, would work against maintenance of tolerance, which relies on persistence of antigen to make tolerant any newly arising B or T cells.

8. ***C*** Group 1 is immune, while group 2 has low zone tolerance of T cells only. Therefore, (2) is obviously correct, since both B and T cells come from immune animals, but (4) is also correct, because immune T cells from group 1 and normal B cells from group 2 should also

reconstitute the recipient. In (1) and (3) tolerant T cells from group 2 would not help either immune or normal B cells.

9. ***B*** Induction of tolerance is favored by intravenous injection of soluble antigens (3), which makes T and B cells tolerant, while large amounts of nonmetabolizable antigens make B cells tolerant by direct binding to receptors (1). Haptens have no ability to affect the response, unless they are coupled to carriers; immune animals (4) are difficult to make tolerant, because they already have expanded clones of mature T and B cells.

10. ***C*** Tolerance is specific for the antigen used for induction and can, under appropriate circumstances, be induced in adults. Hence (1) and (3) are wrong.

CHAPTER

16

AUTOIMMUNITY

INTRODUCTION

When Ehrlich first enunciated his concept of ***"horror autotoxicus"*** at the turn of the century, it was accepted that this mysterious "fear of self-poisoning" was what kept the body from reacting against itself. Since that time, many examples have been found in which an immune response against some "self" antigen is evoked with pathologic consequences. The nature of these responses against self is as varied as the immune response itself, with possible involvement of antibody, complement, immune complexes, and cell-mediated immunity. Many experimental models have been developed to study these phenomena and, in general, these models rely on active immunization with known antigens. However, the inducing agents for most of the well-recognized, naturally occurring autoimmune diseases remain unknown.

Explanations of the causes of autoimmune diseases have changed markedly over the years. At one time, it was thought that autoimmune diseases resulted from the presence of ***"forbidden clones,"*** which had either escaped the self-tolerance process or had arisen de novo by mutation. At present it is generally believed that many self-reactive clones actually exist, but that they are held in check by a variety of control mechanisms. It is the breakdown or failure of the control mechanisms that allows the immune response directed against self and the resultant disease process to appear. Additionally, many autoimmune reactions are thought to be the result of responses to cross-reactive antigens carried by invading microorganisms. In this chapter, some of the more common of the numerous autoimmune diseases are described, together with the mechanisms most probably responsible for them.

EXAMPLES OF AUTOIMMUNE DISEASE

Antibody-Mediated Autoimmune Diseases

AUTOIMMUNE HEMOLYTIC ANEMIA. One of the causes of a reduction in the number of red cells in the circulation is their destruction or removal by antibody directed against an antigen on the surface of the red cell. The destruction of the red cells can be attributed either to activation of the ***complement cascade*** and eventual ***lysis*** of the red cell (the resultant release of hemoglobin may lead to its appearance in the urine—i.e. ***hemoglobinuria***), or to ***opsonization*** by antibody and some of the components of complement. In the latter case, the red cells are bound to, and engulfed by, macrophages of the reticuloendothelial (RE) system, whose receptors for Fc and C3 attach to the antibody-coated red cells.

It is customary to divide the antibodies responsible for autoimmune hemolytic anemia into two groups, based on their physical properties. The first group consists of the ***"warm" autoantibodies***, so-called since they react optimally with the red cells at 37°C. The warm autoantibodies belong primarily to the ***IgG*** class and react with the ***Rh*** antigens on the surface of the red cells. Because activation of the complement cascade requires the close alignment of at least two molecules of IgG, the relatively sparse distribution of Rh antigens on the surface of the erythrocyte does not favor lysis via the complement pathway. IgG antibodies to these antigens are effective in the induction of ***immune adherence*** and ***phagocytosis.*** Thus individuals with autoimmune hemolytic anemia can be identified by a ***Coombs' test,*** which is designed to detect bound IgG on the surface of red cells. The reasons for the formation of the antibody causing the hemolytic anemia are unknown.

A second kind of antibody, the ***cold agglutinins***, attaches to red cells only when the temperature is below 37°C, and dissociates from the cells when the temperature rises above 37°C. Cold agglutinins belong primarily to the ***IgM*** class and are specific for the ***I*** or ***i*** antigens present in ***glycophorin***, a major constituent of the surface of red cells. Since the cold agglutinins belong to the IgM class, they are highly efficient at activating the complement cascade and causing ***lysis*** of the erythrocytes to which they attach. Nevertheless, hemolysis is not severe in patients with autoimmune hemolytic anemia due to cold agglutinins, so long as body temperature is maintained at 37°C. When arms, legs, or skin are exposed to cold and the temperature of the circulating blood is allowed to drop, however, severe attacks of hemolysis may occur. Sometimes, cold agglutinins appear after infection by *Mycoplasma pneumoniae* or viruses, but the reason for their appearance is unknown.

Another form of autoimmune hemolytic anemia is induced by ***drugs*** and is, thus, not strictly autoimmune in origin. However, it bears many of the same characteristics as the autoimmune disorder. A drug like penicillin, for example, may bind to some protein on the surface of red cells and induce formation of antibody, in much the same way as any hapten–carrier complex. The resulting antibody reacts with the drug (hapten) on the surface of the cell, causing ***lysis*** or ***phagocytosis***. In such cases, however, the disease is self-limiting and disappears when use of the drug is discontinued.

MYASTHENIA GRAVIS. Another autoimmune disease, in which antibodies to a well-defined target antigen are implicated, is ***myasthenia gravis***. In this disease, the targets are the ***acetylcholine receptors*** at neuromuscular junctions. Reaction of the receptor with antibody blocks the reception of a nerve impulse normally carried across the junction by acetylcholine molecules. This blockade results in severe ***muscle weakness***, manifested by difficulty in chewing, swallowing, and breathing, and it eventually leads to death from ***respiratory failure***. The disease can be experimentally induced in animals by immunization with acetylcholine receptors purified from torpedo fish or electric eel, which demonstrate significant cross-reactivity with mammalian receptors. The experimental disease, resulting from the formation of antibodies against the foreign receptors, which then bind to the mammalian receptors, mimics almost exactly the natural form of the disease and may be passively transferred with antibody.

The development of myasthenia gravis may somehow be linked to the thymus, since many patients have concurrent ***thymoma***, or hypertrophy of the thymus, and removal of the thymus sometimes leads to regression of the disease. Molecules cross-reacting with the acetylcholine receptor have been found on various cells in the thymus, such as thymocytes and epithelial cells, but whether these molecules are the primary stimulus for the development of the disease is unknown.

Immune Complex-Mediated Autoimmune Diseases

SYSTEMIC LUPUS ERYTHEMATOSUS (SLE). This disease presumably gets its name (literally "red wolf") from a reddish rash on the cheeks, which is a frequent early symptom. However, the distribution of the rash resembles the wings of a butterfly rather than the face of a wolf. The designation "wolf-like" is, thus, far-fetched, but the term "systemic" is quite appropriate since the disease attacks many organs of the body and causes ***fever***, ***joint pain***, and damage to the ***central nervous system***, ***heart***, and ***kidneys***. The kidney lesions are most clearly understood and are the most probable cause of death from SLE.

Despite the almost total mystery concerning the origin of this disease, a fair amount is known about the immunologic mechanisms responsible for the pathology that is observed. For unknown reasons, patients with SLE produce antibodies against several native components of the body. Of most interest are those antibodies produced against ***native double-stranded DNA***, which are a typical and prominent feature of SLE. Antibodies are also produced occasionally to ***denatured***, ***single-stranded DNA*** or to ***nucleohistones***. These antibodies are of particular interest since no known method of immunization with DNA has yet succeeded in inducing such antibodies experimentally.

Whatever their origin, these antibodies are believed to form circulating soluble complexes with DNA derived from the breakdown of normal tissue, such as skin. The abnormal sensitivity of SLE patients to ultraviolet irradiation, which causes prompt exacerbation of symptoms, lends some credence to this idea. The soluble complexes, as in any immune-aggregate disease (see Chapter 13), are filtered out of the blood in the kidneys and get trapped against the basement membranes of the glomeruli. Other complexes may be similarly trapped in arteriolar walls and joint synovial spaces to form the characteristic ***"lumpy-bumpy"*** deposits. These complexes now activate the ***complement cascade*** and attract ***granulocytes***; the subsequent ***inflammatory reaction*** is characterized as ***glomerulonephritis***. The resulting damage to the kidneys leads to a leakage of protein (***proteinuria***), and sometimes hemorrhage (***hematuria***), with symptoms waxing and waning as the rate of formation of immune complexes rises and falls. More recently, an alternative model has been proposed in which antigen alone (double-stranded DNA) becomes trapped in the glomerular basement membrane, through electrostatic interactions with a constituent of the membrane. When the antibody appears, it binds to the antigen in the membrane and activates the same sequence of inflammatory events. This sequence of events could explain the failure, in some instances, to detect any circulating DNA-antibody complexes.

Although, as already mentioned, the antigen that initiates production of these antibodies is unknown, some recent findings suggest a plausible explanation that offers an attractive approach to therapy. Animals immunized with certain strains of encapsulated bacteria, for example Klebsiella, make antibodies that cross-react very strongly with DNA. A common antigenic epitope appears to be the phosphorylated backbone of many of the cross-reacting polysaccharides and DNA. Thus, it is conceivable that SLE is the result of an immune response made by only a few individuals to some common environmental organism. The presence of a genetic component to this disease (discussed later in this chapter), merits further investigation.

RHEUMATOID ARTHRITIS. Rheumatoid arthritis is another example of an autoimmune disease in which inflammatory processes are believed by some to be a consequence of the formation of immune complexes. In this case, an abnormally produced antibody, generally of the ***IgM*** class and called ***rheumatoid factor,*** is specific for a determinant on the Fc portion of the patient's own IgG molecules. Again, it is not understood why these antibodies should form in high quantities in certain people. The complexes between rheumatoid factor and IgG are apparently deposited in the synovia of joint spaces, where they activate the complement cascade to release the chemotactic factors that attract the ***granulocytes***. The ongoing ***inflammatory response***, accompanied by ***increased vascular permeability***, induces ***joint swelling*** and ***pain*** as this exudate accumulates. The ***hydrolytic enzymes*** released by the neutrophils progressively break down the ***collagen*** and ***cartilage*** in the joints, with the eventual destruction of the sliding surfaces needed for proper function. After repeated bouts of inflammatory insult, with deposition of ***fibrin*** and replacement of the cartilage by fibrous tissue, the joint fuses (***ankylosis***), becomes immobile, and the inflammatory process subsides.

T-Cell–Mediated Autoimmune Disease—Hashimoto's Thyroiditis

This disease of the ***thyroid***, primarily found in middle-aged women, leads to the formation of a ***goiter*** (enlarged thyroid), or to ***hypothyroidism*** which results from destruction of thyroid function. Once again, there is no known etiology and the evidence for mediation by T cells is, at best, indirect. The evidence rests, in part, on the histologic picture that accompanies this disease. There is an infiltration of predominantly mononuclear cells into the thyroid follicles, which is characteristic of other T-cell–mediated delayed hypersensitivity reactions. Progressive destruction of thyroid follicles accompanies the presence of these infiltrates, and the gland attempts to regenerate and becomes enlarged. When destruction of follicles reaches a certain level, the output of thyroid hormone declines and the symptoms of hypothyroidism appear: dry skin, puffy face, brittle hair and nails, and a feeling of being cold all the time.

Several target antigens appear to be involved in this disease process, including ***thyroglobulin***, the major hormone made by the thyroid. Microsomal antigens from thyroid epithelial cells have also been implicated, and antibodies to both these types of antigen have been found in patients with Hashimoto's disease.

Further evidence implicating T-cell–mediated responses comes from study of ***experimental autoimmune thyroiditis,*** which may either be induced in animals by immunization with thyroglobulin in complete Freund's adjuvant or passively transferred by clones of T cells specific for thyroglobulin. An important distinction between the experimental and the naturally occurring autoimmune disease is that the former is acute and non-recurring while the latter has a chronic, recurrent course. Thus, the precipitating event in the naturally occurring autoimmune disease is probably some ongoing process, rather than a single immunizing event.

For reasons similar to those described above, ***multiple sclerosis***, which involves demyelinization of central nervous system tissue, has been considered to be a T-cell–mediated, autoimmune disease. The lesions resemble the cellular infiltrates involved in delayed-type hypersensitivity reactions. ***Experimentally induced allergic encephalomyelitis***, which follows immunization with myelin protein in complete Freund's adjuvant is a T-cell–mediated response that resembles, in many of its characteristics, multiple sclerosis. This evidence is, however, far from conclusive in establishing multiple sclerosis as an autoimmune disease.

Autoimmune Diseases Arising From Deficiency in Components of Complement

For unknown reasons, many patients with deficiencies in the early components of complement develop autoimmune diseases such as SLE. In addition, specific allotypes of some complement components predispose to the development of autoimmunity.

ETIOLOGY OF AUTOIMMUNE DISEASE

There must be mechanisms to prevent autoimmune disease from arising in normal individuals, but they are incompletely understood. Burnet's Clonal Selection Theory (see Chapter 9) postulated that autoreactive lymphocytes that made contact with self antigens during ontogeny were deleted or aborted. While this hypothetical mechanism provides some defense against autoimmunity, it cannot be the sole explanation, since normal individuals contain lymphocytes that can be shown to react against self antigens. For example, there are B cells that can bind thyroglobulin or DNA, and T cells that can respond to myelin protein or collagen.

Another protective device is the ***sequestration*** of potential antigens from the lymphoid system. The lens protein of the eye and the antigens of spermatozoa are considered to be examples of sequestered antigens, and when they are introduced to the immune system—by accident or design—an autoimmune response results. However, sequestration cannot explain why so many other self antigens such as thyroglobulin, IgG, and DNA, which circulate freely, are involved in autoimmune disease.

In view of all the potentially self-reactive lymphocytes with access to self antigens, the fact that autoimmune disease is the exception rather than the rule has led to a theory of ***immunoregulation*** that maintains that ***homeostasis*** is attributable to mechanisms, that hold autoreactive cells in check. Several examples of such control mechanisms, and how they may be upset to cause autoimmune disease, are described below.

Absence of Helper T Cells

Since it is known that low doses of antigen can produce tolerance in T cells without provoking an immune response (see Chapter 15), it is possible that some self antigens that circulate at low concentrations (thyroglobulin is an excellent example) render specific T cells tolerant but have no similar effect on B cells. Thus B cells, capable of binding thyroglobulin, exist in normal individuals but are not triggered to make autoantibody because help by appropriate T cells is not available (see Fig. 16.1A).

Several ***bypass mechanisms*** have been suggested, including provision of a new or altered carrier determinant capable of activating helper T cells. Experimentally, such a bypass can be achieved by ***chemical alteration*** of the

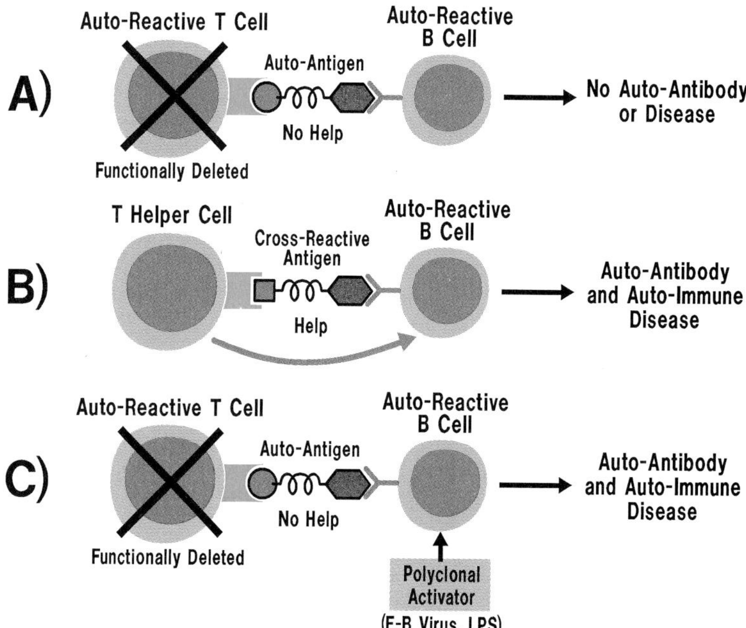

Figure 16.1
Possible mechanisms of induction of autoimmunity.

antigen, or by incorporating it into complete Freund's adjuvant or by using a ***cross-reactive antigen*** from a related species (see Fig. 16.1B). Another possible mechanism involves ***polyclonal activation***, which could nonspecifically trigger many B-cell clones (including the autoreactive ones) to produce antibody (see Fig. 16.1C).

Such conditions are believed to be mimicked to some extent by viral infections or by administration of drugs that may have the capacity to alter the carrier molecule and elicit help from T cells. Many bacterial infections, such as streptococcal infections, elicit antibody that cross-reacts with normal tissue (heart in the case of streptococcal infection), thus producing autoimmune disease. Finally, many bacteria, as well as Epstein-Barr viruses, are known to be powerful adjuvants and to induce polyclonal activation with a potential for eliciting an autoimmune response.

Control by Suppressor T Cells

Normal animals have been shown to control their immune responses by induction of ***suppressor cells*** and, in fact, experimental autoimmune processes have been shown to elicit shut-off mechanisms that involve suppressor T cells (see Chapter 15). This effect may explain why the experimentally induced phenomena tend to be acute and self-limiting. Finally, when activity of suppressor T cells in experimental animals is impaired by a low dose of irradiation or by treatment with cyclophosphamide, autoimmune diseases appear more rapidly and are more severe.

Several ***bypass mechanisms*** have been postulated. In addition to the experimental situations mentioned above, evidence of impaired immunoregulation has been found in several cases of human autoimmune disease, primarily as a deficiency in the functioning of T cells. In some cases, ***antibodies against suppressor T cells*** appear, so that the deficiency of these cells may represent a secondary phenomenon.

Absence of Antigens of the Class II MHC on Accessory Cells

Since helper T cells respond to antigen only when it is presented in association with class II antigens (see Chapter 11), it is possible that certain autoantigens on cells that possess only class I antigens are not presented and do not elicit autoimmune responses.

There are several possible ***bypass mechanisms***. It has been shown experimentally that a number of normal cells, such as the ***endothelial cells*** in blood vessels and ***thyroid epithelial cells***, may be induced by exposure to γ-interferon or lymphokines from activated T cells to express class II antigens on their surface. These activated normal cells now become capable, in the absence of other accessory cells, of presenting their surface antigens (such as thyroglobulin) to appropriate T cells, thus inducing autoimmune responses. Conceivably, therefore, viral infections of various tissues may lead, through the above mechanism, to induction of class II antigens in relevant cells, thus triggering a response to some self antigen that they possess.

GENETIC FACTORS IN AUTOIMMUNE DISEASE

Although the autoimmune diseases discussed here are all very different from one another, they have sufficient features in common to allow them to be considered as an entity. Foremost among these common features is the existence of a ***genetic predisposition*** that has been found to be associated with all the diseases discussed. However, while familial tendencies occur, the pattern of inheritance is generally complex and indicates involvement of several genes. Also, there tends to be considerable overlap of disease symptoms, with some people showing multiple autoantibodies to a variety of self antigens and others showing a different pattern. Although the genes involved may differ for each disease, the strongest evidence is of ***linkage between autoimmune disease and certain HLA haplotypes.*** While the exact mechanisms whereby these HLA haplotypes exert their influence is unknown, they could potentially take several forms, for example as defects in Ir genes. These observations on genetic predisposition are strongly reinforced by the study of autoimmune diseases in inbred strains of animals, such as the NZB $\times$ NZW mice, which develop a disease very similar to human SLE. The NZB mice develop autoimmune hemolytic anemia and glomerulonephritis, while the NZW strain mice have no clinical symptoms. However, when crossed with the NZB mice, the NZW mice produce F_1 offspring that have a much earlier and more severe form of SLE-like glomerulonephritis. The NZW mice must therefore contribute some gene(s) that affect(s) the time of onset and severity of the disease. Similarly, autoimmune disease in humans may involve the interplay of multiple genes.

The study of autoimmune diseases has the potential for a double reward: more successful treatment—or even prevention—of many serious autoimmune diseases and clucidation of the normal control and regulation of the immune response, of which autoimmune disease may represent an aberration.

SUMMARY

1. An autoimmune disease is one in which the body makes an immune response to one of its own constituent antigens, which then causes pathologic damage.

2. A multiplicity of organs and tissues is involved in autoimmune disease, and the type of immune response may take almost any of the known forms of hypersensitivity, which involve antibody, complement, and T cells.

3. Currently, it is believed that many autoreactive clones of T and B cells exist normally but are held in check by homeostatic mechanisms. It is the breakdown, by various mechanisms, of these controls that leads to the activation of autoreactive clones and autoimmune disease.

4. Most autoimmune diseases demonstrate familial occurrence, with a genetic predisposition among family members.

5. A strong association exists between many of these diseases and certain HLA haplotypes, suggesting a variety of mechanisms, which include some form of control by Ir genes.

REFERENCES

Schwartz RS, Roitt IM (1986): Autoimmune disorders. Progress in Immunol 6:477.

Smith HR, Steinberg AD (1983): Autoimmunity—A perspective. Annu Rev Immunol 1:175.

Talal N (1980): Tolerance and autoimmunity, Chapter 4. In Parker C (ed): Clinical Immunology, Vol 1. Philadelphia: W.B. Saunders.

REVIEW QUESTIONS

Questions 1 and 2 are followed by several suggested answers or completions. Select ONE that is BEST in each case.

1. Rheumatoid factor, found in synovial fluid of patients with rheumatoid arthritis, is most frequently found to be
   a) IgM reacting with kappa chains of IgG.
   b) IgM reacting with H chain determinants of IgG.
   c) IgE reacting with bacterial antigens.
   d) antibody to collagen.
   e) antibody to DNA.

2. Autoimmune diseases due to antibody may occur
   a) as a consequence of formation of antigen–antibody complexes.
   b) as a result of antibody blocking a cell receptor.
   c) as a result of antibody-induced phagocytosis.
   d) as a result of antibody-induced complement mediated lysis.
   e) as a result of all of the above.

For questions 3–7, ONE or MORE of the completions given is correct. Choose the appropriate answer:
A) if only *1, 2, 3* are correct
B) if only *1 and 3* are correct
C) if only *2 and 4* are correct
D) if only *4* is correct
E) if *all* are correct

3. The following is/are possible mechanism(s) for the development of autoimmune diseases:
   1) alteration of a self antigen so it is recognized as foreign.
   2) leakage of sequestered self antigen.
   3) loss of suppressor T cells.
   4) infection with a microorganism that carries a cross-reactive antigen.

(Continued on next page)

4. Aging New Zealand black (NZB) mice have
   1) increased frequency of autoimmune antibodies.
   2) increased suppressor T cell function.
   3) glomerulonephritis.
   4) a decrease in MHC-controlled antigens.

5. Autoantibodies to self antigens, such as thyroglobulin, can be induced in mice with tolerant T cells by
   1) immunization with rabbit thyroglobulin.
   2) removal of the thymus.
   3) injection of a polyclonal activator, such as lipopolysaccharide.
   4) blocking of macrophage function.

6. Hemolytic anemia may result from
   1) passive transfer of maternal Rh antibody to the fetus.
   2) production of cold agglutinins after certain viral infections.
   3) production of antibody to certain drugs.
   4) transfusion of autologous stored red cells.

7. Lupus erythematosus
   1) is due to a mutation in double-stranded DNA.
   2) has multiple symptoms and affects many organs.
   3) is an example of a T-cell–mediated autoimmune disease.
   4) results from formation of immune aggregates.

ANSWERS TO REVIEW QUESTIONS

1. ***b*** Rheumatoid factor is generally an IgM antibody that reacts with the determinants on the H chain.

2. ***e*** All are possible causes of antibody-induced, autoimmune disease.

3. ***E*** All are possible causes of autoimmune disease.

4. ***B*** (1) and (3) are correct. There is no known increase in the function of suppressor T cells in these mice and, in fact, this function may actually decrease.

5. ***B*** T cell tolerance may be bypassed by (1) use of a cross-reactive thyroglobulin or (3) by polyclonal activation of B cells. (2) and (4) are irrelevant.

6. ***A*** (1), (2) and (3) are known causes of hemolytic anemia. (4) is not known to cause formation of autoantibody.

7. ***C*** Lupus erythematosus affects skin, kidneys, heart, and joints. Symptoms are due to immune complexes that lodge in these areas and induce damage via activation of complement and infiltration of leukocytes. DNA may be involved as an antigen, but mutation (1) plays no role, and the disease is mediated by antibodies and not by T cells.

CHAPTER

17

TRANSFUSION IMMUNOLOGY

INTRODUCTION

After the discovery of the circulatory system by Harvey in the 17th century, many attempts were made to transfuse blood, first from animals into humans and later from humans into other humans. These transfusions almost always had disastrous consequences. The discovery in 1900 of the ABO blood group antigens by Landsteiner (a Nobel prize winner) established the immunologic basis for transfusion reactions.

The discovery of the ABO blood groups, the subsequent discovery of the Rh antigens, and the tests which were developed to determine the blood group antigen made the transfusion of blood from one human to another a practical and useful clinical procedure.

In this chapter we discuss the major erythrocyte ***alloantigens*** (antigens that differ between individuals of the same species); the problems they can cause; how they are detected; and how today, as a result of blood group typing, most blood transfusions proceed without any significant immunological risk.

THE ABO SYSTEM

Investigations with various human sera and red blood cells (RBC) led Landsteiner to conclude that, on the basis of the substances or antigens present on their surface, human RBC can be divided into four major groups: 1) erythrocytes with ***group A*** substance; 2) erythrocytes with ***group B*** substance; 3) erythrocytes with both ***group A and B*** substances; and 4) erythrocytes with ***neither group A nor group B*** substances. These blood group types were named A, B, AB and O, respectively. Landsteiner further established that individuals with type A blood have serum antibodies that agglutinate type B erythrocytes; people with type B blood have antibodies that agglutinate type A erythrocytes; individuals with type AB blood have no antibodies to these alloantigens; and individuals with type O blood have antibodies that agglutinate type A, B, and AB erythrocytes. The antibodies that agglutinate the alloantigen-bearing cells are referred to as ***isohemagglutinins.***

Subsequent studies on the familial distribution of the blood group antigens established that they are encoded by three alleles, A, B, and O, with A and B being dominant over O and co-dominant with respect to each other. The blood groups, their genotypes, their phenotypes, and the antibodies present in the sera of people with the RBC of a given blood group are shown in Table 17.1.

TABLE 17.1. The Genotype and Phenotype of the ABO Blood Group and the Antibodies Present in the Sera of Individuals With the ABO Blood Groups

Erythrocyte antigens		Distri-	
Genotype	Phenotype	bution (%)*	Antibodies present in sera
AA AO	A	42	anti-B (agglutinate group B and AB RBC)
BB BO	B	9	anti-A (agglutinate group A and AB RBC)
AB	AB	3	no anti-A or anti-B (will not agglutinate A, B, or AB RBC)
OO	O	46	anti-A and anti-B (agglutinate A, B, or AB RBC)

*White, North American population.

While the A and B genes determine the presence of A and B substances respectively, the O gene is totally inactive and does not code for any of the erythrocyte alloantigens. Nevertheless, blood group O erythrocytes do have a glycoprotein on the surface—the ***H substance***—which can be recognized by antisera from different animals. This glycoprotein is not the product of the O gene since it is present on RBC of people who are homozygous for the A or B genes.

The A, B, and H substances are related to each other in the following way: During the synthesis of the blood group molecules, H substance is synthesized first. The H substance is a glycoprotein with L-fucose as the terminal epitope that is recognized by antibodies. The A gene codes for an enzyme that converts the H substance into another glycoprotein—the A substance—by adding a terminal α-N-acetyl-galactosamine group (which becomes the antigenic determinant group of blood group A). Similarly, the B gene codes for an enzyme that converts the H substance into still another glycoprotein—the B substance—by adding a terminal α-D-galactosyl residue (which becomes the antigenic determinant of blood group B). Group O individuals do not make either enzyme and, thus, their erythrocytes have the unmodified H substance on their surface.

Since the H substance is common to groups A, B, AB, and O, none of the individuals in any of the blood groups has antibodies to the H substance. However, there are rare cases in which humans form antibodies to the H substance of O type RBC. Because this rare antibody was first found in Bombay, the individuals who form anti-H antibodies are called ***Bombay type*** individuals. They lack the gene that converts a glycolipid precursor to the H substance. Accordingly, they do not have the H (nor the A or B) substance, and they produce serum isoantibodies to the H substance (as well as to the A and B substances).

From studies performed on blood group alloantigens present in saliva (see below), it appears that the A, B, and H antigens represent different determinants present on the same glycopeptide molecule. This conclusion is based on the observation that antiserum specific to one of these antigens (the H substance) causes the coprecipitation of the A and B antigens as well.

Distribution of A, B, and H Antigens

The ABO blood group substances A, B, and H are present as ***glycoproteins*** on the surface of ***erythrocytes,*** as well as on the surface of many ***epithelial*** cells and most ***endothelial*** cells. The A, B, and H substances are also present as ***mucopolysaccharides*** in secretions (such as saliva, sweat, gastric juices) of approximately 80% of all humans; these people are termed ***"secretors,"*** and their secreted substances are immunologically identical to those present on their erythrocytes. The secretion of these substances is controlled by alleles Se and se, with Se being dominant. Only homozygous recessive individuals (se/se) are non-secretors. Thus, the individual oligosaccharide determinant, which accounts for the designation A, B, or O, may appear on different backbones, but it is recognized by the same antiserum.

Isohemagglutinins

Because of their ability to agglutinate human RBC, and because they are of human origin, antibodies to the A and B antigens are called ***isohemagglutinins***. (It is more correct to call them allohemagglutinins, but the term isohemagglutinins has gained general acceptance.) They occur naturally—i.e. without deliberate sensitization or immunization against them—and they are often referred to as "natural isohemagglutinins." Individuals with type O erythrocytes normally produce IgM isohemagglutinins, directed against A and B blood groups; individuals with type A blood have anti-B IgM isohemagglutinins, and those with type B blood have anti-A IgM. It is still not certain what triggers the synthesis of these antibodies in the absence of prior exposure to the antigens. It is generally believed, however, that the antibodies have been induced by polysaccharides of intestinal bacteria or of other microorganisms that cause occult infections and induce antibodies that cross-react with the A and B blood group substances. Evidence in support of this hypothesis derives from the fact that isoantibodies are not present at birth but develop during the first year of life, as the gut is colonized by various bacteria.

MN BLOOD GROUP

The MN blood group is a ***minor blood group*** that was discovered by use of rabbit antisera raised against human erythrocytes. This blood group is totally independent of the ABO system.

Regardless of the ABO blood type, the erythrocytes of each human individual have M or N, or both, antigens on their surface. These antigens are encoded by the co-dominant M and N alleles. The antigenic activity is related to the glycoprotein ***glycophorin*** (of molecular weight approximately 16,000 daltons), which is present on the membrane of all erythrocytes. There are at least two types of glycophorin molecules, which differ somewhat in their amino acid sequences and in the extent of glycosylation. Only their glycosylated products are related to the M or the N antigenicity.

Ss ANTIGENS

The S and s antigens are associated with the M and N antigens: the S antigen is associated predominantly with M; and the s, with N. The S and s antigens are encoded by two co-dominant alleles. Like the MN group, the Ss group is a ***minor blood group*** that rarely plays a role in blood transfusion.

Rh ANTIGENS

In the 1930s, after the discovery of ABO and MN blood group antigens, Landsteiner and Weiner discovered that rabbit antisera raised against rhesus monkey RBC agglutinated the erythrocytes from approximately 85% of humans tested. These human erythrocytes had, on their surface, an antigen that cross-reacted with antibody to a rhesus erythrocyte antigen and was responsible for the agglutination of rhesus monkey erythrocytes by rabbit antibodies. Consequently, the antigen was called ***Rh antigen*** (for rhesus) and the cells of these individuals were designated Rh^+ cells. The remaining 15% of humans had no such antigen on the surface of their erythrocytes and their cells were, therefore, designated Rh^- cells.

At approximately the same time as these investigatons were undertaken, Levine and Stetson, who were obstetricians, not immunologists, described the case of a woman, who had given birth to a baby with ***hemolytic disease of the newborn, erythroblastosis fetalis,*** and who had suffered a severe transfusion reaction upon receiving blood from her husband, who had the same ABO type. A collaboration between the obstetricians and Landsteiner and Weiner established that the father's RBC and the baby's RBC were Rh^+ but that the mother's RBC were Rh^-. Similarly, in babies with hemolytic disease, in all cases, the disease occurred when the mother was Rh^- and the baby was Rh^+ (fathered by an Rh^+ father).

It was also shown that the serum of the mothers of babies with hemolytic disease contained antibodies to the Rh antigens and that these antibodies were predominantly of the IgG isotype. This isotype passes through the placenta, so that maternal IgG, directed against fetal Rh antigens on fetal RBC, reacts with the fetal erythrocytes and causes hemolysis. In cases of ABO incompatibility, erythroblastosis fetalis is not a problem because the isohemagglutinins belong to the IgM class and do not cross the placenta. However, even in cases where IgG antibodies are made, they tend to be absorbed by placental tissues, which themselves contain AB blood group substances.

The question arises as to how an Rh^- mother becomes sensitized to Rh antigens. Apparently, small numbers of fetal red blood cells enter the maternal circulation during pregnancy, but this number is too low to induce significant titers of anti-Rh antibodies. Indeed, only 1% of the first pregnancies of Rh^- women with Rh^+ babies results in erythroblastosis fetalis. However, during parturition, the mother is exposed to massive numbers of Rh^+ cells from the fetus and becomes immunized by them, producing high levels of anti-Rh IgG, which can affect a subsequent pregnancy. Indeed, the more pregnancies an Rh^- women goes through (with Rh^+ babies), the greater the likelihood of her receiving "booster" exposures to Rh antigens and the higher her anti-Rh titer.

Rh Genetics

From results of experiments with various anti-Rh sera, it now appears that there are more than 30 distinct, antigenic specificities of Rh antigens. The genetics of the Rh antigens is still controversial, but it appears that the Rh specificitics are encoded by a single Rh locus with closely linked genes and with many alleles. The Rh phenotypes and their frequencies are shown in Table 17.2.

It is now clear that the ***D antigen*** is by far the most important of all the Rh antigens. Over 90% of all cases of hemolytic disease of the newborn are attributable to the D antigen. Thus, a mother who is phenotypically dXX is D^- and is therefore considered Rh^-, and potentially capable of making anti-D antibodies.

TABLE 17.2. Rh Phenotypes and Their Frequencies in the United States

Phenotype				
Fisher-Race nomenclature	Weiner nomenclature	Frequency (%)	Reaction with anti-D	Rh group designation
DCe	Rh_1, R_1	54	+	Rh^+
DCE	Rhz_1, Rz	15	+	Rh^+
DcE	Rh_2, R_2	4	+	Rh^+
Dce	Rh_0, R_0	2	+	Rh^+
dce	rh_1, r_1	13	–	Rh^-
dCe	rh^1, R^1	1.5	–	Rh^-
dcE	rh^{11}, R^{11}	0.5	–	Rh^-
dCE	rhy^1, Ry	Very rare	–	Rh^-

Prevention of Rh Disease

The major event that sensitizes the Rh^- mother to D antigen and other Rh^+ antigens appears to occur during parturition, when the mother is exposed to the baby's Rh^+ erythrocytes. Thus, the administration of anti-Rh antibodies (human anti-Rh) within 72 hours of parturition is an effective way to"tie up" and cause the rapid clearance of Rh^+cells from the mother's circulation. One widely used preparation of anti-Rh antibodies is called ***Rhogam*** and consists of human IgG against the D antigen.

THE KELLY AND DUFFY BLOOD GROUPS

The Kelly and Duffy blood groups are ***minor blood groups*** which, nevertheless, on occasion can be responsible for transfusion reactions. The Kelly system consists of two allelic forms, K and k. Approximately 10% of the population carries the K antigen, which is highly immunogenic, on their erythrocytes. Exposure to K antigen during pregnancy or transfusion induces the formation of anti-K IgG, which may cause lysis in the presence of complement.

The Duffy system depends on the presence of Fy antigens. Repeated transfusions (or repeated pregnancies) may induce anti-Fy IgG, which may cause problems during transfusion.

TRANSFUSION REACTIONS

Transfusion reactions occur because of the reaction between the recipient's antibodies and the transfused cells from the donor. The amount of antibody against the recipient's cells, present in the donor's serum, is generally not important in transfusion, because these antibodies are highly diluted by the serum and the large number of red cells of the recipient. However, transfusion reactions have been known to occur when the donor's antibodies against the recipient's antigens were present at very high titers.

There are three types of immunologically mediated transfusion reactions: ***hemolytic reactions, febrile reactions, and allergic reactions.***

Hemolytic Reactions

Hemolytic reactions are the most serious reactions resulting from blood transfusions. They result mainly from a) ABO incompatibility (usually due to clerical or laboratory error); b) Rh incompatibility (the D antigen is the most immunogenic of all blood group antigens, and transfusion of Rh^+ blood into an Rh^- recipient with high anti-D titers can have disastrous consequences); and c) incompatibility in minor blood group antigens, such as Kelly or Duffy.

Severe hemolytic reactions occur within minutes of transfusion. The reaction is accompanied by diffuse muscle pain, headache, nausea, and sometimes vomiting. A rise in temperature is common. The reaction can result in a state of shock, and renal failure may develop. Also, because of the activation of the blood clotting factors by damaged erythrocytes, those factors become depleted and a generalized hemorrhagic tendency develops. Such a transfusion reaction, occurring immediately upon transfusion dictates the immediate discontinuation of the transfusion.

Febrile Reactions

Febrile reactions are often due to reactions with minor blood group antigens. Therefore, repeated transfusions of the same blood type mismatched for minor blood groups, which may lead to higher titers of antibodies directed against the minor blood groups, should be avoided.

Allergic Reactions

Allergic reactions range from mild urticaria to systemic anaphylactic shock. The patient may break out in hives and develop bronchoconstriction with dyspnea and wheezing, which may proceed to a cardiovascular collapse with a drop in blood pressure (symptoms typical of systemic anaphylaxis; see Chapter 13).

SELECTION OF DONORS

In routine ***blood typing,*** tests for only the ABO and Rh (C, D, and E) blood groups of donor and recipient are performed. Mismatch or incompatibility with respect to these antigens precludes transfusion between the pair.

CROSS-MATCHING

As has already been mentioned, high titers of antibodies against minor blood groups may lead to transfusion reactions. Cross-matching of donor and recipient blood group antigens provides a more reliable measure of blood group compatibility than routine ABO and Rh typing. The cross-matching between donor and recipient usually consists of an agglutination test, which involves the mixing of donor's cells with recipient's serum, both in the absence and presence of anti-immunoglobulins (the Coombs' test). This procedure is referred to as major cross-match. A minor cross-match (not generally performed in the United States or Canada) consists of mixing the donor's serum with a sample of the recipient's cells.

In cases of extreme emergency, when cross-matching is not possible, unmatched blood from the universal donor (type O, Rh^-) may be used.

SUMMARY

The major erythrocyte alloantigens of humans, which are responsible for transfusion reactions are as follows:

1. The ABO blood group antigens are present on the surface of erythrocytes (and on the surface of many epithelial and endothelial cells).

2. Isohemagglutinins are "naturally" occurring IgM antibodies directed against the ABO alloantigens. Individuals with type O blood have anti-A and anti-B IgM; individuals with type A blood have anti-B agglutinins; and individuals with type B blood have anti-A agglutinins.

3. MN and Ss antigens constitute minor human blood groups.

4. Rh antigens are present on erythrocytes of 85% of the human population, referred to as Rh^+. The remaining 15% have no Rh antigens on their erythrocytes and are referred to as Rh^-. Rh^- mothers, who are exposed to Rh antigens, make anti-Rh IgG antibodies which pass through the placenta and cause hemolytic disease of the newborn—erythroblastosis fetalis.

Transfusion reactions may result in the destruction of the transferred cells by hemolysis, or by opsonization and increased phagocytosis. They can also result in fever and/or allergic reactions.

To avoid transfusion reactions, the donor and recipient blood groups are cross-matched, primarily for ABO and Rh compatibility.

REFERENCES

Leikola J (1984): Blood banking and immunohematology. In Stites DP, Stobo JD, Fudenberg HH, Wells JV (eds): Basic and Clinical Immunology, Ed 5. Los Altos, California: Lange Med. Pub.

Miller VW (ed) (1981): Technical Manual of the American Association of Blood Banks, Ed 8. Washington, D.C.: American Association of Blood Banks.

Mollison PL (1979): Blood Transfusion in Clinical Medicine, Ed 6. Oxford, England: Blackwell Scientific Publications.

Race RR, Sanger R (1968): Blood Groups in Man. Philadelphia: F.A. Davis.

Wallace J (1977): Blood Transfusion for Clinicians. New York: Churchill Livingstone.

REVIEW QUESTIONS

For questions 1–4, choose the ONE answer that is BEST in each case.

1. Blood from group AB donors can be transfused to a recipient without causing a transfusion reaction if
   a) the recipient is type AB.
   b) the recipient is type A.
   c) the recipient is type B.
   d) the recipient is type O.
   e) the recipient and donor are siblings.

2. Transfusion between donors and recipients with different ABO blood group antigens
   a) should not be attempted.
   b) should be performed only after treatment with immunosuppressive drugs.
   c) should be followed by giving the recipient epinephrine or antihistamines.
   d) will induce a mixed lymphocyte reaction.
   e) will result in a graft versus host reaction.

3. The following statements regarding hemolytic disease of the newborn are correct except
   a) administration of anti Rh globulins to an Rh^- mother soon after delivery of an Rh^+ baby can suppress the induction of anti-Rh globulins by the mother.
   b) it is an example of a type II hypersensitivity reaction.
   c) if the newborn is Rh^- and the mother is Rh^+, the fetus becomes tolerant to Rh antigens.
   d) the mother forms antibodies against Rh antigens which she lacks.
   e) D antigen is the most important Rh antigen in hemolytic disease of the newborn.

4. A type A, Rh^+ woman gave birth to a type O, Rh^- baby. Therefore, all of the following statements are true except
   a) the mother must be heterozygous for Rh antigen.

b) the mother does not have the AA genotype.
c) the father could have the BO, Rh^+ genotype.
d) a type AB, Rh^+ man could not be the father.
e) the baby may have the AO genotype.

For questions 5 and 6, ONE or MORE of the completions given is correct. Choose the appropriate answer:
A) if only *1, 2, 3* are correct
B) if only *1 and 3* are correct
C) if only *2 and 4* are correct
D) if only *4* is correct
E) if *all* are correct

5. Blood group incompatibility poses a transfusion risk because
   1) the donor's immunoglobulins react with the recipient's erythrocytes.
   2) a mixed lymphocyte reaction takes place.
   3) the recipient's T lymphocytes will become activated by the donor's antigens.
   4) the recipient's immunoglobulins react with donor's erythrocytes.
6. The structural units that confer immunologic specificity to ABO blood group substances
   1) contain no galactose.
   2) are oligosaccharides.
   3) are small peptides attached to a polysaccharide backbone.
   4) contain fucose and N-acetylhexosamine.

ANSWERS TO REVIEW QUESTIONS

1. ***a*** If the donor's blood group is AB, donor's blood can be transfused into a type AB recipient because the recipient does not make antibodies against his or her own blood group. Type AB cells cannot be transfused to a type A individual because the recipient has anti-B antibodies. Similarly, type AB cells cannot be transfused into a type B individual because he or she has antibodies against type A. Finally, AB cells cannot be transfused into a type O individual because that individual has both anti-A and anti-B antibodies. Unless they are homozygous twins, even brothers and sisters can have different blood groups.

2. ***a*** Transfusion should not be performed if donor and recipient differ in their ABO blood group antigens. Transfusion of blood into a recipient with different blood group antigens will not cause a GVH reaction because the recipient will reject the donors cells. A GVH reaction due to donor's lymphocytes may occur, if the recipient is immunologically suppressed.

(Continued on next page)

A mixed lymphocyte reaction between donor's and recipient's lymphocytes may occur, but this reaction is not the one responsible for the transfusion reaction, in which recipient's antibodies destroy the donor's erythrocytes.

3. ***c*** All the statements are correct except c: hemolytic disease of the newborn (erythroblastosis fetalis) occurs only when the mother is Rh^- and the fetus is Rh^+; thus, statement c is irrelevant.

4. ***e*** All the statements are true except statement e. A type O individual must be homozygous for O, since both A and B are dominant over O.

5. ***D*** 4 is correct. The transfusion risk arises because the recipient's immunoglobulins (the isohemagglutinins which are IgM, or the IgG antibodies if the recipient has been previously transfused with cells that contain the donor's antigens) react with the donor erythrocytes. The reaction of the donor immunoglobulins with the recipient erythrocytes is usually not of clinical significance because of the dilution of the donor antibodies in the recipient blood. However, if the donor contains high titers of antibodies against recipient's erythrocytes, a transfusion reaction may occur in which the donor antibodies destroy recipient erythrocytes.

   Although donor blood contains lymphocytes, which may participate in a mixed lymphocyte reaction with recipient lymphocytes, this reaction poses no transfusion risk. Also, the possibility that the recipient lymphocytes will become activated by donor antigens does not pose a potential transfusion risk, when donor and recipient are incompatible.

6. ***C*** 2 and 4 are correct. The structural units of ABO blood group antigens are oligosaccharides, which contain fucose and N-acetylhexosamine. Also, the A and B substances contain galactose. There are no peptides involved in the immunological specificity of the ABO blood groups.

CHAPTER

18

TRANSPLANTATION IMMUNOLOGY

INTRODUCTION

The immune response has evolved as a way of discriminating between *"self"* and *"non-self."* Once "foreignness" has been established, the immune response proceeds toward its ultimate goal of destroying the foreign material: a microorganism or its product, a substance present in the environment, a drug, or a tumor cell. The triggering of the immune system in response to such foreign substances is, of course, of great survival value.

The transplantation of cells or organs from one individual to another for therapeutic purposes has become, in some cases, commonplace. For example, transfusions of blood are routine, and over 10,000 kidneys are transplanted per year worldwide. More spectacular, and frequently widely publicized, even transplantations of the heart are becoming more common. Except for monozygotic twins, all cells of individuals from a given species (and, of course, from different species) carry on their surfaces many molecules that differ between individuals. Thus, if cells from a given individual are transferred or transplanted into another individual, they will be recognized by the recipient as foreign and will trigger an immune response aimed at destroying those foreign cells.

Transfusion refers to the transfer of blood from one individual to another. The transfer of any other tissue or organ is referred to as ***transplantation***. Transfusion immunology was dealt with in Chapter 17; transplantation immunology is the subject of this chapter.

RELATIONSHIP BETWEEN DONOR AND RECIPIENT

Various situations of transplantation from donor to recipient are shown in Figure 18.1 and are described below.

1. An ***autograft*** is a graft or transplant from one area to another on the same individual. An autograft is exemplified by the transplantation of skin from one area of an individual to a burned area of skin on the same individual. The graft is recognized as ***autochthonous*** ("self"), and no immune response is induced against it. Barring technical difficulties in the transplantation process, the graft will survive or "***take***" in its new location.

2. An ***isograft*** or ***syngraft*** is a graft or transplantation of cells, tissue, or organ from one individual to another individual who is ***syngeneic*** (genetically identical) to the donor. An example of an isograft is the transplantation of a kidney from one identical (homozygotic) twin to the other.

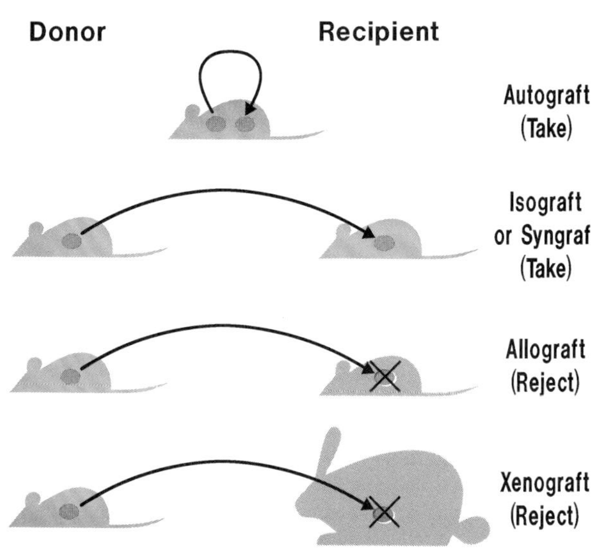

Figure 18.1.
Situations of tissue transplantation.

As in the case of an autograft, the recipient who is genetically identical to the donor recognizes the donor's tissue as "self" and does not mount an immune response against it. The two individuals, i.e. donor and recipient, are described as ***histocompatible***.

3. An ***allograft*** is a graft, or transplant, from one individual to a genetically dissimilar individual of the same species. Since all individuals of a given outbred species, except monozygotic twins, are ***allogeneic*** (genetically dissimilar), regardless of how closely they may be related, the graft is recognized by the recipient as "foreign" and is immunologically rejected. The donor and recipient, in this case, are ***non-histocompatible*** or ***histoincompatible.***

4. A ***xenograft*** is a graft between a donor and a recipient from different species. The transplant is recognized as foreign, and the immune response mounted against it will destroy or reject the graft. Donor and recipient are again described as ***histoincompatible***.

IMPLICATION OF THE IMMUNE RESPONSE IN GRAFT REJECTION

There are many lines of evidence to prove that graft rejection is mediated by immunologic mechanisms.

First and Second Set Rejections

The most direct evidence for the involvement of the immune response is provided by experiments in which skin is transplanted from one individual to a genetically different individual of the same species—i.e. between allogeneic donor and recipient. Mouse skin with black hair transplanted onto the back of a white-haired mouse appears normal for one or two weeks. However, after approximately two weeks, the transplant begins to be rejected, and is completely sloughed off within a few days. This process is called ***first set rejection.*** If, after the rejection, the recipient is transplanted with another piece of skin from the same initial donor, the process of ***rejection is accelerated***, and the graft is sloughed off much more quickly, within about a week of the second transplant. This accelerated rejection is termed a ***second set rejection.*** The second set rejection is an expression of ***immunologic memory.***

Adoptive Transfer

The capacity to mount a second set rejection can be transferred from one individual to another by the ***transfer of lymphoid cells***. Also, second set rejection exhibits immunologic specificity, since a second set rejection occurs only when the transplanted tissue is derived from the individual that served as donor of tissue for the first transplantation. If an individual that exhibits a second set rejection is transplanted with tissue from yet another individual that is genetically different from the original donor, this transplant will be rejected as a first set rejection.

Histopathology

In addition to the evidence just described, many other lines of evidence point to the immunologic nature of graft rejection. For example, 1) histologic examination of the site of the rejection reveals ***lymphocytic and monocytic cellular infiltration*** reminiscent of the delayed-type hypersensitivity reaction; 2) individuals that lack T lymphocytes (such as athymic, or "nude," mice or humans with DiGeorge syndrome—see Chapter 12) do not reject allografts or xenografts; and 3) the process of rejection slows down considerably or does not occur at all in immunosuppressed individuals.

Antibodies and Cell-Mediated Immunity Against Allotransplant

It has been conclusively demonstrated that specific ***T cells*** and ***circulating antibodies*** are induced to an allograft or a xenograft after transplantation. However, although antibodies are responsible for the rejection of red blood cells during the transfusion reaction (see Chapter 17), T cells constitute the major immunologic component responsible for the rejection of most other tissues. In fact, it has been demonstrated in many instances that certain antibodies that are not effective in the process of graft rejection compete with T cells for the transplantation antigens, thereby ***blocking*** the process of rejection mediated by T cells and enhancing the survival of the graft. Because of this phenomenon, these antibodies are described functionally as ***enhancing antibodies*** (see Fig. 18.2).

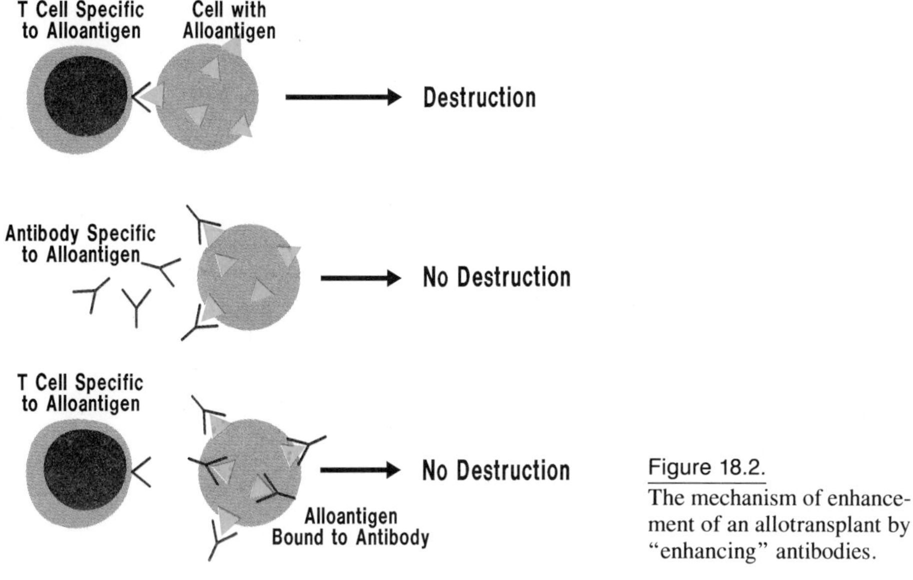

Figure 18.2.
The mechanism of enhancement of an allotransplant by "enhancing" antibodies.

CLINICAL CHARACTERISTICS OF ALLOGRAFT REJECTION

Clinically, allograft rejections fall into three major categories: 1) ***hyperacute rejection***, 2) ***acute rejection***, and 3) ***chronic rejection***. The following are descriptions of the rejection reactions as might be observed, for example, after transplantation of a kidney.

Hyperacute Rejection

Hyperacute rejection occurs within a few minutes to a few hours of transplantation. It is a result of destruction of the transplant by ***preformed antibodies*** to the graft, synthesized as a result of previous transplantations, blood transfusions, or pregnancies. These antibodies activate the ***complement*** system, causing ***swelling*** and ***interstitial hemorrhage*** in the transplanted tissue, which decrease the flow of blood through the tissue. ***Thrombosis*** with ***endothelial injury*** and ***fibrinoid necrosis*** are often seen in cases of hyperacute rejection. The recipient may have ***fever***, ***leukocytosis*** and produce ***little or no urine.*** The urine may contain various cellular elements, such as erythrocytes.

At present there is no therapy for successful prevention or termination of hyperacute rejection.

Acute Rejection

Acute rejection is seen in a recipient who has not previously been sensitized to the transplant. It is the common type of rejection experienced by individuals for whom the transplanted tissue is a mismatch, or who receive an allograft and insufficient immunosuppressive treatment to prevent rejection. For example, an acute rejection reaction may begin a few days after transplantation of a kidney, with a complete loss of kidney function within 10–14 days.

Acute rejection of a kidney is accompanied by a rapid ***decrease in renal function***. ***Enlargement and tenderness*** of the grafted kidney, a ***rise in serum creatinine levels***, a ***fall in urine output***, ***decreased renal blood flow***, and presence of blood ***cells*** and ***proteins in the urine*** are characteristic. Histologically, there is an intense ***mononuclear infiltration*** of the cortical interstitium.

The acute rejection reaction may be reduced by immunosuppressive therapy, for example with antilymphocytic serum, corticosteroids or other drugs (see below).

Chronic Rejection

Chronic rejection occurs in allograft transplantation months after the transplanted tissue has assumed its normal function. In cases of kidney transplantation, chronic rejection is characterized by ***slow, progressive, renal failure***. Histologically, the chronic reaction is accompanied by ***proliferative inflammatory lesions*** of the small arteries, ***thickening of the glomerular basement membrane***, and ***interstitial fibrosis***. Because the damage caused by immune injury has already taken place, immunosuppressive therapy at this point is useless, and little can be done to save the graft.

HISTOCOMPATIBILITY ANTIGENS

The antigens that evoke the immune response associated with graft rejection are referred to as ***transplantation antigens,*** or ***histocompatibility antigens*** (H antigens for short). The histocompatibility antigens are cell surface molecules encoded by histocompatibility genes (H genes) situated at a histocompatibility locus (H locus). Since different alleles encoding allelic forms of the histocompatibility antigens exist at each H locus in different individuals, the antigens are also referred to as ***alloantigens.***

If there were only one H locus with two alleles, for example A and B, the possible genotypes and phenotypes of the alloantigens would be:

Genotype	Phenotype
AA	A
AB	AB
BB	B

Transplantation between individuals with the above genotypes would be accepted or rejected as follows:

	Donor		Recipient	Accept/Reject	Reason
1)	AA	→	AA	Accept	A recognized as self
2)	BB	→	AA	Reject	B recognized as foreign
3)	AB	→	AA	Reject	B recognized as foreign
4)	AA	→	BB	Reject	A recognized as foreign
5)	BB	→	BB	Accept	B recognized as self
6)	AB	→	BB	Reject	A recognized as foreign
7)	AA	→	AB	Accept	A recognized as self
8)	BB	→	AB	Accept	B recognized as self
9)	AB	→	AB	Accept	A and B recognized as self

The above example applies to a single H locus with two alternative genotypes. In reality, there are many H loci containing many alleles. For example, in mice there are about 40 H loci, the most important of which is ***H-2*** (see Chapter 11). The H-2 locus is the most important because differences at this locus always lead to rapid graft rejection; differences at any of the other loci lead to slower rejection (although multiple differences at minor H loci can cumulatively lead to rapid rejection). The H-2 locus in the mouse consists of a segment of the chromosome 17 (see Fig. 11.1A). This segment contains genes that encode several important products associated with immunologically related phenomena, such as ***the major histocompatibility antigens (class I encoded by K and D genes and class II encoded by I region genes),*** and genes that code for ***components of the complement*** system (see Chapter 11). Because of its importance in graft rejection, this segment of the chromosome of the mouse is called the ***major histocompatibility complex*** or ***MHC.***

The loci at the MHC are generally closely linked. The particular combination of alleles present at linked loci on one chromosome is termed the ***haplotype.*** In a sense, the haplotype is the genotype of linked loci on each of the parental chromosomes.

In humans, the strong histocompatibility antigens are encoded by genes situated on a segment of chromosome 6. Analogous to the segment on chromosome 17 of mice, this segment, known as ***human leukocyte antigens (HLA),*** constitutes the major histocompatibility complex or MHC of humans. This segment contains genes that encode the strong, ***human histocompatibility antigens,*** as well as genes that encode ***the complement components*** and ***class II antigens,*** which participate in immune responses and are analogous to the Ir gene product in mice (see Chapter 11).

The human HLA gene complex (see Fig. 11.1B) consists of several closely linked genes (loci), known as A, B, C, and D, with the ***D locus*** consisting of DP, DQ, and DR genes (formerly called SB, DC, and DR). Each locus has many different alleles. As in the mouse, the particular combination of alleles at the same locus on the same chromosome is termed the haplotype; two haplotypes, one from each parent, constitute the genotype of the individual.

The A, B and C loci code for ***class I antigens*** (see Chapter 11), which are present on all nucleated cells and can be detected serologically. These antigens are therefore designated ***serologically defined antigens (SD).*** Antigens encoded by the DP, DQ, and DR genes of the D locus have a more limited cellular distribution and are detected primarily by an assay that employs a mixed lymphocyte culture (see below). They are, therefore, designated ***lymphocyte-defined antigens (LD).*** However, the D-related or DR antigens can also be detected serologically.

Class I Antigens

The A, B and C genes of humans, and the K and D genes of mice, encode antigens that are found on the surface of ***all the nucleated cells*** of the body, including T and B lymphocytes and macrophages, but excluding erythrocytes. These antigens are called class I antigens. Each of the loci encodes a polypeptide chain with a molecular weight of approximately 45,000 daltons. On the cell membrane, each such polypeptide is linked, non-covalently, with a lighter chain, a β_2***-microglobulin*** (molecular weight 12,000 daltons), which is encoded by a gene on another chromosome. Thus, the resulting class I molecule has a ***heavy chain*** encoded by the MHC and a ***light chain*** encoded elsewhere (see Fig. 11.3).

The light chain (β_2-microglobulin) of various individuals within a species is identical. Thus, the diversity or polymorphism exhibited by class I molecules of different individuals within a species is attributable to variations in the heavy chain encoded by the genes of the MHC. The heavy chain is usually glycosylated, with about 10% of its molecular weight made up by carbohydrate. However, deglycosylation of the chain does not alter its antigenic properties, so that the diversity in antigenic specificities exhibited by the various class I molecules is attributable solely to the heavy chain polypeptide encoded by genes of the MHC. Although class I molecules of different individuals within a species are different, there is over 80% homology in the amino acid sequences of class I molecules of various individuals, suggesting that all class I molecules are encoded by genes of common ancestry.

Class I antigens readily induce formation of antibodies and cytotoxic T lymphocytes. Thus, cells bearing class I antigens on their surface constitute the targets involved in the rejection of tissue, which is mediated by antibodies and complement and by cytotoxic T lymphocytes. Antigens encoded by the A and B loci evoke a strong immune response; antigens encoded by the C locus evoke a weak response.

Class II Antigens

The ***D region genes*** of man and the ***I region genes*** of the mouse encode glycoproteins found on the surface of ***B lymphocytes***, ***monocytes***, ***Langerhans' cells*** of the skin, and ***endothelial cells***. These glycoproteins, known as ***class II molecules***, differ from individual to individual within a species. They are associated with various processes that take place during an immune response, notably ***presentation*** of antigen to T cells by macrophages and by B cells (see Chapter 11).

The structure of class II molecules is different from that of class I molecules (see Fig. 11.3). Class II molecules consist of two chains of approximately the same size, an ***alpha chain*** (molecular weight 33,000 daltons), and a ***beta chain*** (molecular weight approximately 28,000 daltons), which are noncovalently linked. Both chains show some variability due to the variability in the genes that encode them. However, that exhibited by the alpha chain is limited, whereas the beta chains exhibit significant variability.

There is a high degree of homology in amino acid sequence between the polypeptide chains of class II antigens, indicating that they are encoded by genes that arose (by duplication) from a common ancestral gene. Moreover, there is a high degree of homology between class I and class II antigens, as well as between those antigens and domains of the immunoglobulin molecule, a link that is strongly suggestive of a common ancestry for all these stuctures.

The D antigens of the HLA play the most important role in tissue rejection. They are the antigens that ***activate helper T cells*** (see Chapter 11). There is good agreement among transplant immunologists that the better the match (or parity) in HLA-D, the higher the probability of survival of the graft. If the donor and recipient share both DR haplotypes, then the probability of graft survival is significantly increased, compared to a situation where only one DR haplotype is shared. In general, the graft does not survive if the donor and recipient do not share any DR haplotype.

TESTS FOR HISTOCOMPATIBILITY ANTIGENS

The analysis of histocompatibility antigens of donor and recipient allows a determination of the degree of foreignness between the two individuals, and serves to predict the outcome of a transplantation.

There are several ways to determine the degree of parity or disparity between transplantation antigens. One way is by utilization of various antisera to detect cell surface antigens. Another way is by measuring the reaction between leukocytes from the donor and recipient.

Serological Detection of Transplantation Antigens

The ***serologically defined (SD)*** antigens are usually classified by use of a panel of antisera against transplantation antigens. These antisera are obtained from people who have had multiple transplantations or transfusions, and from multiparous women. Recently, monoclonal antibodies have become useful for defining SD antigens. These antisera and monoclonal antibodies are used in a ***lymphocytotoxicity test*** in which the sera, in the presence of complement, are monitored for ability to damage the target cells, which are lymphocytes. Thus, lymphocytes of the donor and recipient, which carry class I and class II antigens, are reacted with a panel of antibodies. The reaction with the various antibodies establishes the ***serologic type*** of each transplantation antigen on the cells. Identity of donor and recipient transplantation antigens is indicated by identity in the specific antisera with which the two sets of cells react (or do not react).

Serologic ***tissue typing*** provides a fairly reliable measure of parity (or disparity) between transplantation antigens of the donor and the recipient. However, because the number of antisera available for such a test is finite, there is always the possiblity that, although the panel of sera shows a "match"—i.e. the identity of antigens on the donor's and recipient's leukocytes—differences would be found if the panel of antisera were enlarged.

Detection of Transplantation Antigens by the Mixed Leukocyte Reaction

In the ***mixed leukocyte reaction (MLR),*** leukocytes from donor and recipient are cultured together for several days. The donor leukocytes contain T cells with specificity directed against the alloantigens on the recipient cells, and those ***T cells*** will therefore be triggered to ***proliferate*** in the presence of these antigens. The same is true for recipient leukocytes, which will proliferate in the presence of alloantigens on the donor cells. The proliferation is usually measured by introducing a radioactively labeled precursor to DNA, such as ***^{3}H-thymidine,*** into the culture. The greater the extent of proliferation, the more DNA is synthesized by the proliferating cells, and the more radioactivity is incorporated into the cells' DNA. The radioactivity incorporated in DNA is then calculated to provide a measure of the proliferative response.

In comparison to the serological test, which defines the specific antigens of the MHC of the donor and recipient, the MLR measures the total parity (or disparity) between donor and recipient cells, a parameter that is of utmost importance for transplantation: the stronger the MLR (the greater the extent of proliferation), the higher the disparity between donor and recipient. Conversely, a mixed lymphocyte culture, in which cellular proliferation is not induced, indicates complete parity or histocompatibility between donor and recipient. Histocompatibility is revealed when the MLR is performed on cells from identical twins.

In most cases, it is essential to ascertain whether the recipient lymphocytes will react against the donor histocompatibility antigens (rather than whether the donor lymphocytes will react against the recipient alloantigens). For this purpose, a mixed lymphocyte culture is set up in which the donor cells have been treated with mitomycin C or X-irradiation to prevent their proliferation. In this way, the only cells with the ability to proliferate are the recipient leukocytes. Such a reaction is called a ***one-way mixed leukocyte reaction***.

The one-way MLR is also performed when immunocompetent cells are to be transplanted into an immunosuppressed individual. It is essential that such transplantation be performed between extremely well-matched individuals in order to avoid a reaction by the transplanted immunocompetent cells directed against the recipient's tissue. Such a reaction, termed a ***graft versus host reaction (GVH reaction),*** is of particular concern when bone marrow, which contains immunocompetent T cells, is transplanted into an immunologically incompetent host.

Although MLR testing for histocompatibility is a highly effective indicator of the degree of parity between donor and recipient, it is a lengthy procedure and requires several days, whereas the serological test takes only a few hours. Thus, the use of MLR and/or serological testing is dictated by the speed with which an organ must be transplanted after its removal from the donor. While transplantation of organs from a living donor can await the results of the MLR test, sufficient time for this test may not be available in cases of organs obtained from recent cadavers.

PROLONGATION OF ALLOGRAFTS

Unless transplantation is performed between identical twins, allotransplantation always carries the risk of allograft rejection. The higher the degree of disparity between donor and recipient, the faster will be the rejection of the graft.

There are several measures taken during allotransplantation that are aimed at prolonging allograft survival. These measures employ drugs that suppress the immune response.

Anti-Inflammatory Agents

Adrenocortical steroids, such as prednisone, prednisolone, and methyl prednisolone, are anti-inflammatory agents. The immunosuppressive action of these steroids is due to their ability to stabilize lysosomal membranes, thus preventing the release of harmful lysosomal enzymes. These steroids may also interfere with the processing and presentation of antigen to T cells by antigen-presenting cells (see Chapter 10).

Antimetabolites

Antimetabolites that suppress the immune response include the purine antagonists ***azathioprine*** and ***mercaptopurine***, which interfere with the synthesis of RNA. ***Chlorambucil*** and ***cyclophosphamide***, compounds that alkylate DNA, also have antimetabolic activity and interfere with the metabolism of DNA.

Cytotoxic Agents

Among the cytotoxic agents that suppress the immune response are many that are cytotoxic to lymphocytes. Such agents include ***antilymphocytic serum (ALS)*** or ***antilymphocytic globulins (ALG), steroids, alkylating agents, X-rays,*** and ***antibiotics*** such as actinomycin D. All these agents are cytotoxic, but they are particularly effective against proliferating cells, such as the lymphocytes, which proliferate in response to alloantigens.

Cyclosporine is a compound that is becoming important for immunosuppression during allotransplantation. It is a product of a fungus, and it greatly enhances graft survival, presumably by suppressing helper T cells or by increasing the activity of suppressor T cells.

It is important to note that, when immunosuppression is induced by the methods mentioned, it is not antigen-specific. In fact, it results in a generalized suppression of the whole immune response, including the response against infectious microorganisms. Thus, the immunosuppressed individual is highly susceptible to infections. Furthermore, because immunosuppression is associated with an increased incidence of lymphoproliferative disorders, management of the transplant patient must take into account the immunosuppressed state of the individual.

Enhancement by Antibodies

In most cases of tissue or organ transplantation, rejection is largely a result of cell-mediated immunity, in which T lymphocytes are the key participants. Cells recognize specific alloantigens, become activated, and release lymphokines, which recruit inflammatory cells to the site of the reaction. In general, antibodies have not been demonstrated to be efficient in mediating the rejection of tissue allografts (except, of course, in the destruction of blood cells in transfusion reactions). In fact, as mentioned earlier in this chapter, under many experimental conditions, antibodies against the foreign tissue have been found to bind with the foreign tissue and to prevent its destruction by the mechanisms of cell-mediated immunity (Fig. 18.2). The prevention of rejection or the prolongation of survival of the graft by specific antibodies is called ***enhancement,*** and the antibodies responsible for it are called ***enhancing antibodies.*** The relevance of enhancing antibodies in clinical situations of organ or tissue transplantation remains to be established.

MHC AND DISEASE

A striking feature of the HLA system is that a particular haplotype (such as HLA-A1-B8) occurs in the general population with a much higher frequency than would be expected from a random association of genes. This indicates that there is a ***linkage disequilibrium*** between certain alleles. This linkage disequilibrium implies that there is a certain advantage to be gained by the absence of recombinational events at a given site in a gene segment and by the linkage of particular genes, or alternatively, that there is an advantage to be gained by preservation of a certain linkage. The finding that some diseases are associated with a particular combination of HLA genes is probably associated with the phenomenon of linkage disequilibrium. The subject of the association of MHC and diseases is discussed in Chapter 11.

GRAFT VERSUS HOST REACTIONS

Transplantation of immunocompetent lymphocytes from a donor to a genetically different recipient can result in a reaction mounted by the grafted lymphocytes against the recipient's tissue. This ***graft versus host (GVH)*** reaction (also described in Chapter 14) is particularly important in cases where immunocompetent lymphoid cells are transplanted into individuals who are ***immunologically incompetent*** and therefore cannot reject the transplanted cells. This situation is best exemplified in cases where immunocompetent cells are transferred into individuals with various immunodeficiency disorders. In experimental animals, a GVH reaction may lead to a ***wasting syndrome*** in the recipient; in humans, GVH reactions may produce ***splenomegaly*** (enlarged spleen), ***enlarged liver and lymph nodes***, ***diarrhea***, ***anemia***, ***weight loss***, and other disorders in which the underlying causes are inflammation and destruction of tissue. The graft versus host reaction is initiated by the transferred T lymphocytes from the donor, which recognize the recipient’s tissue as foreign. However, most of the inflammatory cells that participate in the reaction, and that are mainly responsible for destruction of tissue, are host cells recruited to the site of the reaction by lymphokines released by the donor’s lymphocytes.

SUMMARY

1. Transplantation rejection is immunologically mediated.

2. Both T cells and circulating antibodies are induced against allografts or xenografts. While antibodies are responsible for rejection of erythrocytes, T cells are mainly responsible for the rejection of most other tissue.

3. The most important transplantation antigens, which cause rapid rejection of the allograft, are found on cell membranes and are encoded by genes in the major histocompatibility complex (MHC), which is called H-2 in mice and HLA in humans. The structures encoded by these genes are of great importance in the discrimination between “self” and “non-self” and in cellular interaction. These structures are referred to as class I and class II antigens.

4. In case of minor mismatches, survival of allografts may be prolonged by anti-inflammatory agents, cytotoxic agents, and antimetabolites.

5. There appears to be a correlation beteen the MHC and disease, with several diseases strongly correlated with a particular histocompatibility type.

REFERENCES

Bach FH, Van Rood JJ (1976): The Major Histocompatibility Complex — Genetics and Biology, Parts 1–3. N Engl J Med 295:806, 872, 927.

Batchelor JR, Chiu YL (1986): Transplantation: Achievements and challenges outstanding. Progress in Immunol 6:1002.

Daussett J, Svejgard A (1977): HLA and Disease. Copenhagen: Munksgaard Press.

Good RA (1983): Immunologic reconstruction: Achievements and potentials. In Dixon FA, Fisher DW (eds). The Biology of Immunologic Disease. Sunderland, Massachusetts: Sinauer.

Kimball JW (1983): Introduction to Immunology. New York: MacMillan.

Najarian JS (1983): Immunologic aspects of transplantation. In Dixon FA, Fisher DW (eds): The Biology of Immunologic Disease. Sunderland, Massachusetts: Sinauer.

Simmons RL, So SKS (1984): Clinical transplantation. In Stites DP, Stabo JD, Fudenberg HH, Wells VW (eds): Basic and Clinical Immunology, Ed 5. Los Altos, California: Lange Medical Publications.

REVIEW QUESTIONS

For questions 1–4, select the ONE answer or completion that is BEST.

1. Kidney transplantation was performed using a kidney from a donor who was matched to the recipient by serological tissue typing. However, within a few months the kidney was rejected. Assuming no technical problems from the surgical procedure, one reason for the rejection may be that
a) there was insufficient blood supply to the graft.
b) there could have been a mismatch, which would have been detected by a mixed lymphocyte reaction.
c) the recipient developed blocking antibodies.
d) the recipient also suffered from Wiscott-Aldrich syndrome.
e) the donor was agammaglobulinemic.

2. Currently, the best indicator for predicting compatibility for transplantation of tissue from donor (A) to recipient (B) is obtained by
a) one-way mixed lymphocyte reaction between B cells and mitomycin C-treated A cells.
b) one-way mixed lymphocyte reaction between A cells and mitomycin C-treated B cells.
c) serological typing and cross-matching of A and B cells.
d) two-way mixed lymphocyte reaction between A and B cells.
e) matching for blood group antigens.

3. The MHC complex contains all of the following except
a) genes that encode transplantation antigens.
b) genes that encode immunoglobulins.
c) genes that regulate immune responsiveness.
d) genes that encode some components of complement.
e) genes that encode class I and class II antigens.

4. The most common serological test used for the detection of HLA antigens on lymphocytes is
a) the complement fixation test.
b) double gel diffusion.
c) complement-dependent cytotoxicity test.
d) mixed lymphocyte reaction.
e) radioimmunoassay.

For questions 5–8, ONE or MORE of the completions given is correct. Choose the appropriate answer:
A) if only *1, 2, 3* are correct
B) if only *1 and 3* are correct
C) if only *2 and 4* are correct
D) if only *4* is correct
E) if *all* are correct

5. GVH disease
   1) requires histocompatibility differences between donor and recipient.
   2) requires immunocompetent donor cells.
   3) may result from infusion of blood products that contain viable lymphocytes into an immunologically incompetent recipient.
   4) requires suppressor T cells.

6. Transplantation reaction may involve the following:
   1) cell-mediated immunity.
   2) type 3 (immune aggregate) hypersensitivity.
   3) complement-dependent cytotoxicity.
   4) the release of MAF (macrophage activating factor).

7. Which of the following statements concerning the mixed lymphocyte reaction (MLR) are correct:
   1) Specific responding cells are B lymphocytes.
   2) MLR results in clonal expansion of specific, alloantigen-reactive cells.
   3) MLR between unrelated individuals who differ according to HLA serology are usually negative.
   4) Stimulation of proliferation is controlled primarily by the HLA-D region alleles.

8. In clinical transplantation, cytotoxic antibodies
   1) cause delayed rejection of the transplant.
   2) are responsible for hyperacute rejection.
   3) cause rejection when present in the donor.
   4) may be directed against HLA antigens.

(Continued on next page)

ANSWERS TO REVIEW QUESTIONS

1. ***b*** The most probable reason for the rejection is that, although serologically the donor and recipients were matched, this was an incomplete measure. The accuracy of serological matching is predicated on the number of sera used in the test. There is always the possibility that a mismatch would have been detected if additional sera had been used. The mixed lymphocyte reaction is more reliable, since it can detect mismatches that may not be detected serologically. Answer (a) is not correct, since it is stated that there were no problems due to the surgical procedure. Answer (c) is incorrect since blocking antibodies developed by the recipient would be expected to enhance the survival of the transplant. Answer (e) is incorrect because the immune status of the kidney donor is, in this case, irrelevant to the outcome of the transplantation.

2. ***a*** Compatibility can be reliably predicted by the one-way mixed lymphocyte reaction between the recipient's B cells and mitomycin C-treated cells from the donor. In this way, the test measures only the reactivity of the recipent cells against the donor antigens, which is of practical importance in the transplantation. The reverse—i.e. reaction between A cells and mitomycin C-treated recipient B cells—is of no practical importance, because A is not the recipient. Serological typing and cross-matching of A and B are of value, since those tests are more rapid than the MLR reaction. However, there is always the possibility that the panel of antisera used is not complete, and that if more antisera were used a mismatch would be found. The two-way MLR is important in assessing the total degree of parity (or disparity) in transplantation antigens, but it does not determine if the reaction is that of the donor to the recipient cells, or that of the recipient to donor cells, or both. Matching for blood group antigens is imperative but not sufficient.

3. ***b*** The MHC complex contains all genes mentioned except genes that encode immunoglobulins. They are on a different chromosome.

4. ***c*** The most common serological test used for detection of HLA antigens on lymphocytes is the complement-dependent cytotoxicity test. The mixed lymphocyte reaction, especially the one-way MLR, is an excellent test for HLA-D antigens, but it is a test based on cellular reactions and not on the reaction of serum antibodies.

5. ***A*** 1, 2, and 3 are correct. The GVH disease is caused by the destruction of cells or tissue of an immunoincompetent recipient by immunocompetent lymphoid cells transferred from a histoincompatible donor. The GVH reaction does not require suppressor T cells.

6. ***E*** All are correct. The important process in the rejection of an allotransplant is cell-mediated immunity. Here, T cells, which recognize the alloantigens, become activated; the T cells release lymphokines, one of which is MAF; they recruit and activate other phagocytic cells that, together with cytotoxic T cells, destroy the graft. However, the reaction to the allotransplant may also involve antibodies (IgM and IgG), which can cause damage to tissue via activation of complement and the recruitment of polymorphonuclear cells to the site of the reaction. The polymorphonuclear cells would damage the graft by the release of their lysosomal enzymes.

7. ***C*** 2 and 4 are correct. The MLR reaction results in the clonal expansion of specific T cells, which recognize the alloantigens in the D region of the HLA. Although clones of B cells may also expand, the major cellular expansion is that of the T cells. The MLR between unrelated individuals who differ according to HLA serology are usually positive (rather than negative).

8. ***C*** 2 and 4 are correct. Cytotoxic antibodies, such as IgM and IgG, cause hyperacute rejection by complement-mediated cell lysis or by opsonization and subsequent destruction of the transplant by phagocytic cells. The cytotoxic antibodies may be directed against blood group antigens or HLA antigens on transferred cells (e.g. leukocytes). The presence of cytotoxic antibodies in the donor is usually of no clinical importance since, even if they are transferred to the recipient with the donor's blood, they become highly diluted in the recipient.

CHAPTER 19

TUMOR IMMUNOLOGY

INTRODUCTION

The existence of an immune response directed against a tumor is based on changes in the surface components of the tumor cell, that do not occur in its nonmalignant counterpart, and that give rise to structures that may be antigenic. In 1943 Gross observed that when tumor cells were transplanted into the skin of syngeneic (genetically identical), histocompatible mice, the cells formed nodules that grew for a few days and then regressed. When identical tumor cells were reinjected into the mice, they did not produce nodules or grow. These findings were interpreted to mean that the mice that rejected the tumor did so because they had become immunologically resistant—or immune—to the tumor. Subsequently, ***tumor-specific transplantation antigens (TSTAs)***, which have the ability to induce anti-tumor immune responses, have been demonstrated for many tumors in a variety of animal species, including humans.

The goals of tumor immunology are 1) to elucidate the immunological relationship between the host and the tumor and 2) to utilize the immune response to tumors for the purpose of ***diagnosis, prophylaxis,*** and ***therapy.*** In the present chapter we shall discuss various aspects of these goals.

TUMOR ANTIGENS

Some antigens on the surfaces of malignant cells may constitute new structures, unique to the cancerous cells and ***absent*** from their normal counterparts. Other antigens may represent structures that are common to both malignant and normal cells, but that are ***"masked"*** on the normal cell and become ***"unmasked"*** on the malignant cell. Still other antigens on malignant cells represent structures that are present on ***fetal or embryonic cells*** but not on normal adult cells. These latter antigens are referred to as ***oncofetal*** or ***oncodevelopmental*** antigens.

CLASSIFICATION OF TUMOR ANTIGENS

Tumor antigens may be classified into four major categories. The categories differ both in the mechanisms that induce the malignancy and in the immunochemical properties of the tumor antigens. The four categories of tumor antigens are discussed in the sections that follow.

Antigens of Tumors Induced by Chemical or Physical Carcinogens

Antigens of tumors induced by chemical carcinogens exhibit ***little or no immunological cross-reactivity***; each tumor exhibits a ***distinct antigenic specificity***. Thus, cells of a given tumor, arising from a single transformed cell, all share common antigens, while different tumors, even if induced by the same carcinogen, are antigenically distinct from one another. For example, if the chemical carcinogen methylcholanthrene is applied in an identical manner to the skin of two genetically identical animals, or on two similar sites on the same animal, the cells of the developing tumors (sarcomas) will exhibit antigens unique to each tumor, with no immunological cross-reactivity between the tumors.

As with chemically induced tumors, there is little or no cross-reactivity between physically induced tumors, such as those induced by ultraviolet light or by X-irradiation.

Random mutations induced by the chemical or physical carcinogen are probably responsible for the absence of immunological cross-reactivity between the different tumors induced by any one of these carcinogens.

Many human and animal tumors are attributed to chemical and physical environmental factors such as radiation, smoke, and tar. Unfortunately, since tumors induced by chemical and physical carcinogens do not exhibit immunological cross-reactivity, the utilization of the immune response for the diagnosis, prophylaxis, and therapy of such tumors is difficult, if not impossible.

Antigens of Virally Induced Tumors

Tumors induced by DNA or RNA oncogenic viruses exhibit ***extensive immunological cross-reactivity***. Any particular oncogenic virus induces the expression of the same antigens in a tumor, regardless of the tissue of origin or the animal species.

For example, DNA viruses such as polyomas, SV40, and Shope papilloma virus induce tumors that exhibit extensive cross-reactivity within each group. Many leukemogenic viruses, such as Raucher leukemia virus, induce the formation of tumors that exhibit cross-reactivity not only within each group, but also between some groups. In this connection, there is considerable evidence to suggest that several human cancers, such as ***Burkitt's lymphoma***, ***nasopharyngeal carcinoma***, and ***T cell leukemia***, are caused by viruses. Thus, although the viral etiology of these cancers remains to be conclusively established, the immunological cross-reactivity in these, as well as in some other human malignancies, is similar to the cross-reactivity seen in animal tumors induced by viruses. For example, cross-reactivity is well established for cell surface antigens of Burkitt's lymphomas or of neuroblastomas from different patients. ***Colon carcinoma*** cells obtained from different patients also exhibit immunological cross-reactivity, as do melanoma cells from different patients.

The antigens of virally induced tumors are encoded by the virus, but they are distinct from virion antigens and are referred to as ***tumor associated antigens*** (TAA). Occasionally, virally induced tumors may express oncofetal antigens, encoded by the host genome. These are normally shut off during maturation but get reexpressed as a result of deregulation of genes on the host's genome by the oncogenic virus during the malignant transformation.

Oncodevelopmental Tumor Antigens

Many tumors express on their cell surfaces, or secrete into the blood, products that are normally present during embryonic and fetal development, but that are either not present or present at very low levels in normal adult tissue. These structures are not immunogenic in the autochthonous (native or original) host. Their presence can be detected by antisera prepared against them in allogeneic or xenogeneic animals. One such oncofetal antigen is the ***carcinoembryonic antigen CEA,*** which is found primarily in serum of patients with ***cancers of the gastrointestinal tract***, especially cancer of the colon. CEA antigens may be shed into the circulation and can be found in sera of patients with a variety of neoplastic diseases. Elevated levels of CEA (above 2.5 ng/ml) have been detected in the circulation of patients with colon cancer, some types of lung cancer, pancreatic cancer, and some types of breast and stomach cancer. However, CEA has also been detected in the circulation of patients with non-neoplastic diseases, such as emphysema, ulcerative colitis, and pancreatitis, as well as in the sera of alcoholics and heavy smokers.

Another oncodevelopmental antigen is ***alpha-fetoprotein (AFP),*** which is present at high concentrations in normal fetal serum and in maternal serum but absent from serum of normal individuals. AFP is rapidly secreted by cells of a variety of cancers and is found in the sera of patients with ***hepatomas*** and ***testicular teratoblastomas***.

The association of oncodevelopmental antigens with a wide variety of tumor types strongly suggests that their presence is the result of the derepression of normal genes that are usually repressed in the normal adult individual.

Antigens of Spontaneous Tumors

Spontaneous tumors are those tumors that are induced by unknown causes. Until recently, for most spontaneous tumors, it was difficult to discern an immunological response in the autochthonous host, and antigens on the surface of cells from spontaneous tumors were detected only with the aid of allogeneic or xenogeneic antiserum. However, with the recent advent of sensitive detection techniques, antibodies to autochthonous tumors have been detected in patients with some tumors, most notably malignant melanoma. In some cases, the antigens do not exhibit immunological cross-reactivity, in other cases they do. Thus, immunochemically defined antigens of spontaneous tumors resemble those of chemically or virally induced tumors.

THE IMMUNE RESPONSE TO TUMORS

Most of what is known about the host's immune response to tumors has been derived from experiments with transplantable tumors in animals. Moreover, most of the information concerning humoral and cellular anti-tumor immune effector mechanisms and their capacity to destroy tumor cells has been derived from experiments in vitro. Nevertheless, there is now ample presumptive evidence to suggest that the immune response plays an important role in the relationship between the host and the tumor, in humans as well as in other animals.

Humoral and ***cellular*** immune effector mechanisms capable of destroying tumor cells in vitro are summarized in Table 19.1. In general, destruction of tumor cells by these mechanisms is more efficient in the case of ***dispersed tumors***—i.e. when the target tumor cells are in suspension. It is difficult to demonstrate destruction of tumor cells in the case of solid tumors.

TABLE 19.1. Humoral and Cellular Effector Immune Mechanisms in Tumor Cell Destruction

A. Humoral mechanisms
  1. Lysis by antibody and complement
  2. Antibody and complement-mediated opsonization
  3. Antibody-mediated loss of tumor cell adhesion

B. Cellular mechanisms
  1. Destruction by cytotoxic T cells
  2. Antibody-dependent, cell-mediated cytotoxicity (ADCC)
  3. Destruction by activated macrophages
  4. Destruction by natural killer (NK) cells

Humoral Responses

LYSIS OF TUMOR CELLS MEDIATED BY ANTIBODY AND COMPLEMENT. Both ***IgM*** and ***IgG*** antibodies have been shown to destroy tumor cells in vitro in the presence of complement. Several studies conducted with mice indicate that, in the presence of complement, anti-tumor antibodies are effective in vivo in destroying leukemia and lymphoma cells, and in reducing metastases in several other tumor systems. Other studies in vivo and in vitro, however, show that the same antibodies, in the presence of complement, are ineffective in destroying the cells of the same tumor in a solid form.

DESTRUCTION OF TUMOR CELLS BY OPSONIZATION AND PHAGOCYTOSIS. Destruction of tumor cells by phagocytic cells has been demonstrated in vitro, but only in the presence of anti-tumor immune serum and complement. The relevance of this finding in vivo is unknown.

ANTIBODY-MEDIATED LOSS OF ADHESIVE PROPERTIES OF TUMOR CELLS. It appears that metastatic activity of certain kinds of tumors requires the adhesion of the tumor cells to each other and to the surrounding tissue. Antibodies directed against tumor cell surfaces may interfere with the adhesive properties of the tumor cells. The relevance of this mechanism in vivo is also unknown.

Cell-Mediated Responses

DIRECT DESTRUCTION OF TUMOR CELLS BY CYTOTOXIC T LYMPHOCYTES. Destruction of tumor cells in vitro by specific immune T lymphocytes has been demonstrated numerous times for a variety of tumors, both dispersed and solid. Moreover, from many studies with experimental animals (primarily but not exclusively mice), there is good evidence that tumor-specific, cytotoxic T cells are responsible for destruction of tumor in vivo. Although helper T cells participate in the induction and regulation of cytotoxic T cells, the destruction of the tumor cell is achieved by the ***cytotoxic T lymphocytes (CTL)*** with specificity for the antigens on the surface of the tumor cell.

ANTIBODY-DEPENDENT, CELL-MEDIATED CYTOTOXICITY. ***Antibody-dependent, cell-mediated cytotoxicity (ADCC)*** involves 1) the binding of tumor-specific antibodies to the surface of the tumor cells; 2) the interaction of various cells, such as granulocytes, macrophages, and ***K cells*** ("killer" lymphocytes without T or B cell surface markers), which possess surface receptors for the Fc portion of the antibody attached to the tumor cell; and 3) the destruction of the tumor cells by substances that are released from these cells that carry receptors for the Fc portion of the antibody. The importance of this mechanism in the destruction of tumor cells in vivo is still not clear.

DESTRUCTION OF TUMOR CELLS BY ACTIVATED MACROPHAGES. Macrophages may become highly cytotoxic when they become "activated" by lymphokines, most notably by a specific ***macrophage activating factor (MAF)*** that is identical to ***γ-IFN*** and produced by an activated population of T lymphocytes which, by themselves, are not cytotoxic. These T lymphocytes ($T4^+$ in humans, $L3T4^+$ in mice) are antigen-specific; they release MAF after activation by antigen. Other lymphokines released by these antigen-activated T lymphocytes attract macrophages to the area of the antigen, and still others, like ***migration inhibitory factor (MIF)*** prevent migration of macrophages away from the antigen. The mechanism of activation of macrophages by T cells specific for tumor antigen, leading to destruction of tumor cells, is similar to mechanisms involved in delayed type hypersensitivity reactions or in the killing of microorganisms: antigen-specific T cells become activated by antigen, and they release lymphokines, which attract and activate macrophages. These activated macrophages are cytotoxic to the microorganisms, to tumor cells, and even to "self" cells in the vicinity of the activated macrophages.

Mounting evidence to indicate that destruction of tumor cells by activated macrophages occurs in vivo includes the following observations: 1) resistance to a tumor can be abolished by specific depletion of macrophages; 2) increased resistance to tumor accompanies an increase in the number of activated macrophages; and 3) activated macrophages are frequently found at the site of regression of a tumor.

DESTRUCTION OF TUMOR BY NATURAL KILLER CELLS. ***Natural killer (NK) cells*** are lymphoid cells found in spleen, lymph nodes, bone marrow, and peripheral blood of nonimmune rodents and normal humans. These cells can lyse a variety of target cells, such as virally infected cells, antibody-coated cells, undifferentiated cells, and cells from a number of different tumors. The NK cells lack most of the characteristic cell surface markers of mature T lymphocytes, B lymphocytes, or macrophages. They can be functionally distinguished from ***K cells*** (killer cells), since the activity of NK cells is not increased after immunization, and it is not dependent on the presence of antibody. The level of activity of NK cells is different in different strains of mice and can be augmented by exposure to bacterial adjuvants, tumor cells, virally infected cells, and interferon. Activation of NK cells does not involve immunological memory, and activation is inhibited by prostaglandin E.

It appears that NK cells identify their target via recognition of, and binding with, the ***glycosphingolipid asialo-GM$_1$***. However, the exact mechanism by which NK cells recognize and kill their targets is still not understood.

There is circumstantial evidence to suggest that NK cells play an important role in the host–tumor relationship and may be particularly important in the host's defense against early stages of tumor growth, before the development of killer T cells and T-cell–mediated activated macrophages.

The humoral and cellular effector immune mechanisms that participate in the destruction of tumors are summarized in Table 19.1.

ROLE OF THE IMMUNE RESPONSE IN THE RELATIONSHIP BETWEEN HOST AND TUMOR

The foregoing discussion dealt with immune effector mechanisms, which have been demonstrated in vitro, and in some instances in vivo, to destroy tumor cells. However, a question may be raised about the degree to which the immune response plays a role in the host-tumor relationship. There are several phenomena that strongly indicate that the immune response has a profound effect on that relationship. These are described below.

Tumors in Immunosuppressed Individuals

There is evidence that tumors occur more frequently in immunosuppressed individuals than in their normal counterparts. Such tumors are predominantly but not exclusively ***lymphoproliferative*** malignancies. The almost 100-fold increase in the incidence of lymphoproliferative tumors in victims of radiation or in patients subjected to deliberate immunosuppression, and the elevated incidence of a wide range of tumors in older individuals whose immune response is reduced strongly suggest that the immune response plays an important role in the relationship between a tumor and its host.

Tumors in the Immunocompetent Host

An involvement of the immune response in the host–tumor relationship is suggested by the correlation between the appearance of various immunological effector mechanisms and the state of resistance to transplanted tumors in experimental animals. Furthermore, there is a correlation between the appearance of immune components at the site of the tumor and the regression of tumors in animals and humans. Moreover, there are examples in experimental animals to indicate that the primary tumor may induce a state of acquired "concomitant immunity" in the host. ***Concomitant immunity*** is expressed by the host's ability to reject newly arising or transplanted tumors of the same type, despite the progression of the primary tumor.

Immune Surveillance

The ***theory of immune surveillance***, proposed by Thomas in the 1950's and expanded by Burnet (a Nobel prize winner) later in the same decade, suggests that the immunological mechanisms that operate in the rejection of an allograft, in particular cell-mediated immunity, have evolved as a primary and specific defense against neoplastic cells, which arise continually in the normal organism as a result of somatic mutations. There are many examples, both experimental and clinical, that support the theory of immune surveillance, in particular those cases in which the incidence of cancer is high in the immunodeficient or immunosuppressed host. However, doubt is cast on the validity of the theory of immune surveillance by the finding that the incidence of tumors in athymic mice is no higher than in their normal counterparts. It should be noted, however, that such athymic mice have increased numbers of NK cells. Furthermore, surface antigens on tumor cells of "spontaneous" tumors are generally of weak immunogenicity. Thus, to date, the theory remains controversial and unproven.

Limitations of the Effectiveness of the Immune Response Against Tumors

Whether or not the theory of immune surveillance is correct, there is no question that an immune response can be induced against tumors. Then, why, in spite of the immune response, does the tumor continue to grow in the host? Several possible mechanisms may be operational; either alone or in combination with each other (Table 19.2). Factors that may influence the escape of tumor cells from destruction by the immune system are described in the paragraphs that follow.

TABLE 19.2. Limitations of the Effectiveness of the Immune Response to Tumors

1. Tumor resides in immunologically privileged site
2. Antigenic modulation of tumor antigens
3. Presence of enhancing or "blocking" factors
4. Suppressor T lymphocytes
5. Immune suppression by tumor cell products
6. Excessive tumor mass

PRIVILEGED SITES. Certain areas of the body, such as parts of the eye and tissues of the central nervous system, are immunologically "privileged" sites: they are inaccessible to effector cells of the immune response or their products. Consequently, tumors arising in such immunologically privileged sites escape destruction by the immune response.

ANTIGENIC MODULATION. Tumor cells may change their antigenic characteristics or lose their antigens altogether, thus escaping destruction by the immune response. In fact, it is conceivable that the immune response destroys all the antigen-bearing tumor cells, thereby selecting for non-antigenic tumor cells.

ENHANCING AND BLOCKING FACTORS. On theoretical grounds, destruction of tumor cells by immune components may be ***"blocked"*** by circulating, ***soluble antigens*** derived from the tumor, which would bind with tumor-specific antibodies or cells and would prevent the binding of these antibodies and cells with the same antigens present also on the surface of the tumor cell. In addition, various immune components may interfere with each other. For example, protection of tumor cells and enhancement of tumor growth may be achieved in vivo by first reacting the tumor cells with ***tumor-specific antibodies***. If these antibodies do not destroy the tumor, they can, in fact, inhibit its destruction by tumor-specific T lymphocytes directed against the same or adjacent antigens on the surface of the tumor cell. Thus, antibodies, as well as circulating antigen, and also ***antigen–antibody complexes*** may constitute "**blocking**" factors, which prevent the destruction of the tumor and may even enhance its growth. Moreover, some studies have indicated that some tumor-specific immune responses may even enhance the metastasis of a tumor.

SUPPRESSOR T LYMPHOCYTES. Antigen-specific, ***suppressor T cells*** play an important role in the regulation of the immune response to that antigen. Tumor-specific, suppressor T cells have been demonstrated in many experimental systems. In humans, a generalized decrease of immune competence has been observed during advanced malignancy. Whcther this decrease can be attributed to immunological mechanisms or to suppression mediated by tumor cells (see below) is unknown.

SUPPRESSION MEDIATED BY TUMOR CELLS. Certain types of tumors synthesize various compounds, such as ***prostaglandins***, which reduce many aspects of immune responsiveness. However, the role of this mechanism in the escape of tumors from destruction by the immune response is still unclear.

LARGE TUMOR MASS. The immune response and its various components have a finite capacity for the effective destruction of tumors (or, for that matter, of invading microorganisms). Thus, while immunization may result in effective protection against an otherwise lethal dose of tumor cells, it is ineffective if the dose of tumor cells is sufficiently large. The progression of the growth of a tumor in an immunocompetent host, in the face of an immune response, may be due to a rapid increase in the mass of the tumor, which outstrips the increase in immune responsiveness, until the large mass of the tumor overwhelms any effects of the immune response.

IMMUNODIAGNOSIS

Immunodiagnosis of tumors may be performed to achieve two separate goals: 1) the immunological detection of ***antigens*** specific to tumor cells and 2) the assessment of the host's ***immune response*** to the tumor (Table 19.3). Obviously, immunodiagnosis is predicated upon immunological cross-reactivity, and immunological methods may be used to detect tumor antigens and other "markers" in cases where tumor antigens exhibit similarities from individual to individual. In the presence of such immunological cross-reactivity, antibody or lymphocytes from individuals with the same type of tumor would be expected to react with the cross-reactive tumor antigens, regardless of the individual from which they have been derived.

TABLE 19.3. Tumor Immunodiagnosis

A. Detection of tumor cells and their products by immunological means
  1. Myeloma and Bence-Jones proteins (e.g. plasma cell tumors)
  2. Alphafetoprotein (AFP) (e.g. liver cancer)
  3. Carcinoembryonic antigen (CEA) (e.g. gastrointestinal cancers)
  4. Immunlogical detection of other tumor cell "markers" (e.g. enzymes and hormones)
  5. Detection of tumor-specific antigens (in the circulation or by immunoimaging).

B. Detection of anti-tumor immune response
  1) Anti-tumor antibodies
  2) Anti-tumor cell-mediated immunity

Immunologic Detection of Tumor Antigens

Tumor cells may express cytoplasmic, cell surface or secreted products that are different in nature and/or quantity from those produced by their normal counterparts. Because of the generally weak antigenicity of the tumor-specific markers, most such differences, either qualitative or quantitative, have been demonstrated by the use of antibodies produced in xenogeneic animals. In the past few years, the use of ***monoclonal antibodies*** has greatly enhanced the specificity of immunodiagnosis of tumor cells and their products. Some of the most widely used and reliable immunodiagnostic procedures for the detection of malignancies are as follows:

DETECTION OF MYELOMA PROTEINS PRODUCED BY PLASMA CELL TUMORS. Abnormally high concentration in serum of monoclonal immunoglobulins of a certain isotype, or the presence of light chains of these immunoglobulins (***Bence-Jones proteins***) in the urine, is indicative of ***plasma cell tumors***. The concentration of these ***myeloma proteins*** in the blood or urine is a reflection of the mass of the tumor. Consequently, the effectiveness and duration of therapy for this tumor may be determined by the measurement of the concentration of myeloma proteins in the serum and urine.

DETECTION OF ALPHAFETOPROTEIN. Alphafetoprotein (AFP) is a major protein in fetal serum. After birth, the level of AFP falls to ~20 ng/ml. Levels of AFP are elevated in patients with ***liver cancer***, but they are also elevated in noncancerous, hepatic disorders such as cirrhosis and hepatitis. Nevertheless, concentrations of AFP of 500–1000 ng/ml are generally indicative of the presence of a tumor that is producing AFP.

CARCINOEMBRYONIC ANTIGEN. Carcinoembryonic antigen (CEA) is a term applied to a glycoprotein produced normally by cells that line the gastrointestinal tract, in particular the colon. If the cells become malignant, their polarity may change, so that CEA is released into the blood instead of the colon. Concentrations in the blood of CEA exceeding 2.5 ng/ml are generally indicative of malignancy. Here again, however, higher than normal levels of CEA in blood may be due to noncancerous diseases, such as cirrhosis of the liver and inflammatory diseases of the intestinal tract and lung.

There are other "markers" associated with malignancies such as enzymes and hormones that can be detected by immunological methods. Qualitative as well as quantitative determinations of all tumor markers are useful in monitoring the extent of malignancy and the effect of therapy upon it.

The immunological detection of tumors has recently been improved by the availability of highly specific, antitumor, monoclonal antibodies. Monoclonal antibodies are currently being tested for their efficacy not only in the detection of antigens and products associated with the presence of tumor cells, but also for their efficacy in the localization and imaging of tumors. Injection of ***radiolabeled***, tumor-specific antibodies into the tumor-bearing individual permits ***visualization*** by computer assisted tomography (CAT) of the radiolabeled antibodies attached to the tumor. This method allows the detection of small metastases as well as the primary tumor mass.

Assessment of the Host's Immune Response to Tumor

It has been demonstrated in experimental animals and in humans, that individuals with certain tumors have cell-mediated immunity and/or antibodies directed against tumor antigens. For example, antibodies to ***Epstein-Barr virus (EBV)*** have been demonstrated in patients with Burkitt's lymphoma, and antibodies reacting with melanoma-specific or sarcoma-specific antigens have been detected in patients with the respective malignancies.

To date, immunodiagnosis of cancer does not constitute a reliably accurate method of choice for the early detection of malignancy. It is, however, proving useful clinically in monitoring the progression (or regression) of certain tumors.

TUMOR IMMUNOPROPHYLAXIS

Immunization against an oncogenic virus would be expected to provide prophylaxis ***against the virus*** and, hence, against the subsequent induction of tumor by the virus. Indeed, this approach has been successful in the protection of chickens against ***Marek's disease***, and a significant degree of protection against ***feline leukemia*** and ***feline sarcoma*** has been achieved by immunization with the respective oncogenic viruses. Immunization ***against the tumor*** itself requires that the tumor possess specific antigens and that these antigens cross-react immunologically with any prepared vaccine. There are literally thousands of reports of effective immunization against transplantable animal tumors, using as immunogens, 1) sublethal doses of live tumor cells; 2) tumor cells in which replication has been blocked; 3) tumor cells with enzymatically or chemically modified surface membranes; and 4) extracts of antigens from the surface of tumor cells, either unmodified or chemically modified. In spite of these reported successes in the protection of experimental animals against transplantable tumors, the efficacy of immunoprophylaxis for protection of humans and animals against spontaneous tumors has not been sufficiently evaluated. This lack of complete study relates to the need for appropriate immunogens and the danger of inducing the production of immunological elements that may be detrimental to the host, such as the blocking factor or factors that enhance metastasis, as mentioned above.

IMMUNOTHERAPY

Numerous attempts have been made in the past twenty years to treat cancers in animals and humans by immunologic means. Although some reports of successful immunotherapy in experimental animals, and of seemingly successful immunotherapy of human cancers, are sparsely scattered in the literature, to date cancer immunotherapy has not been proved to be an effective treatment of cancer, either when used as the sole treatment or as an adjunct to other forms of therapy such as chemotherapy, radiotherapy, or surgery.

Attempts at immunotherapy of animal and human malignancy were aimed at the augmentation of specific anticancer immunity, utilizing various preparations of tumor antigens, or at the nonspecific enhancement of the immune response, particularly of macrophages, using *BCG (Bacillus Calmette Guérin)* or *Corynebacterium parvum.* Trials are also in progress on the effects of various ***lymphokines***, such as ***interferon***, ***interleukin-2***, and ***tumor necrosis factor (TNF)*** on tumor regression. As of 1987, these trials are mostly inconclusive. A very recent development is the use of so-called ***lymphokine-activated killer cells*** (***LAK***). These cells are produced in vitro by cultivation of the patient's own peripheral lymphocytes (or those removed from the tumor) with interleukin-2 (IL-2). Upon reinfusion into the patient, dramatic improvement has been recorded in a number of cases.

With the advent of monoclonal antibodies, trials of cancer immunotherapy are underway in which toxins, such as ricin, or radioactive isotopes are attached to tumor-specific monoclonal antibodies, which deliver the toxins or the radioactivity to the tumor cells. The extent to which these "***immunotoxins***" will prove effective in the treatment of cancer remains to be established.

SUMMARY

1. Tumor immunology deals with the 1) immunological aspects of the host–tumor relationship and 2) utilization of the immune response for diagnosis, prophylaxis, and treatment of cancer.

2. Tumor antigens of chemically or physically induced tumors do not cross-react immunologically. Extensive cross-reactivity is exhibited with virally induced tumor antigens; antigens of some spontaneous tumors show cross-reactivity while others do not. Several types of tumors produce oncofetal substances, which are normally present during embryonic development.

3. In the immune response to tumors, both humoral and cellular immune responses and their effector mechanisms are expressed. Destruction of tumor cells may be achieved by 1) antibodies and complement; 2) phagocytes; 3) loss of the adhesive properties of tumor cells caused by antibodies; 4) cytotoxic T lymphocytes; 5) antibody-dependent, cell-mediated cytotoxicity (ADCC); and 6) activated macrophages and NK cells.

4. The role of the immune response to tumors appears to be important in the host-tumor relationship, as indicated by increased incidence of tumors in immunosuppressed hosts and by the presence of immune components at sites of tumor regression. However, the immune response to a tumor may not be effective in eliminating the tumor because of a variety of possible mechanisms, which include the effects of enhancing and blocking factors, rapid growth of tumor, and large tumor mass.

5. Immunodiagnosis may be directed toward the detection of tumor antigens or the host's immune response to the tumor.

6. Immunoprophylaxis may be directed against oncogenic viruses or against the tumor itself.

7. Immunotherapy of malignancy employs various preparations for the augmentation of tumor-specific as well as non-specific immune responses. "Immunotoxins" made with monoclonal antibodies are currently being tested. To date immunotherapy of cancer has proved to be unsuccessful in most cases.

REFERENCES

Baldwin RW, Byers VS (1986): Monoclonal antibody targeting of cytotoxic agents for cancer therapy. Progress in Immunol 6:695.

Benjamini E, Rennick DM, Sell S (1984): Tumor Immunology. In Stites DP, Stobo JD, Fudenberg HH, Wells JV (eds): Basic and Clinical Immunology. Los Altos, California: Lange Medical Pub.

Herberman RB (ed) (1983): Basic and Clinical Tumor Immunology. Boston, Massachusetts: Martinus Nijhoff.

Reisfeld RA, Cheresh DA (1987): Human tumor antigen. Advances in Immunol 40:323.

Terry WD, Windhorst D (eds) (1978): Immunotherapy of Cancer: Present Status of Trials in Man, Vol 6. Progress in Cancer Research and Therapy. New York: Raven Press.

Waters H (ed) (1978): The Handbook of Cancer Immunology. New York: Garland STPM Press.

Weiss DW (1980): Tumor Antigenicity and Approaches to Tumor Immunotherapy. Berlin: Springer Verlag.

REVIEW QUESTIONS

For questions 1–2, choose the ONE BEST answer or completion.

1. The appearance of many primary, lymphoreticular tumors in man has been correlated with
   a) hypergammaglobulinemia.
   b) acquired hemolytic anemia.
   c) BCG treatment.
   d) resistance to antibiotics.
   e) impairment of cell-mediated immunity.

2. Tumor antigens have been shown to cross-react immunologically in cases of
   a) tumors induced by chemical carcinogens.
   b) tumors induced by RNA viruses.
   c) all tumors.
   d) tumors induced by irradiation with ultraviolet light.
   e) tumors induced by the same chemical carcinogen on two separate sites on the same individual.

For questions 3–6, ONE or MORE of the completions given is correct. Choose the appropriate answer:
A) if only *1, 2, 3* are correct
B) if only *1 and 3* are correct
C) if only *2 and 4* are correct
D) if only *4* is correct
E) if *all* are correct

3. Blocking factors formed during tumor growth
   1) bind with T lymphocytes and induce lysis of tumor cells.
   2) block the stimulation of tumor-specific B cells.
   3) block cell growth of tumor cells in vitro.
   4) block the action of cytotoxic T lymphocytes on tumor cells in vitro.

4. Rejection of a tumor may involve which of the following?
   1) T-cell–mediated cytotoxicity.
   2) ADCC.
   3) complement-dependent cytotoxicity.
   4) destruction of tumor cells by phagocytic cells.

5. Tumor growth is enhanced by
   1) cytotoxic T lymphocytes.
   2) suppressor T lymphocytes.
   3) presence of interferon.
   4) presence of "blocking" factors.

6. Immunotoxins are
   1) toxic substances released by macrophages.
   2) lymphokines.
   3) toxins complexed with the corresponding anti-toxins.
   4) toxins coupled to antigen-specific immunoglobulins.

ANSWERS TO REVIEW QUESTIONS

1. ***e*** There is a nearly 100-fold increase in the incidence of lymphoproliferative tumors in individuals with impaired immunity, in particular with impaired cell-mediated immunity. Hypergammaglobulinemia, acquired hemolytic anemia, or resistance to antibiotics are not correlated with increases in lymphoproliferative tumors; neither is BCG treatment, which in some instances has even been shown to influence favorably the course of some leukemias.

2. ***b*** Immunologic cross-reactivity has been demonstrated only in cases of virally induced tumors (caused by either RNA or DNA viruses). Tumors induced by chemical or physical carcinogens do not exhibit cross-reactivity, even if induced by the same carcinogen on separate sites on the same individual.

3. ***D*** Only 4 is correct. Blocking factors, formed during tumor growth, may consist of free circulating antigen, circulating antitumor antibodies, or antigen–antibody complexes. Blocking by tumor antigens is achieved through the binding of these antigens with tumor-specific T lymphocytes, thereby preventing the binding of the lymphocytes to antigens on the tumor cells. Tumor-specific antibodies may combine with tumor antigens on the tumor cells, thereby blocking the binding of cytotoxic T lymphocytes to these cells. Similar types of blocking can be achieved by circulating antigen–antibody complexes. The blocking factors do not perform any of the functions listed in options 1, 2, and 3.

4. ***E*** All are correct. Destruction of tumor cells may be mediated by T-cell–mediated cytotoxicity; by antibody-dependent, cell-mediated cytotoxicity (ADCC); by complement-mediated cytotoxicity; and by phagocytic cells, which are attracted to the tumor by T cell lymphokines and/or complement components, and which become activated by the lymphokines or perform enhanced phagocytosis as a result of the presence of opsonins on the target cells.

5. ***C*** Tumor growth may be enhanced by suppressor T cells, which suppress the immune response to the tumor. Growth

(*Continued on next page*)

can also be enhanced by blocking factors, such as circulating tumor antigens, antitumor antibodies, or antigen–antibody complexes, all of which may compete with effector elements, such as cytotoxic T lymphocytes, for the tumor antigen on the tumor cell. The presence of interferon will not prevent the effector elements from destroying the tumor cell.

6. ***D*** Immunotoxins consist of toxic substances (or radioactive atoms) conjugated to immunoglobulin molecules specific for tumor cells or other target cells.

CHAPTER 20

IMMUNOPROPHYLAXIS AND IMMUNOTHERAPY*

INTRODUCTION

Protection against infectious diseases by ***immunoprophylaxis*** (immunization) represents an immense, if not the greatest, accomplishment of biomedical science. One disease, smallpox, has been totally eliminated by the use of immunization, and the incidence of other diseases has been significantly reduced, at least in areas of the world where immunization can be practiced correctly.

If a large enough number of individuals can be immunized to achieve "herd immunity," the transmission of communicable diseases between persons is interrupted. Although deliberate immunization alone can sometimes reduce the incidence of a disease to a very low level, successful immunization programs require the intelligent practice of other measures, both hygienic and sanitary, which contribute to general improvements in public health.

Immunoprophylaxis results from either ***active*** or ***passive*** immunization. In active immunization, an individual generates an immune response after direct exposure to antigen. Passive immunization results when an individual receives antibody or other cellular product from another, actively immunized

*Contributed by Demosthenes Pappagianis, University of California, Davis.

individual. The transfer of immunocompetent cells into a host who previously was incompetent is termed ***adoptive transfer.*** Active and passive immunizations are further exemplified as shown in Table 20.1.

TABLE 20.1. Examples of Active and Passive Immunization

Type of immunity	How acquired
Active	
Natural (unintended)	Infection
Artificial (deliberate)	Vaccination
Passive*	
Natural	Transplacental or colostral transfer of antibody, mother to infant
Artificial	Administration of immune human globulin

*Passive immunity is generally of shorter duration than active immunity.

OBJECTIVES OF IMMUNIZATION

Preexposure protection is generated prior to possible exposure to an infectious agent, as in the case of the usual active immunizations in childhood, or the passive protection supplied by injections of immune globulin to protect a traveler against "infectious hepatitis" (hepatitis A virus) in countries where that disease is common. Protection against development of disease can also be afforded by postexposure protection, for example, by administration of rabies vaccine and immune globulin against rabies virus, toxoid and antitoxin against diphtheria and tetanus toxins, antitoxin against the botulinus toxin, and immune serum globulins against hepatitis A and B viruses.

HISTORICAL ASPECTS OF IMMUNIZATION

The protective active immunity (immunoprophylaxis) that may result from natural, unintended, or deliberate exposure to infectious agents or their components was evident to the ancients of Asia, who intentionally exposed people to the scabs and fluid from the lesions of smallpox, a disease known in the Western World as "variola major." The practice, termed ***variolation,*** was applied in the Western World in the early 1700s. The wife of the British ambassador in Constantinople had noticed that the most prized women in the harems were those who had been spared the disfiguring effects of smallpox by prior variolation. She was instrumental in the introduction of variolation into England in 1721 (the practice was introduced in the British colonies in America in the same year).

Successful protection against smallpox was dependent on the presence of antigens of inactive and active virus in the lesions. The crudeness of the preparation assured the presence of active (and virulent) virus in sufficient concentration to produce smallpox, so that some unfortunate individuals died of the disease. Such undesirable consequences are always a risk when active or viable infectious agents are used. Because of the morbidity and mortality associated with variolation, the practice was soon discontinued in the West.

Later in the 18th century it was noted that milkmaids who were exposed to cowpox, a disease of cattle, appeared to escape infection with smallpox. It was then that Jenner, an English physician, showed that deliberate administration of lymph from a cow with vaccinia to humans led to protection against smallpox. It is evident from this cross-protection by vaccinia that the viruses of smallpox and cowpox share an antigen(s). (The vaccinia virus used in modern times is known to differ genetically from the cowpox virus.)

Approximately a century later (1879) Roux, working in Pasteur's laboratory, demonstrated that bacteria that caused chicken cholera or anthrax could be weakened (attenuated) by certain cultivation practices in the laboratory, so that they could no longer cause disease but still retained enough antigenicity to induce immunity. He also showed that storage in the laboratory of tissue infected with rabies virus yielded an agent that was markedly less virulent than the parent rabies virus, but still antigenic. Pasteur termed these protective antigens "***vaccines***" in commemoration of Jenner's work on the use of vaccinia to protect against smallpox.

Toward the end of the 19th century, it was discovered that certain bacteria cause disease (diphtheria, tetanus) through their release of potent exotoxins. Fortuitously, it was demonstrated that treatment of these (protein) ***exotoxins*** with formaldehyde and other chemicals eliminated their toxicity but left their antigenic properties unaffected. These modified toxins, or "***toxoids***" (see Chapter 3), have been the mainstays of immunization for many decades.

Although the existence of viruses was recognized in the late 19th century, successful cultivation in the laboratory, separate from the intact mammal, was not achieved until the 1930s, when tissue-culture techniques permitted replication and modification of the yellow fever virus so that it could be used for a vaccine. The most significant advance, however, followed the discovery, in 1949 by Enders, that poliomyelitis virus could be grown in vitro in human embryonic cells or monkey kidney cells. Recovery of sufficient quantities of virions permitted preparation of inactivated (noninfective) polio vaccine and, later, modified, attenuated viral vaccines. "Subunit" vaccines, which contain particular fractions of viruses (or bacteria) have been introduced more recently.

ACTIVE IMMUNIZATION

Recommended Immunizations

The present, customary, active immunizations are indicated below (additional specific examples will be cited later):

UNIVERSAL APPLICATION. The usual recommended schedule for active immunization at various ages is shown in Table 20.2.

TABLE 20.2. Recommended Usual Schedule for Active Immunization at Ages Shown

Age	Vaccine
2 months	Diphtheria, tetanus, pertussis (DTP-1)*, trivalent oral polio (TOP-1)
4 months	DTP-2, TOP-2
6 months	DTP-3, TOP-3
15 months	Measles, mumps, rubella
18 months	DTP-4, TOP-4
4–6 years	DTP-5, TOP-5
14–16 years (and each 10 years thereafter)	Td (tetanus, reduced adult dose of diphtheria toxoid)
18–24 years	Measles, mumps†, rubella
25–64 years	Measles‡, mumps†, rubella**
>65 years	Influenza, pneumococcus

*DTP is administered with alum *adjuvant* (Chapter 3).
†Especially for susceptible males.
‡For persons born after 1956.
**Mainly for females up to 45 years of age.
For specific details see: Morbidity and Mortality Weekly Report, 1983, 32:1–8, 13–17; Morbidity and Mortality Weekly Report, Supplement 28, Sept. 1984, 33; Nov. 1.

SELECTIVE APPLICATION. In addition to the usual schedule of immunizations shown in Table 20.2, some individuals receive additional vaccination as follows (see also Table 20.4):

Viral. ***Influenza virus*** (inactivated) is given to persons over 60 years of age and to those with cardiorespiratory ailments. ***Hepatitis B*** (inactivated), is given to medical personnel who are exposed to human blood. ***Varicella*** (attenuated) is given to patients with acute lymphocytic leukemia. (Vaccination against smallpox, no longer recommended for civilians, is still given to military personnel in several countries.)

Bacterial. A polyvalent vaccine made from capsular polysaccharides of several types of *Streptococcus pneumoniae* is given to individuals with ***cardiorespiratory ailments***, to anatomically or functionally ***asplenic individuals***, and to patients with ***sickle cell anemia***, ***renal failure***, ***alcoholic cirrhosis***, or ***diabetes mellitus***. *Haemophilus influenzae* (type B capsular polysaccharide), is recommended for ***2- to 3-year-old children*** in daycare centers, and for anatomically or functionally ***asplenic individuals***. *Neisseria meningitidis* vaccine (several serogroups of capsular polysaccharide) is given to ***military recruits*** and to ***children in high-risk regions***.

BASIC MECHANISMS OF PROTECTION

Anatomical Location of Host Immune Response

There are differences in the intravascular–extravascular distribution of immunoglobulins. Local synthesis of secretory IgA in the lamina propria, beneath a mucous membrane, yields antibody at the epithelial surface (respiratory or intestinal), an area through which certain pathogens may enter. IgA is the predominant Ig in secretions of the nasal, bronchial, intestinal, and genitourinary tracts, and in saliva, colostrum, and bile. ***Oral administration*** of attenuated (Sabin) polio vaccine leads to demonstrable antipolio IgA in nasal and duodenal secretions, whereas ***parenteral injection*** of inactivated (Salk) polio vaccine does not. The local antibodies generated by the Sabin vaccine provide obvious advantages in the interception of a pathogen at the portal of entry. However, IgG and IgM may also be found in local secretions, so that serum Ig may also play a role at an epithelial surface. Furthermore, the hematogenous (viremic or bacteremic) stage of several infections, that are acquired through a mucous membrane leads to an encounter between agent and antibody in the circulating and extravascular fluid.

While IgM appears to have restricted access to extravascular areas, both IgG and IgM can be found in exudates. (In the cerebrospinal fluid, these immunoglobulins may be found as a result of local production in the central nervous system due to the stimulus of infectious agents.) There are some unique, but still poorly understood, differences in the partitioning of immunoglobulins in serum and secretions. For example, while IgG_4 represents only 3.5% of the plasma IgG, it constitutes 15% of IgG in colostrum.

Significance of Primary and Secondary Responses

The rapidity of the ***anamnestic response*** to a re-encounter with antigen provides the host with potential protection upon repeated exposures to an infectious agent. This anamnestic response is relevant in at least two significant ways in the application of immunoprophylaxis. First, it may be of particular importance in those infections with a relatively long incubation period (greater than 7 days), as is illustrated in Figure 20.1, where the theoretical relationship

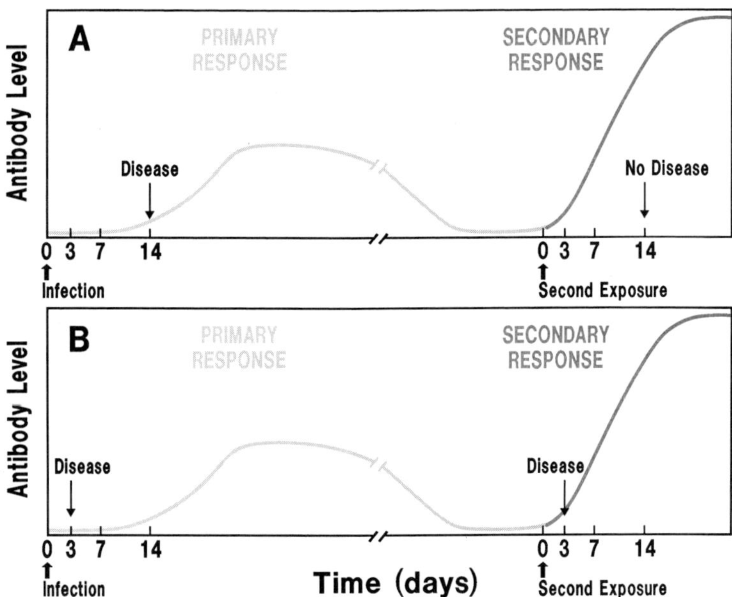

Figure 20.1.
The relationship between the primary and secondary immune responses and disease. (After Macleod CM, J Immunol 70:421, 1953.)

between incubation period and effectiveness of the anamnestic response is shown. Thus, assuming that an individual is infected by an agent, B, which causes disease after a 3-day incubation period, that individual would have sufficient antigenic stimulus to induce a *primary* immune response some time—e.g. 7–14 days, after onset of the infection. Upon a second encounter with agent B, the individual may again develop disease, because an anamnestic response may not be sufficiently rapid to inhibit agent B (Fig. 20.1B). The individual infected with an agent, A, which causes disease after a 14-day-incubation period would produce a primary response, for example some 7–14 days after infection. Upon a second encounter with agent A, the anamnestic response occurring within 7 days would be sufficient to reduce or prevent the disease with the 14-day-incubation period (Fig. 20.1A).

The second influence of the anamnestic response concerns the ***level*** to which the immune response has been raised. In the example cited above, agent B, which causes disease in 3 days, may be prevented from causing disease after a re-exposure if there is a high enough level of antibody. Such a level can be achieved deliberately by a series of immunizations (especially applicable with nonviable antigens). Thus, it is customary to give several injections of tetanus toxoid (as DTP) over a period of 6 months, in childhood immunizations. Such a "primary series" of injections generates anamnestic secondary responses that successively raise the concentration of antitoxin to protective levels, which are sustained in the serum for 10-20 years.

Protective Effect of the Immune Response

Acquired immune responses may exert their effects essentially independently of certain innate defense mechanisms—e.g. neutralization of bacterial exotoxin by antitoxic antibody. Alternatively, these acquired responses may function in concert with other components of the host defense apparatus—e.g. when antibody functions to opsonize infectious particles, or when antibody interacts with complement and an infectious agent leading to lysis of the agent.

ANTITOXIC IMMUNITY. Antitoxic immunity is predominantly associated with ***IgG***, although IgA may also neutralize exotoxins such as cholera enterotoxin. Because the exotoxins bind firmly to their target tissue, they generally cannot be displaced by subsequent administration of antitoxin. Hence, in those diseases mediated by exotoxins, prompt administration of antitoxins is necessary to prevent attachment of (additional) exotoxin and the damage caused by the exotoxin. In guinea pigs, antitoxin given 1 hour before injection of diphtheria toxin affords complete protection, but antitoxin given 1 or 2 hours after injection of the toxin is ineffective. This can also be illustrated by the effectiveness of antitoxin given at varying times as protection against the lethal effects of diphtheria toxin in humans (Table 20.3).

TABLE 20.3. Protection of Humans by Diphtheria Antitoxin Given on Indicated Day of Disease

Day	Number of cases	Fatality rate (%)
1	225	0
2	1,441	4.2
3	1,600	11.1
4	1,276	17.3
5 (or later)	1,645	18.7

From Pappenheimer AM Jr (1965): The diphtheria bacilli and the diphtheroid [sic]. In: "Bacterial and Mycotic Infections of Man," Ed 4. RJ Dubos and JG Hirsch (eds). J.B. Lippincott Co., Philadelphia, p 480.

Exotoxic enzymes, e.g. the lecithinase of the bacterium *Clostridium perfringens* or of snake venom, may be neutralized by antibody. However, the enzymatically active sites of some enzymes may not be inhibited by enzyme-specific antibody.

The presence of antitoxic activity in IgG means that an adequately immunized mother can transmit antitoxin to her fetus and thus afford protection to the infant in its first days or weeks after birth. This protection is extremely important in areas of the world where unclean obstetric environments can lead to ***tetanus neonatorum*** (of the newborn).

ANTIVIRAL IMMUNITY. The antiviral response can be complex, with several factors involved, such as the route of entry, site of attachment, and other aspects of pathogenesis by the infecting virus; induction of interferon; antibody response; and cell-mediated immunity. Thus, intracellular infection of the epithelium of the respiratory tract by influenza virus leads to production of virus in epithelial cells and spread of the virus to adjacent epithelial cells. An appropriate and sufficient immune response would involve action of antibody at the epithelial surface. This action might be effected through locally secreted ***IgA***, or ***IgG*** or ***IgM*** extravasated locally. On the other hand, some viral diseases, e.g. measles or poliomyelitis, begin by infection at a mucosal epithelium (respiratory or intestinal, respectively) but exhibit their major pathogenic effects after being spread hematogenously to other target tissues. Antibody at the epithelial surface could be enough to protect against the virus, but circulating antibody could do likewise.

Interferons are antiviral proteins or glycoproteins produced by several different types of cell in the mammalian host, in response to viral infection (or other inducers such as double stranded RNA). Interferons appear before detectable activated macrophages or antibody. They serve, therefore, as an early protective device, by causing host cells to produce antiviral proteins different from antibodies.

The antibody response to viruses can be demonstrated, ***in vitro***, to involve Igs that 1) ***neutralize*** (impede) infectivity of viruses for susceptible host cells; 2) ***fix complement***, and 3) ***inhibit adherence to and agglutination of erythrocytes*** by some viruses (hemagglutination inhibition). As in the case of antitoxic immunity, IgG appears to be the most significant of the antiviral antibodies, but once a virus has attached to a host cell, it is not displaced by antibody.

The effects of ***antiviral Ig in vivo*** include 1) ***neutralization***; 2) ***complement-mediated lysis of infected host cells***, which carry viral antigen on the cell membrane; 3) ***inhibition of critical viral enzymes*** (e.g. neuraminidase of influenza virus); and 4) ***opsonization***. Opsonization represents a convergence of humoral and cellular immune mechanisms. IgG, which has combined, through its Fab portion, with viral antigens on the surface of infected host cells, links also to Fc receptors on macrophages, polymorphonuclear cells (PMNs), or killer (K) cells. These cells then can phagocytose and/or damage the virus-infected cell—a phenomenon termed ***antibody-dependent cellular cytotoxicity (ADCC)*** (see Chapter 5).

Cell-mediated immune responses usually precede the antibody-mediated mechanisms. T cells interacting with virus may produce lymphokines, e.g. ***macrophage chemotactic factor (MCF)*** or ***migration inhibition factor (MIF),*** which cause accumulation of macrophages, which inhibit the formation of intercellular bridges and, thus, the intercellular transfer of viruses. In addition, such macrophages can phagocytose antibody-coated viruses (the phagocytosis may not lead to destruction of the virus, but may rather serve as means of disseminating the virus, as happens in the case of measles virus and HIV, the human T cell lymphotrophic virus associated with acquired immune deficiency syndrome [AIDS]). ***Cytotoxic cells*** may act directly against viral antigen associated with class 1 molecules of the MHC on the surface of host cells.

ANTIBACTERIAL IMMUNITY. Antibacterial immune responses include ***lysis,*** via antibody and complement; ***opsonization;*** and ***phagocytosis,*** with elimination of phagocytosed bacteria by the liver, spleen, and other components of the reticuloendothelial system.

Opsonization and phagocytosis, especially of gram-positive bacteria, involve the action of ***IgG*** and ***IgM*** alone or in concert with ***C3b***, which promotes phagocytosis of bacteria by PMN. The ***alternative complement pathway*** may be triggered nonspecifically by the lipopolysaccharide endotoxin found in the walls of gram-negative bacteria, or by the polysaccharide capsule of gram-negative and gram-positive bacteria acting on C3. This alternative pathway leads to formation of the chemotactic molecules C3a and C5a, and the opsonin C3b. In addition, the activation of the alternative pathway may result in ***immune adherence*** and bacteriolytic action of C5, 6, 7, 8, C9. Because the opsonized and phagocytosed bacteria are cleared by the spleen, anatomically or functionally asplenic patients are particularly vulnerable to encapsulated bacteria, even though the alternative complement pathway may be activated by the bacteria. The classical lytic complement pathway operates in conjunction with IgM against gram-negative bacteria.

Cell-mediated immunity is also active against certain bacteria, characterized by their intracellular habitat, e.g. *Mycobacterium tuberculosis*.

ANTI-FUNGAL, ANTI-PROTOZOAL, AND ANTI-HELMINTHIC IMMUNITY. Immune responses to fungi, protozoa, and helminths involve humoral and/or cellular immunity, as is the case for immunity to viruses and bacteria. There are also, however, unique aspects of the response to these organisms dependent on the various stages of their life cycles.

AGE AND TIMING OF IMMUNIZATIONS

The various mechanisms involved in protection described in the preceding section, can be affected by several factors—e.g. nutritional status; presence of underlying disease, which affects levels of globulin or cell-mediated immunity; and age.

In utero, the human fetus normally appears well insulated from antigens and most infectious agents, although certain pathogens (e.g. rubella virus) can infect the mother and seriously injure the fetus. The immunity of the mother protects the fetus by permitting interception and removal of infectious agents before they can enter the uterus, or it protects the newborn by virtue of transplacental or mammary gland antibody.

The fetus and neonate have poorly developed lymphoid organs, with the exception of the thymus, which at the time of birth is largest in size relative to body size. The fetus appears capable of synthesizing mainly IgM, which becomes apparent after 6 months of gestation. Levels of IgM gradually increase to about 0.1 mg/ml of serum at the time of birth, which is about 10% of the adult level.

Immunoglobulin (IgG) becomes detectable in the fetus at about the second month of gestation, but it is IgG of maternal origin. The level of IgG increases significantly at about 4 months' gestation, and at the time of birth the concentration of IgG (about 10–12 mg/ml serum) slightly exceeds the maternal concentration of IgG. Thus, the fetus is provided with maternally synthesized IgG antibodies, which can provide antitoxic, antiviral and some kinds of antibacterial protection. The levels of these maternal antibodies gradually decline as the infant begins to synthesize its own antibodies, so that total IgG at 2–3 months of age is only about 50% of the level at birth. The serum concentrations of immunoglobulins during human development are shown in Figure 20.2.

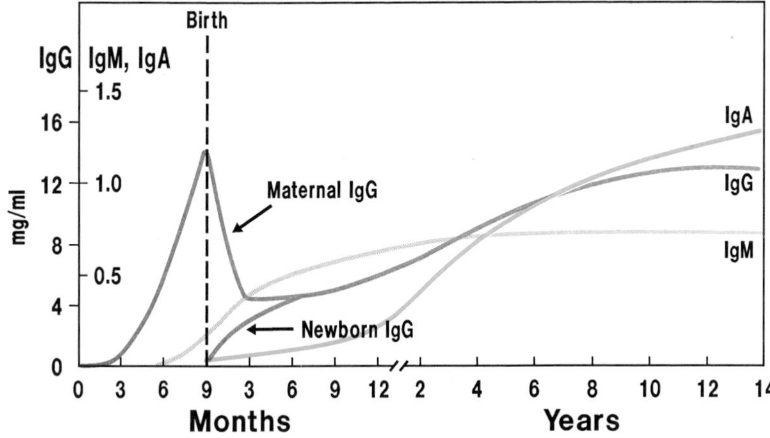

Figure 20.2.
Concentration of immunoglobulins in the serum during human development. (After Bennich H, Johanssen SGO. Adv Immunol 13:1, 1971.)

In general, the newborn has weak immune responses, which increase in effectiveness with age. The newborn is developmentally prepared to produce IgM preferentially and, thus, the response is influenced by the nature of the antigen available. The newborn can respond to toxoids, parenterally administered inactivated poliomyelitis virus or orally administered attenuated poliomyelitis virus, and others. However, administration of pertussis vaccine (whole, killed bacteria) very soon after birth not only fails to induce a protective response but also creates an impaired response (tolerance?) to the vaccine when it is given again later in infancy.

Maternal antibody, while capable of providing protection to the neonate against a variety of infectious agents or their toxins, may also reduce the response to antigen. For example, a sufficient quantity of maternal measles antibody persists in the one-year-old infant to interfere with the active response of the infant to the vaccine, so that vaccination against measles is now carried out at 15 months of age rather than at 12 months. However, administration of the measles vaccine by the respiratory route causes an increase in levels of circulating antibody, despite the presence in the child of maternal antibody which apparently thwarts production of antibody only in response to injection of vaccine.

Children less than 2 years of age have a general inability to produce adequate levels of antibody in response to injection of bacterial capsular polysaccharides, e.g. those of *Haemophilus influenzae* type b, various subgroups of *Neisseria meningitidis*, and *Streptococcus pneumoniae* serotypes. It has been suggested that this inability arises because infants do not respond to T-cell–independent antigens, despite their early capacity to generate IgM. Linkage of such antigens to T-dependent antigens, like diphtheria or tetanus toxoid would be expected to enhance the response to polysaccharides.

At the other end of the age spectrum, i.e. in people older than 60 years of age, there also appears to be a reduced capability to mount a primary response to some antigens, but the elderly appear to retain the ability to mount a secondary response to antigens to which they have been previously exposed. The elderly respond well to bacterial polysaccharides, so that administration of pneumococcal polysaccharide vaccine can usually induce protective levels of antibody. Other groups, besides the elderly, who are especially susceptible to pneumococcal pneumonia (e.g. those with sickle cell disease, Hodgkin's disease, multiple myeloma, chronic cardiorespiratory or chronic metabolic disease, such as diabetes mellitus and renal failure) should also be immunized. Inasmuch as influenza damages the respiratory epithelium and predisposes to bacterial pneumonia, influenza vaccine should be provided to the same groups as those who have enhanced susceptibility to the encapsulated respiratory pathogen *Streptococcus pneumoniae*, and to persons at high risk of exposure (e.g. residents of nursing homes and medical personnel).

USE OF MIXED, MULTIPLE ANTIGENS

Routine immunization against some infectious agents is simplified by their having a single antigenic type (e.g. the toxins of diphtheria and tetanus, and various viruses such as measles, mumps, and rubella). However, immunization against other agents (e.g. poliovirus and pneumococci) must provide protection against several antigenic types. The host can be vaccinated simultaneously with several antigens and still generate adequate responses, although in some instances the generation of sufficient immunity requires repeated (booster) administration of antigen(s). The usual, initial immunization of children entails the injection of diphtheria and tetanus toxoids, whole killed cells of *Bordetella pertussis*, and the oral administration of attenuated polioviruses types 1, 2, and 3 (Sabin vaccine). The estimated 10^{12} lymphoid cells in the human body appear to be capable of responding to a huge array of antigens without significant competition. Although there is a possibility that a live viral vaccine may inhibit the immune response to a second live viral vaccine given a few days later, this interference does not appear to be of practical importance. Thus, it has been ascertained that simultaneous injection of ***measles***, ***mumps***, and ***rubella*** vaccines provides a protective response to all three of these viruses.

Because of some unique needs or limited efficacy, some vaccines are recommended only under limited circumstances. These vaccines and appropriate circumstances are described in Table 20.4.

TABLE 20.4. Vaccines Recommended Under Limited Circumstances

Occupational or other exposure	Vaccine
Health care personnel	Hepatitis B
Health care personnal in close contact with tuberculosis patients	BCG (bacille Calmette Guérin)
Veterinarians*, animal handlers*, and victims of certain animal bites	Rabies
Handlers of imported animal hides, furs, bonemeal, wool, and animal bristles	Anthrax
Military personnel	Meningococcus, yellow fever
Homosexual males, illicit drug users	Hepatitis B
Travel to certain areas	Meningococcus, yellow fever, cholera†, typhoid fever†, plague

*In some parts of the world (e.g. USSR) attenuated *Brucella* vaccine is administered to humans.
†The duration and efficacy of these is limited.
For tabulation of available vaccines see Table 20.7.

PRECAUTIONS

Site of Administration of Antigen

The usual site of ***parenteral*** (intradermal, subcutaneous, intramuscular) administration of vaccines is the arm, in particular the deltoid muscle. Recent studies have shown a suboptimal response to hepatitis B vaccine when given by intragluteal injection, as compared with injection in the arm. The parenteral administration of inactivated polio vaccine may induce a higher antibody response in the serum than the attenuated oral polio vaccine, but the response to the latter, which includes secretory IgA, affords adequate protection.

Some vaccines may provide a greater antibody response when given by the ***respiratory*** route than when given by injection (e.g. attenuated measles vaccine) but administration via the respiratory route has not yet supplanted parenteral administration.

Hazards

There are potential hazards associated with the use of some vaccines. Vaccines made from ***attenuated*** organisms (e.g. measles, mumps, rubella, oral polio, bacille Calmette Guérin) have the potential for causing ***progressive disease*** in the ***immunocompromised*** patient, or in the patient on ***steroid therapy***. (In rare cases, reversion of attenuated poliovirus type III to virulence in the intestine of the vaccinated individual has caused paralytic polio; for this reason, some workers favor the ***inactivated*** polio vaccine.)

The attenuated organisms should ordinarily not be given to pregnant women because of potential damage to the fetus. (The virions in rubella vaccine have been transmitted to the fetus, although without any recognized injurious effect.)

Vaccination against smallpox is no longer carried out (except in some military personnel) since the disease has been eradicated; however, if this vaccine should be required in the future as a carrier of other antigens, care must be taken because this virus can cause serious problems, not only in immunocompromised individuals, but also in individuals with certain cutaneous lesions. Contact must be avoided until the vaccinia lesions have healed.

Of the ***inactivated*** vaccines, the whole killed *B. pertussis* bacterial vaccine occasionally causes serious side effects, e.g. encephalopathy in the infant. Controversy surrounds the pertussis vaccine, but its use has continued, since the complications of whooping cough outweigh the risks of immunization.

Obviously, pertussis vaccine should not be given to infants with a history of neurologic problems, such as convulsions. Tetanus and diphtheria toxoids may provoke local hypersensitivity reactions. Because an adequate initial series of immunizations in childhood appears to give immunity that lasts some 10 years, the use of "booster" injections of tetanus toxoid should be guided by the nature of an injury and the history of immunization. The increased hypersensitivity to diphtheria toxoid of adolescents and adults necessitates use of a smaller dose of diphtheria toxoid than is used for children. (Usually the diphtheria toxoid is given with tetanus toxoid (T), the lower dose of diphtheria toxoid being indicated by a lowercase d, as in Td). Since untoward reactions follow repeated injections of pneumococcal polysaccharide vaccine, only a single injection of the currently used 23-valent vaccine is recommended. Increased incidence of neurologic complications ***(Guillain-Barré syndrome)*** followed use of the 1976 swine influenza vaccine, but they are not a significant problem with the influenza vaccines currently in use. Because the virus is cultivated in chick embryos, allergy to egg protein is a contraindication to vaccination against influenza. Whole influenza virus vaccine is used in adults but gives side effects in children, so that a split-virus component vaccine is recommended for persons under 13 years of age.

Some vaccines contain ***preservatives***, e.g. the organomercurial compound thimerosal ("Merthiolate") or antibiotics (e.g. neomycin or streptomycin), to which the vaccinated individual may be allergic.

The potential for use of vaccines to prevent certain cancers in man has been discussed in Chapter 19. For example, the association between primary carcinoma of the liver and infection by Hepatitis B virus (HBV) is strong enough to suggest that use of the inactivated HBV vaccine in highrisk groups may provide protection against development of hepatoma, as well as hepatitis due to this virus.

RECENT APPROACHES TO PRODUCTION OF VACCINES

Recent advances in ***recombinant DNA*** technology and in the technology of rapid, automated ***synthesis of peptides*** hold promise for improvements in available vaccines and new approaches to the production of vaccines. In addition, the developing concepts and technology directed toward the use of ***anti-idiotypes*** of certain specificities as immunogens, to mimic the structure of particular epitopes, offers another approach for the developments of novel vaccines.

Because of their greater purity, synthetic vaccines may afford protection that is associated with fewer side effects. Production of vaccines against hepatitis B from yeast by recombinant DNA technology may simplify the production of greater quantities of a safer vaccine than the vaccine prepared from blood plasma of humans.

PASSIVE IMMUNIZATION

Passive immunity results from the transfer of antibody or immune cells to one individual from another individual who has already responded to direct stimulation by antigen. It can be divided into ***natural*** and ***artificial*** passive immunity.

Natural Passive Immunity

MATERNAL IMMUNITY VIA THE PLACENTA. The presence of maternal antibody confers passive protection to the fetus, which is effective in those circumstances when ***IgG*** suffices, for example as an antitoxic and antiviral antibody, or as an anti-bacterial antibody, e.g. against *Haemophilus influenzae* (type b) or *Streptococcus agalactiae* (group b). Adequate active immunization of the mother constitutes a simple and effective means of providing passive protection to the fetus and infant in the first few months of life.

MATERNAL IMMUNITY VIA COLOSTRUM. Human milk contains a variety of factors that may influence the response of the nursing infant to infectious agents. Some of these factors are natural selective factors that can affect the intestinal microflora—i.e. by enhancement of growth of desirable bacteria and by nonspecific inhibition of some microbes, by the action of ***lysozyme***, ***lactoferrin***, ***interferon***, and ***leukocytes*** (macrophages, T cells, B cells, and granulocytes). ***Antibodies*** are found in breast milk, the concentration being higher in the ***colostrum*** (first milk) immediately postpartum (Table 20.5). The production of antibody in the mammary gland is related to antigens that enter the maternal intestine and movement of antigen-stimulated cells from intestinal lamina propria to the breast (the "enteromammary system"). Thus, organisms colonizing or infecting the alimentary tract of the mother may lead to production of colostral antibody, which affords protection to the nursing infant against pathogens that enter via the intestinal tract. Antibody to the enteropathogens *E. coli*, *Salmonella typhimurium, Shigella* species, poliomye-

TABLE 20.5. Levels of Immunoglobulin in Colostrum*

	Day postpartum				Approximate normal adult level (mg/dl)
	Day 1	Day 2	Day 3	Day 4	
IgA†	600	260	200	80	200
IgG‡	80	45	30	16	1,000
IgM	125	65	58	30	120

*After Michael JG, Ringenback R, Hottenstein S (1971): J Infect Dis 124:445.
†80% of this is secretary sIgA.
‡IgG_4 represents 15% of colostral IgG; 3.5% of serum IgG.

litis virus, coxsackie and ECHO viruses have been demonstrated. (Antibodies to nonalimentary pathogens have also been demonstrated in colostrum—e.g. tetanus and diphtheria antitoxins, and antistreptococcal hemolysin).

Tuberculin-sensitive T lymphocytes are also transmitted to the infant through the colostrum, but the role of such cells in passive transfer of cell-mediated immunity is uncertain.

Artificial Passive Immunity

HETEROLOGOUS VERSUS HOMOLOGOUS ANTIBODY. World War I afforded unusually suitable if regrettable circumstances for the testing of the value of passive immunization with tetanus antitoxin. In 1914 the British Army was incurring 30 cases of tetanus per 1,000 wounded soldiers. In 1915 antitoxin produced in the horse was used to treat the wounded British troops. Almost immediately, the incidence of tetanus fell to one or two cases per 1,000 wounded. This experience allowed the determination of the minimum concentration of antitoxin needed to provide protection—0.01–0.1 unit/ml of serum—and also showed that the period of protection was brief. The basis for the latter fact is shown schematically in Figure 20.3. (The half-life of $IgG_{1,2,4}$ is 23 days; IgG_3 has a half-life of 7 days.) The peak level in blood is reached about two days after subcutaneous injection.

Homologous human antibody would naturally be expected to last longer than the ***heterologous*** equine antibody. The fate of homologous and of heterologous antibody is depicted by the diagram in Figure 20.4. Four phases are involved in the diminution of the level of heterologous antibody: dilution, catabolism, formation of immune complex, and elimination.

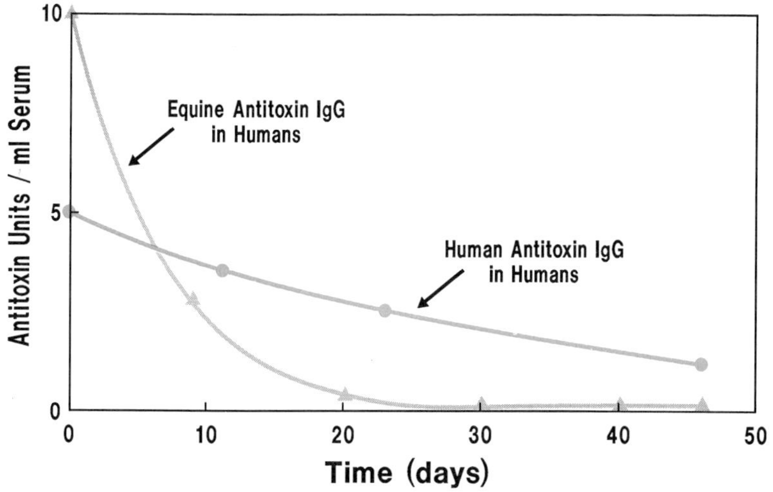

Figure 20.3.
Serum concentrations of human and equine IgG antitoxin following administration into humans.

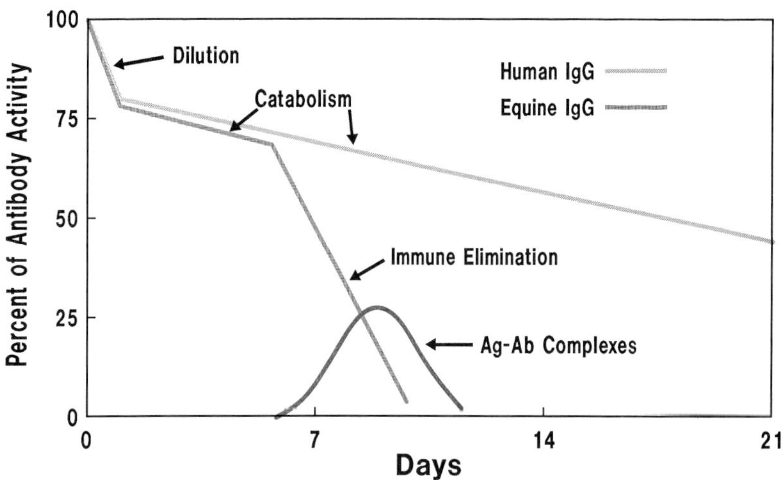

Figure 20.4.
The fate of human and equine IgG following administration into humans.

Heterologous antibody, such as that from the horse, can cause at least two kinds of hypersensitivity reaction: ***type I*** (immediate, anaphylaxis), or ***type III*** (serum sickness from immune complexes). If necessary, it is possible to desensitize the individual to type I reactions by administration of gradually increasing but minute amounts of the foreign serum, given repeatedly over several hours.

USE OF HUMAN IMMUNE SERUM GLOBULIN. The use of globulin from human serum apparently began in the early 1900's, when serum of patients convalescing from measles was given to children who had been exposed to measles but had not yet developed symptoms. Additional attempts in 1916, and later, showed that early administration of measles convalescent serum could protect against emergence of clinically apparent measles. In 1933 human placentae were also recognized as a source of measles antibody.

In the early 1940s Cohn and colleagues devised a method for separation of the "gamma globulin" fraction from human serum by precipitation with cold ethanol. This ***"Cohn fractionation"*** represented a practical and safe method for production of homologous human antibody for clinical use. Nevertheless, there are still some preparations of heterologous antibody (e.g. equine diphtheria antitoxin and antilymphocyte serum (ALS)) used in humans.

PREPARATION AND PROPERTIES OF HOMOLOGOUS IMMUNE SERUM GLOBULIN. Plasma is collected from healthy donors or placentae. If obtained from donors with no special attention paid to prior immunization or convalescence from an infection, the plasma or serum from several donors is pooled and the preparation is termed ***immune serum globulin (ISG) or human normal immunoglobulin (HNI).*** If the plasma or serum is from donors who are specially selected after an immunizing or booster dose of antigen, or after convalescence from a specific infection, the globulin preparation is designated accordingly—e.g. tetanus immune globulin (TIG), hepatitis B (HBIG), varicella zoster (VZIG), and rabies (RIG). Large quantities can be obtained by ***plasmapheresis.*** The fraction containing antibody globulin(s) is precipitated by cold ethanol. The resultant preparation: 1) is free of hepatitis virus and the HIV of AIDS; 2) concentrates many of the antibodies about 25-fold (preparations contain about 16.5 g/dl globulin, mainly IgG); 3) is stable for years; and 4) can provide peak levels in blood approximately two days after intramuscular injection (newer preparations, which appear to be safe when given intravenously, involve additional treatment—e.g. reduction by dithiothreitol and stabilization in 10% maltose).

The commercially available immune globulin contains higher concentrations of Ig than those in whole serum (see Table 20.6), but there is a relative deficiency of IgA and IgM. Deficiency of the latter could be significant if protection is required against lipopolysaccharide endotoxin or whole gram-negative bacteria, which are adversely affected by IgM plus complement.

TABLE 20.6. Composition of Human Immune Serum Globulin

Source	Immunoglobulin (mg/dl)		
	IgG	IgA	IgM
Whole serum	1,200	180	200
Immune serum globulin	16,500	100–500	25–200
Placental immune serum globulin	16,500	200–700	150–400

INDICATIONS FOR USE OF IMMUNE GLOBULINS

Specific Immune Globulin. Antibody (Rhogam) to RhD antigen is given to mothers within a 72-hour perinatal period to protect against their immunization by fetal Rh^+ erythrocytes;

Tetanus immune globulin (TIG) (antitoxin) is used to provide passive protection after certain wounds and in the absence of adequate active immunization with tetanus toxoid (usually given simultaneously with toxoid but in the opposite arm);

Varicella-zoster immune globulin (VZIG) is given to leukemics at risk within 72 hours after exposure to chickenpox;

Rabies immune globulin (RIG) is given together with active immunization with human diploid cell rabies vaccine (human RIG is not universally available so equine antibody may be necessary in some areas);

Hepatitis B immune globulin (HBIG) may be given in the perinatal period to a child born of a mother with evidence of hepatitis B infection; to medical personnel after accidental stick with a hypodermic needle; or after sexual contact with an individual with hepatitis B. (ISG may also be used against hepatitis B—see below);

Vaccinia immune globulin is given to eczematous or immunocompromised individuals with intimate exposure to vaccinia (used to vaccinate military personnel in the United States).

Immune Serum Globulin (ISG). ISG is used in certain circumstances: hepatitis A: ISG can be used for both pre- and post-exposure protection; hepatitis B: ISG preparations in recent years have been regarded as sufficiently potent to substitute for HBIG in some circumstances; non-A–non-B hepatitis: ISG may offer protection against this blood-associated disease; measles: ISG is used for the protection of infants exposed to measles prior to vaccination with attenuated measles virus, or to children with immunosuppressive conditions; hypogammaglobulinemia: repeated injections of ISG are required; idiopathic thrombocytopenic purpura (ITP): presumably the higher dose of IgG in the ISG can block the Fc receptors on phagocytic cells and prevent them from phagocytosing and destroying platelets coated with autoantibodies.

PRECAUTIONS. As indicated above, the usual preparation of globulin is given by the ***intramuscular route***, since ***intravenous*** administration is contraindicated because of possible ***anaphylactoid*** reactions. During the fractionation by ethanol precipitation, ***aggregates of Ig*** form which can ***activate complement*** to yield anaphylatoxins (IgG_1, IgG_2, IgG_3, and IgM by the classical pathway; IgG_4 and IgA by the alternative pathway). Newer preparations (see above) are available and safe for intravenous administration.

One unique contraindication to the use of immune globulin preparations is in cases of congenital deficiency of IgA. Since they have never seen IgA, such individuals recognize it as a foreign protein and respond to it with an anaphylactic reaction.

Table 20.7 is a compilation of available vaccines and antisera.

IMMUNOTHERAPY

Immunotherapy has been attempted but has ***limited applicability***. Thus, except for the post-exposure immunization described above, there is little applicability of immunotherapy to the treatment of infectious diseases. Some efforts were made to treat bacterial meningitis by intrathecal and other parenteral routes of administration of heterologous antibody. The success of this approach was questionable and the advent of antimicrobial agents (sulfonamides and antibiotics) lessened the zeal for studying immunotherapy in cases of bacterial meningitis and other infections. Restoration of immune capability—e.g. in treatment of burn patients who incur serious infections—is receiving attention, and prospects for combined use with chemotherapy are generating renewed interest in immunotherapy.

Nonspecific Immunostimulation

Attempts to arrest growth of tumors have involved nonspecific immunostimulation with the vaccine of attenuated *Mycobacterium bovis* (BCG—bacille Calmette-Guérin), killed *Propionibacterium acnes (Corynebacterium parvum)*, thymosin, levamisole, lentinan (β1,3-glucan from a mushroom of the genus

TABLE 20.7A. Immunizing Preparations (Vaccines and Antisera) Useful in Humans

Vaccines	Type of vaccine
Bacterial	
Anthrax	Alum-precipitated antigen from culture filtrate
Cholera	Killed *Vibrio cholerae*
Haemophilus influenzae	Type b polysaccharide
Meningococcal meningitis	Polysaccharide, group A,C,Y,W135 of *Neisseria meningitidis*
Pertussis	Killed *Bordetella pertussis*
Plague	Killed *Yersinia pestis* (attenuated strain in some parts of the world)
Pneumococcal infection	Polysaccharide (capsule) of 23 serotypes of *Streptoccocus pneumoniae*
Tetanus	Toxoid
Tuberculosis	Attenuated live bacille Calmette-Guérin (BCG)
Typhoid	Killed *Salmonella typhi* (attenuated, see Table 20.7B)
Botulism	Toxoid, limited use in research workers
Brucellosis	Attenuated live *Brucella abortus* strain 19 (limited use in humans outside the United States)
Rickettsial	
Typhus fever	Formalin-inactivated *Rickettsia prowazekii* (attenuated, live; shows promise)
Rocky Mt. spotted fever	Inactivated *Rickettsia rickettsii*
Viral	
Hepatitis B	Inactivated HB surface antigen
Influenza	Inactivated; whole or "split" virus
Measles	Attenuated
Mumps	Attenuated
Polio	Attenuated or inactivated
Rabies	Inactivated
Rubella	Attenuated
Varicella	Attenuated
Antisera	
Botulism	Human immune globulin; equine immune globulin
Diphtheria	Equine immune serum
Hepatitis A	Pooled human serum globulin (ISG)
Hepatitis B	Specific anti-HB (HBIG) or ISG
Hypogammaglobulinemia	Pooled human ISG
Measles	Pooled human ISG
Rabies	Human immune globulin, RIG, equine immune serum
Rh_0 (D)	Immune (human) globulin vs Rh_0 (D) factor
Tetanus	Human immune globulin (TIG)
Vaccinia	Vaccinia immune globulin
Varicella zoster	Zoster immune globulin (VZIG)
Antilymphocyte serum	Equine
Black widow spider	Equine antivenin
Coral snake bite	Equine antivenin
Crotalid snake bite	Polyvalent equine antiserum

TABLE 20.7B. Experimental Vaccines Under Evaluation

Vaccines	Type of vaccine
Bacterial	
Mycoplasma pneumoniae	Live; temperature sensitive
Salmonella typhi	Attenuated
Viral	
Adenovirus types 4,7	Live oral, and subunit
Cytomegalovirus	Attenuated
Hepatitis B recombinant DNA in yeast	Inactivated
Influenza	Active; temperature sensitive
Togavirus (arbovirus)	Attenuated or inactivated
Japanese B encephalitis	Attenuated or inactivated
Venezuelan equine encephalyomyelitis	Attenuated
Western equine encephalomyelitis	Inactivated

Lentinus), and dialyzable leukocyte-transfer factor. Induction of local contact hypersensitivity with dinitrochlorobenzene (DNCB) at the site of a tumor can occasionally, on subsequent topical application of DNCB, lead to diminution in the size of some cutaneous malignancies.

Specific Immunostimulation

Evidence of immunostimulation by specific leukocyte-***transfer factor*** has been reported in the following infectious diseases: 1) chronic mucocutaneous candidiasis, 2) coccidioidomycosis, 3) lepromatous leprosy, 4) tuberculosis, and 5) vaccinia gangrenosa (through transfusion of leukocytes). However, despite several years of study, no clear and unequivocal therapeutic role has emerged for transfer factor.

Plasmapheresis

While ***plasmapheresis*** (the separation of blood cells from plasma) is used for collection of specific, antibody-rich plasma for use as ISG, etc., it has also been used to remove detrimental antibody to afford clinical improvement. For example:

1. In ***myasthenia gravis,*** an antibody to the acetyl choline receptor protein leads to muscle weakness. Plasmapheresis of some patients leads to short-term improvement.

2. In ***Goodpasture's syndrome,*** there is autoimmune antibody to renal glomerular basement membrane. Improvement has followed plasmapheresis.

3. In one type of ***autoimmune hemolytic anemia,*** plasmapheresis has yielded improvement.

It is evident that the cellular production of autoantibodies would continue in all cases and that plasmapheresis can only provide transient benefits. However, transient benefits may provide time for more durable therapeutic interventions.

Leukapheresis

Selective removal of leukocytes from patients' blood has also been used therapeutically—e.g. in some otherwise unresponsive cases of rheumatoid arthritis.

SUMMARY

1. Protection against diseases may be achieved by active as well as passive immunization.

2. Active immunization may result from previous infection or from vaccination, while passive immunization may occur by natural means, such as the transfer of antibodies from mother to fetus, via the placenta, or to her infant, via the colostrum; or by artificial means such as by the administration of immune globulins.

3. Active immunization may be achieved by administration of one immunogen or a combination of immunogens.

4. The incubation period of a disease and the rapidity with which protective antibody titers develop both influence the efficacy of vaccination or the anamnestic effect of a booster injection.

5. The site of administration of a vaccine may be of great importance; many routes of immunization lead to the synthesis predominantly of serum IgM and IgG; oral administration of some vaccines leads to the induction of secretory IgA in the digestive tract.

6. Immunoprophylaxis has had striking success against subsequent infection; immunotherapy has had limited success.

REFERENCES

American College of Physicians (1985): Guide for Adult Immunization, Ed 1. Philadelphia: American College of Physicians.

Fulginiti VA (1982): Immunization in Clinical Practice. Philadelphia: Lippincott.

McClelland DBL, Yap PL (1984): Clinical use of immunoglobulins. Clin Haematol 13:39–74.

Peter G, Giebink GS, Hall CB, Plotkin SA (eds) (1986): Report of the Committee on Infectious Diseases, Ed 20. Elk Grove Village, Illinois: American Academy of Pediatrics.

U.S. Department of Health and Human Services (1983): General Recommendations of Immunization. Morbidity and Mortality Weekly Report (Jan. 14) 32:1–17. Washington, D.C.: U.S. Department of Health and Human Services.

U.S. Department of Health and Human Services (1984): Adult Immunization. Recommendations of the Immunization Practices Advisory Committee (ACIP). Morbidity and Mortality Weekly Report (Suppl. Sept. 28) 33:1S. Washington, D.C.: U.S. Department of Health and Human Services.

(*Continued on next page*)

REVIEW QUESTIONS

For questions 1–6, select the ONE answer or completion that is BEST in each case.

1. The best way to provide immunologic protection against tetanus neonatorum (of the newborn) is to
   a) inject the infant with human tetanus antitoxin.
   b) inject the newborn with tetanus toxoid.
   c) inject the mother with toxoid within 72 hours of the birth of her child.
   d) immunize the mother with tetanus toxoid before or early in pregnancy.
   e) give the child antitoxin and toxoid for both passive and active immunization.

2. Active, durable immunization against poliomyelitis can be accomplished by oral administratation of attenuated vaccine (Sabin) or by parenteral injection of inactivated (Salk) vaccine. These vaccines are equally effective in preventing disease because
   a) both induce adequate IgA at the intestinal mucosa, the site of entry of the virus.
   b) antibody in the serum protects against the viremia that leads to disease.
   c) viral antigen attaches to the anterior horn cells in spinal cord, preventing attachment of virulent virus.
   d) both vaccines induce formation of interferon.
   e) both vaccines establish a mild infection that can lead to formation of antibody.

3. The administration of vaccines is not without hazard. Of the following, which is least likely to affect adversely an immunocompromised host?
   a) Measles vaccine.
   b) Pneumococcal vaccine.
   c) Bacille Calmette Guérin.
   d) Mumps vaccine.
   e) Sabin poliomyelitis vaccine.

4. The administration of foreign (e.g. equine) antitoxin for passive protection in humans can lead to serum sickness, which is characterized by all of the following except:
   a) production by host antibody to foreign antibody.
   b) onset in 24–48 hours.
   c) use of homologous antitoxin.
   d) deposition of antigen–antibody complexes at various sites in the host.
   e) although delayed, the reaction is not a cell-mediated, delayed, type IV, immune response.

5. The pneumococcal polysaccharide vaccine should be administered to all except:
   a) individuals with chronic cardiorespiratory disease.
   b) elderly (over 60 years of age) persons.
   c) children (under 2 years of age).
   d) persons with chronic renal failure.
   e) individuals with sickle cell disease.

6. The following statements about human immune serum globulin (ISG) are true except:
   a) the source is human placenta.
   b) the globulins are obtained by precipitation with cold ethanol.
   c) the concentration of IgG is more than 10-fold greater than in plasma.
   d) IgA and IgM are present in concentrations slightly lower than in plasma.
   e) The ethanol precipitation does not render preparation of globulin free of hepatitis virus.

ANSWERS TO REVIEW QUESTIONS

1. ***d*** The simplest and most effective way to protect the newborn infant against exotoxic disease, such as tetanus and diphtheria, is to induce antibody in the mother. The antitoxic IgG passing through the placenta will provide the necessary protection. While tetanus antitoxin could be used to provide short-term, passive protection, it would be more costly and require an otherwise unnecessary and painful injection. Injection of toxoid in the mother within 72 hours of delivery of the child would not allow time for induction of antibody. While antitoxin and toxoid could provide immediate passive and future active protection, the latter would have to be accompanied by future injections of toxoid and the former is expensive; both would require undesirable injections.

2. ***b*** Both attenuated and inactivated vaccines lead to formation of circulating antibody, which would provide protection by intercepting the infecting virus before it reaches the target tissue in the central nervous system. While the Sabin vaccine induces mucosal gut IgA that may intercept virus at the portal of entry, the parenterally injected Salk vaccine is not effective in inducing mucosal IgA. Viral antigen in the vaccine might attach to the anterior horn cells in the nervous system, but it probably would not provide durable immunity. Induction of interferon would represent potentially only brief protection. Only the Sabin vaccine, being attenuated and "live," would induce a mild infection.

3. ***b*** The pneumococcal vaccine consists of capsular polysaccharides from *Streptococcus pneumoniae* and represents a nonviable vaccine, which cannot lead to infection. Measles, mumps, and Sabin polio vaccines contain attenuated viruses, and BCG is an attenuated bacterium. These attenuated organisms are capable of proliferating in the human host. The normal host limits their repli-

(Continued on next page)

cation, but the immunocompromised host may not be able to do so, and progressive infection may occur.

4. ***b*** The reactions that comprise serum sickness follow administration of the foreign substance within 6–12 days. During this time, the host produces antibody that reacts with the foreign substance(s), which persists in the host and leads to antigen–antibody complexes that can be deposited in joints, lymph nodes, skin, and elsewhere. The manifestations of the immune reaction, although appearing later, nevertheless are classified as type III rather than cell-mediated, delayed (type IV) hypersensitivity because they involve antibodies rather than T cells.

5. ***c*** Children under 2 years of age do not respond adequately to immunization with pure bacterial capsule polysaccharide vaccine. Therefore, vaccinating them may be useless. The various other individuals listed are particularly vulnerable to infection with *Streptococcus pneumoniae*. While some of them may mount a suboptimal response to the vaccine, they should nevertheless be vaccinated.

6. ***e*** The potential hazard of hepatitis viruses in human plasma is overcome by the separation of ethanol-precipitated globulins. The concentration of IgG is about 16,500 mg/dl compared with 1,200 mg/dl in plasma. Whereas the IgG thus becomes highly concentrated in ISG, IgA and IgM are relatively depleted, and their concentration in the ethanol-precipitated ISG is close to their original concentration in the plasma.

GLOSSARY

Accessory cell: Cell required for, but not actually mediating, a specific immune response. Often used to describe antigen-presenting cells (APC; see below).

Adjuvant: A substance, given with antigen, which enhances the response to the injected antigen.

Adoptive transfer: The transfer of the capacity to make an immune response by transplantation of immunocompetent cells.

Affinity: A measure of the binding constant of a single antigen-combining site with a monovalent antigenic determinant.

Agglutination: The aggregation of particulate antigen by antibodies. Agglutination applies to red blood cells as well as to bacteria and inert particles covered with antigen.

Allelic: Relating to one of a series of two or more alternate forms of a gene that occupy the same position or locus on a specific chromosome.

Allelic exclusion: The ability of heterozygous lymphoid cells to produce only one allelic form of antigen-specific receptor when they have the genetic endowment to produce both. Genes other than those for the specific receptors are usually expressed co-dominantly.

Allergen: An antigen responsible for producing allergic reactions by inducing IgE formation.

Allergy: A term covering immune reactions to nonpathogenic antigens, which lead to inflammation and deleterious effects in the host.

Allogeneic: Having a genetic dissimilarity within the same species.

Allograft: A tissue transplant (graft) between two genetically non-identical members of a species.

Allotypes: Antigenic determinants that are present in allelic (alternate) forms. When used in association with immunoglobulin, allotypes describe allelic variants of immunoglobulins detected by antibodies raised between members of the same species.

Alternate pathway: The mechanisms of complement activation that does not involve activation of the Cl, C4, C2 pathway by antigen–antibody complexes.

Anamnestic: Literally, means "does not forget"; it is used to describe ***immunologic memory,*** which leads to a rapid increase in response after re-exposure to antigen.

Anaphylaxis: Immediate hypersensitivity response to antigenic challenge, mediated by IgE and mast cells. It is a life-threatening allergic reaction, caused by the release of pharmacologically active agents.

Anaphylatoxin: Substance capable of releasing histamine from mast cells.

Antibody: Serum protein formed in response to immunization; antibodies are generally defined in terms of their specific binding to the immunizing antigen.

Antibody-dependent, cell-mediated cytotoxicity (ADCC): A phenomenon in which target cells, coated with antibody, are destroyed by specialized killer cells (K cells), which bear receptors for the Fc portion of the coating antibody (Fc receptors). These receptors allow the killer cells to bind to the antibody-coated target.

Antigen: Any foreign material that is specifically bound by antibody; also used loosely to describe materials used for immunization. Compare to ***immunogen.***

Antigen-binding site: The part of an immunoglobulin molecule that binds antigen specifically.

Antigenic determinant: A single antigenic site or ***epitope*** on a complex antigenic molecule or particle.

Antigen-presenting cell (APC): A specialized type of cell, bearing cell surface class II MHC (***major histocompatibility complex***) antigens, involved in processing and presentation of antigen to inducer, or ***helper, T cells***.

Antigen receptor: The specific antigen-binding receptor on T or B lymphocytes; these receptors are transcribed and translated from rearrangements of V genes.

Arthus reaction: A hypersensitivity reaction produced by local formation of antigen–antibody aggregates that activate the complement cascade and cause thrombosis, hemorrhage, and acute inflammation.

Atopy: A term used by allergists to describe IgE-mediated anaphylactic responses in man, usually genetically determined.

Autochthonous: Pertaining to "self."

Autograft: A tissue transplant from one site to another on a single individual.

Autoimmunity (autoallergy): An immune response to "self" tissues or components. Such an immune response usually has pathological consequences leading to autoimmune diseases.

Autologous: Derived from the same individual, "self."

Avidity: The summation of multiple affinities, for example when a polyvalent antibody binds to a polyvalent antigen.

Bence-Jones protein: Dimers of immunoglobulin light chains in the urine of patients with multiple myeloma.

B Lymphocyte (B cell): The precursors of antibody-forming plasma cells; these cells carry immunoglobulin and class II MHC (***major histocompatibiity complex***) antigens on their surfaces.

Bursa of Fabricius: An outpouching of the cloaca in birds, site of development of B cells in birds.

Carcinoembryonic antigen (CEA): Antigen present during embryonic development which normally disappears but reappears in malignant tissue.

Carrier: A large, immunogenic molecule or particle to which an antigenic determinant is attached, allowing the determinant to become ***immunogenic***.

Cell-mediated immunity (CMI): Immune reaction mediated by T cells; in contrast to humoral immunity, which is antibody-mediated. Also referred to as delayed type hypersensitivity.

Cell-mediated cytotoxicity (CMC): Killing (lysis) of a target cell by an effector lymphocyte.

Chemotaxis: Migration of cells along a concentration gradient of an attractant.

Chimera: A mythical animal possessing the head of a lion, the body of a goat, and the tail of a snake. Refers to an individual containing cellular components derived from another genetically distinct individual.

Class switch: See ***isotype switch***.

Classical pathway: The mechanism of complement activation initiated by antigen–antibody aggregates and proceeding by way of C1, C4, and C2.

Clonal deletion: The loss of lymphocytes of a particular specificity due to contact with either "self" or artificially introduced antigen.

Clonal selection theory: The prevalent concept that specificity and diversity of an immune response are the result of selection by antigen of specifically reactive clones from a large repertoire of preformed lymphocytes, each with individual specificities.

Class I, II, and III MHC antigens: Antigens encoded by genes in the ***major histocompatibility complex***.

Combinatorial joining: The joining of segments of DNA to generate essentially new genetic information, as occurs with Ig genes during the development of B cells. Combinatorial joining allows multiple opportunities for 2 sets of genes to combine in different ways.

Complement: A series of serum proteins involved in the mediation of immune reactions. The complement cascade is triggered classically by the interaction of antibody with specific antigen.

Complete Freund's Adjuvant (CFA): An adjuvant used for immunization consisting of an emulsion of aqueous antigen in mineral oil with added mycobacteria.

Congenic (also co-isogenic): Describes two individuals who differ only in the genes at a particular locus and are similar at all other loci.

Constant region (C region): The invariant carboxyl terminal portion of an antibody molecule, as distinct from the variable region which is at the amino terminal of the chain.

Coombs' test: A test named for its originator, R.R.A. Coombs, used to detect non-agglutinating antibodies on red blood cells by addition of an anti-immunoglobulin antibody.

Cross-reactivity: The ability of an antibody, specific for one antigen, to react with a second antigen; a measure of relatedness between two different antigenic substances.

D gene: A small segment of immunoglobulin heavy chain DNA, coding for the third hypervariable region of most antibodies.

Delayed type hypersensitivity (DTH): A T-cell–mediated reaction to antigen, which takes 24–48 hours to develop fully, and which involves release of lymphokines and recruitment of monocytes and macrophages. Also called cell-mediated immunity.

Determinant: Part of the antigen molecule which binds to an antibody-combining site or to a receptor on T cells (see ***hapten*** and ***epitope***).

Differentiation antigen: A cell surface antigenic determinant found only on cells of a certain lineage and at a particular developmental stage; used as an immunologic marker.

Domain: A compact segment of an immunoglobulin molecule, made up of about 110 amino acids around an S–S bond, and encoded by a unique segment of DNA, surrounded by non-translated sequences.

DR antigens: MHC class II antigens found on B cells and antigen-presenting cells of humans.

Enzyme-linked immunosorbent assay (ELISA): An assay in which an enzyme is linked to an antibody and a colored substrate is used to measure the activity of bound enzyme and, hence, the amount of bound antibody.

Eosinophil chemotactic factor of anaphylaxis (ECF-A): A substance released from mast cells during anaphylaxis which attracts eosinophils.

Epitope: An alternative term for ***antigenic determinant***.

Equivalence zone: In a precipitin reaction, the region in which the concentration of antigen and antibody leads to maximal precipitation.

Exon: The region of DNA coding for a protein or a segment of a protein.

Fab: Fragment of antibody containing the antigen-binding site, generated by cleavage of the antibody with the enzyme papain, which cuts at the hinge region.

Fc: Fragment of antibody without antigen-binding sites, generated by cleavage with papain; the Fc fragment contains the C terminal domains of the heavy immunoglobulin chains.

Fc receptor (FcR): A receptor on a cell surface with specific binding affinity for the Fc portion of an antibody molecule. Fc receptors are found on many types of cell.

Fluorescent antibody: An antibody coupled with a fluorescent dye, used with a fluorescence microscope to detect antigen on cells, tissues or microorganisms.

Genotype: All of the genes possessed by an individual; in practice it refers to the particular alleles present at the loci in question.

Germline: Refers to genes in germ cells as opposed to somatic cells, that is, genes in their unrearranged state rather than those rearranged for production of a protein.

Graft versus host reaction (GVH): The pathologic consequences of a response initiated by transplanted immunocompetent T lymphocytes into an allogeneic, immunologically incompetent host. The host is unable to reject the grafted T cells and becomes their target.

Haplotype: A particular combination of alleles present at linked loci on a chromosome.

H-2 complex: The major histocompatibility complex situated on chromosome 17 of the mouse; contains subregions K, I, and D.

HLA complex: The major histocompatibility complex situated on chromosome 6 in man is called HLA, which stands for "human leukocyte antigens." It contains several subregions, called A, B, C, etc.

Hapten: A compound, usually of low molecular weight, that is not itself immunogenic but that, after conjugation to a carrier protein or cells, becomes immunogenic and induces antibody, which can bind the hapten alone in the absence of carrier.

Heavy chain (H chain): The larger of the two types of chain that comprise a normal immunoglobulin or antibody molecule.

Helper T cells: A class of T cells which help trigger B cells to make antibody against thymus-dependent antigens. Helper T cells also help generate cytotoxic T cells.

Heterophile antigen: A cross-reacting antigen that appears in widely ranging species such as humans and bacteria.

Hinge region: A flexible, open segment of an antibody molecule that allows bending of the molecule. The hinge region is located between Fab and Fc and is susceptible to enzymatic cleavage.

Histocompatibility: Literally, the ability of tissues to get along; in immunology, it means identity in all transplantation antigens. These antigens, in turn, are collectively referred to as histocompatibility antigens.

Humoral immunity: Any immune reaction that can be transferred with immune serum is termed humoral immunity (as opposed to cell-mediated immunity). In general, this term refers to resistance that results from the presence of specific antibody.

Hybridoma: A hybrid cell that results from the fusion of any antibody-secreting cell with a malignant cell; the progeny secrete antibody without stimulation and proliferate continuously both in vivo and in vitro.

Hypersensitivity: State of reactivity to antigen that is greater than normal for the antigenic challenge; hypersensitivity is the same as ***allergy*** and denotes a deleterious outcome rather than a protective one.

Hypervariable regions: Portions of the light and heavy immunoglobulin chains that are highly variable in amino acid sequence from one immunoglobulin molecule to another, and that, together, constitute the antigen-binding site of an antibody molecule.

Ia: "Immune response-associated" proteins, found on B cells and antigen-presenting cells of mice, which are MHC (***major histocompatibility complex***) type II proteins.

Idiotype: The combined antigenic determinants (***idiotopes***) found on antibodies of an individual that are directed at a particular antigen; such antigenic determinants are found only in the variable region.

Immune complex: Antigen bound to antibody.

Immunogen: A substance capable of inducing an immune response (as well as reacting with the products of an immune response). Compare to ***antigen***.

Immunoglobulin (Ig): A general term for all antibody molecules. Each Ig unit is made up of two heavy chains and two light chains and has two antigen-binding sites.

Interferon: A group of proteins enhancing and modifying the immune response.

Interleukin-1: A macrophage-secreted protein that promotes T-cell proliferative responses and is also an endogenous inducer of fever.

Interleukin-2: Soluble substance released by T cells which promotes proliferation of other T cells (also called TCGF, T-cell growth factor).

Intron: A segment of DNA that does not code for protein; the intervening sequence of nucleotides between coding sequences or ***exons.***

Immune response (Ir) gene: A gene controlling an immune response to a particular antigen; most genes of this type are in the MHC (***major histocompatibility complex***), and the term is rarely used to describe other types of Ir gene.

Isohemagglutinins: Antibodies to major red blood cell antigens present normally as a result of inapparent immunization by cross-reactive antigens in bacteria, food, etc.

Isotypes: Classes of antibody that differ in the constant regions of their heavy chains (Fc portion); distinguishable also on the basis of reaction with antisera raised in another species. These differences also result in different biological activities of the antibodies.

Isotype switch: The shift of a B cell or its progeny from the secretion of antibody of one isotype or class to antibody with the same V regions but a different heavy chain constant region and, hence, a different isotype (class switch).

J gene: A gene segment coding for the J or joining segment in immunoglobulin DNA; V genes translocate to J segments in L chains, and to D and J segments in H chains.

J chain (joining chain): A polypeptide involved in the polymerization of immunoglobulin molecules IgM and IgA.

K cell: An effector lymphocyte with ***Fc receptors*** which allow it to bind to and kill antibody-coated target cells.

Killer T cell: A T cell with a particular immune specificity and an endogeneously produced receptor for antigen, capable of specifically killing its target cell after attachment to the target cell by this receptor. Also called cytotoxic cell.

Light chain (L chain): The light chain of immunoglobulin is a structural feature that occurs in two forms: kappa and lambda.

Lymphocyte: Small cell with virtually no cytoplasm, found in blood, in all tissue, and in lymphoid organs, such as lymph nodes, spleen, and Peyer's patches.

Lymphokines: Soluble substances secreted by lymphocytes, which have a variety of specific and nonspecific effects on other cells.

Macrophage: A large, phagocytic cell of the mononuclear series.

Macrophage activating factor (MAF): Actually several lymphokines, including γ-interferon, released by activated T cells, which together induce activation of macrophages, making them more efficient in phagocytosis and cytotoxicity.

Migration inhibition factor (MIF): A lymphokine that inhibits the motility of macrophages in culture.

Major histocompatibility complex (MHC): A cluster of genes encoding cell surface antigens that are polymorphic within a species, and that code for antigens that lead to rapid graft rejection between members of a single species which differ at these loci. Several major classes of protein such as MHC class I and II proteins are encoded in this region.

Memory: In the immune system, memory denotes an active state of immunity to a specific antigen, such that a second encounter with that antigen leads to a larger and more rapid response.

MHC restriction: The ability of T lymphocytes to respond only when they are presented with the appropriate antigen in association with either "self" class I or class II MHC proteins.

Minor histocompatibility antigens: These antigens, encoded outside the MHC, are numerous, but do not generate rapid graft rejection or primary responses of T cells in vitro. They do *not* serve as restricting elements in cell interactions.

Mitogen: A substance that non-specifically stimulates the proliferation of lymphocytes.

Mixed lymphocyte reaction (MLR): When lymphocytes from two individuals are cultured together, a proliferative response is generally observed, as the result of reactions of T cells of one individual to MHC antigens on the other individual's cells.

Monoclonal: Literally, coming from a single clone. A clone is the progeny of a single cell. In immunology, monoclonal generally describes a preparation of antibody that is homogeneous, or cells of a single specificity.

Myeloma: A tumor of plasma cells, generally secreting a single species of immunoglobulin.

NK cell: Naturally occurring, large, granular, lymphocyte-like cells that kill various tumor cells; they may play a role in resistance to tumors; their immunologic specificity, if any, is unknown, and their number does not increase by immunization with tumors.

Null cells: A population of lymphocytes bearing neither T cell or B cell differentiation antigens.

Opsonization: Literally means "preparation for eating." The coating of a bacterium with antibody and complement that leads to enhanced ***phagocytosis*** of the bacterium.

Paratope: An antibody-combining site that is complementary to an epitope.

Passive cutaneous anaphylaxis (PCA): The passive transfer of anaphylactic sensitivity by intradermal injection of serum from a sensitive donor.

Phenotype: The physical expression of an individual's genotype.

Pinocytosis: Ingestion of liquid or very small particles by vesicle formation in a cell.

Plasma cell: End-stage of differentiation of a B cell to an antibody-producing cell.

Polyclonal activator: A substance that non-specifically induces activation of many individual clones of either T or B cells.

Polymorphism: Literally, "having many shapes"; in genetics polymorphism means occurring in more than one form within a species, the existence of multiple alleles at a particular genetic locus.

Primary response: The immune response to a first encounter with antigen. The primary response is generally small, has a long induction phase or lag period, consists primarily of IgM antibodies, and generates immunologic memory.

Prophylaxis: Protection.

Prozone: A region of diminished agglutination or precipitation of antigen-antibody complexes in a titration curve due to excess antibody.

Radioallergosorbent test (RAST): A solid phase radioimmunoassay for detecting IgE antibody specific for a particular allergen.

Radioimmunoassay (RIA): A widely used technique for measurement of primary antigen–antibody interactions, and for the determination of the level of important biological substances in mixed samples, taking advantage of the specificity of the antigen–antibody interaction and the sensitivity that derives from measurement of radioactively labeled materials.

Reagin: Allergist's term for IgE antibodies.

Rheumatoid factor: An autoantibody (usually IgM) which reacts with the individual's own IgG. Present in rheumatoid arthritis.

Second-set rejection: Accelerated rejection of an allograft in an already immune recipient.

Secretory component: A surface receptor on epithelial cells lining mucosal surface which binds dimeric IgA and transports it through the cell into mucosal secretions.

Serum sickness: A hypersensitivity reaction consisting of fever, rashes, joint pain, and glomerulonephritis, resulting from localization of circulating, soluble, antigen–antibody complexes, which induce inflammatory reactions. Serum sickness was originally induced following therapy with large doses of antibody from a foreign source—e.g. horse serum.

Slow reacting substance of anaphylaxis (SRS-A): A group of leukotrienes released by mast cells during anaphylaxis which induces a prolonged constriction of smooth muscle. This prolonged constriction is not reversible by treatment with antihistamines.

Suppression: A mechanism for producing a specific state of immunologic unresponsiveness by the induction of suppressor T cells. This type of unresponsiveness is passively transferable by suppressor T cells or their soluble products.

Syngeneic: Literally, genetically identical.

T-dependent antigen: In contrast to ***T-independent antigen,*** a T-dependent antigen is an immunogen that is able to elicit an antibody only when helper T cells are present.

Titer: The reciprocal of the last dilution of a titration giving a measurable effect; e.g., if the last dilution giving significant agglutination is 1:128, the titer is 128.

Tolerance: Diminished or absent capacity to make a specific response to an antigen, usually produced as a result of contact with that antigen under non-immunizing conditions.

Unresponsiveness: Inability to respond to antigenic stimulus. Unresponsiveness may be specific for a particular antigen (see ***tolerance***), or broadly non-specific as a result of damage to the entire immune system, for example after whole-body irradiation.

Vaccination: Originally referred to immunization against smallpox with the less virulent cowpox (vaccinia) virus; more loosely used for any immunization against a pathogen.

Xenogeneic: Originating from a foreign species.

INDEX